AN INTRODUCTION TO

Medical Terminology for Health Care

Senior Content Strategist: Alison Taylor
Content Development Specialist: Carole McMurray with Martin Mellor Publishing Services Ltd
Project Manager: Umarani Natarajan
Designer: Christian Bilbow
Illustration Managers: Teresa McBryan and Brett MacNaughton
Illustrator: Antbits Ltd
Marketing Manager: Deborah Watkins

AN INTRODUCTION TO

Medical Terminology for Health Care

FIFTH EDITION

ANDREW R. HUTTON BSc MSc FRSSA

Retired Lecturer in Life Science, Edinburgh, UK

ELSEVIER

EDINBURGH   LONDON   NEW YORK   OXFORD   PHILADELPHIA   ST LOUIS   SYDNEY   TORONTO 2016

ELSEVIER

First edition 1993
Second edition 1998
Third edition 2002
Fourth edition 2006

Notices

ISBN: 978-0-7020-4495-3

Printed in China

Last digit is the print number: 9 8 7 6 5 4 3 2 1

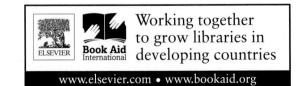

CONTENTS

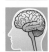

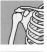

ABOUT THIS BOOK

This book is designed to introduce medical terms to students who have little prior knowledge of the language of medicine. Included in the text are simple, non-technical descriptions of pathological conditions and symptoms, medical instruments and clinical procedures. The medical terms are introduced within the context of a body system or medical specialty, and each set of exercises provides the student with the opportunity to learn, review and assess new words. Each unit includes a case history exercise that outlines the presentation, diagnosis and treatment of a specific medical condition. Once complete, the exercises will form a valuable reference text.

No previous knowledge of medicine is required to follow the text and, to ensure ease of use, the more complex details of word origins and analysis have been omitted. The book will be of great value to anyone who needs to learn medical terms quickly and efficiently.

Andrew R. Hutton
Edinburgh 2016

Acknowledgements

The pathology notes included in Units 2 to 17 were selected with reference to Gary A. Thibodeau and Kevin T. Patton, 2002, *Anatomy and Physiology* (5th edition), Mosby, ISBN 0-323-01628-6.

HOW TO USE THIS BOOK

Before you begin working through the units, read through the introduction that explains the basic principles of reading, writing and understanding medical terms. Once you have understood the elementary rules of medical word building, complete Units 1 to 21, which are based on different medical topics. The units can be studied in sequence or independently. For ease of use, each unit has the same basic plan and is arranged into:

WORD EXERCISES

AN ANATOMY EXERCISE

A CASE HISTORY

PATHOLOGY NOTES

ASSOCIATED WORDS

A WORD CHECK

SELF-ASSESSMENT

The Word Exercises should be completed using the Exercise Guide at the beginning of each unit or with knowledge acquired during the course of this study. Each word exercise enables you to analyze and understand the meaning of medical terms associated with a specific word root. The answers to the word exercises are on pp. 333–358.

The Anatomy Exercise enables you to relate the combining forms of medical roots to their position in the body. Check the meaning of the root words using the Quick Reference box within the respective chapter.

The Case History presents a patient's medical history associated with a particular body system or medical speciality.

The purpose of this exercise is to understand the medical terms associated with disease presentation, investigation, diagnosis and treatment. Some of the case histories may seem difficult to follow because of the terminology used when doctors write formal reports. To assist your understanding, a Word Help box is included with each case, listing the meanings of difficult or unfamiliar words. For each case history, try to gain an overall picture of the health care required for a successful treatment. Answers to the exercise that accompanies each case can be found with the answers to the word exercises on pp. 333–358.

The Pathology Notes section provides additional information relating to diseases and disorders associated with the body system being studied. Use this section for reference only.

The Associated Words section lists additional words that are relevant to the topic being studied. Use this section for reference only.

The Word Check lists all prefixes, combining forms and suffixes in each unit. Try to write the meaning of each component from memory and then correct any errors you have made. Errors can be corrected using the Exercise Guide or the Quick Reference box that follows each Case History. The glossary on pp. 383–410 can also be used.

The Self-Assessment at the end of each unit consists of a set of exercises that test your knowledge of the meaning of word components and their association with the anatomy or with a medical specialty. Aim to complete the assessment tests using knowledge gained from studying each unit and record your score in the box next to each test. Check your answers on pp. 359–368. Unit 22 contains 18 final self-assessment tests that enable you to test your knowledge of medical word components used throughout the package.

INTRODUCTION

OBJECTIVES

Once the introduction is complete, you should be able to do the following:

- name and identify components of medical words
- split medical words into their components
- build medical words using word components

Students beginning any kind of medical or paramedical course are faced with a bewildering number of complex medical terms. Surprisingly, it is possible to understand many medical terms and build new ones by learning relatively few words that can be combined in a variety of ways. Even the longest medical terms are easy to understand if you know the meaning of each component of the word. For example, you may never have heard of **laryngopharyngitis**, but if you learn that **-itis** always means inflammation, **laryng/o** refers to the larynx or voice box and **pharyng/o** refers to the throat or pharynx, its meaning becomes apparent, ie, inflammation of the larynx and pharynx. Laryngopharyngitis is an inflammation of the upper respiratory tract with symptoms of sore throat and loss of voice.

Doctors do not usually use unfamiliar medical terminology when conversing with patients as they may become concerned rather than reassured by a complex description of their illness. However, specific medical terms are used when medical records and letters are completed. They are also used when doctors discuss a patient and when medical material is published.

The terms you will use in this book describe common diseases and disorders, instruments, diagnostic techniques and therapies.

The components of medical words

In this introduction, you will learn how to split medical terms into their components and deduce their meanings. Skills developed here will enable you to derive the meanings of unfamiliar medical words and improve your ability to understand medical literature.

Let us begin by using a medical word associated with an organ with which you are familiar, the stomach:

Example 1   Gastrotomy

First, we can split the word and examine its individual components:

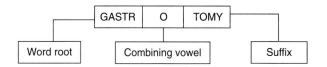

The word root

Roots are the basic medical words. Most are derived from Greek and Roman (Latin) words. Others have their origins in Arabic, Anglo-Saxon and German words. Some early Greek words have been retained in their original form, whilst others have been Latinized. In their migrations throughout Europe and America, many words have changed their spelling, meaning and pronunciation.

In our first example, we have used the root **gastr**, which always means stomach.

The combining vowel

Combining vowels are added to word roots to aid pronunciation and to connect the root to the suffix; a combining vowel has no meaning of its own. In our first example the combining vowel **o** has been added to join the root and suffix.

All the combining vowels **a**, **e**, **i**, **o** and **u** are used, but the most commonly used is **o**. In our first example, we have added the combining vowel **o** to the root **gastr**.

The suffix

The suffix follows the word root and is found at the end of the word. It also adds to or modifies the meaning of the word root.

In our first example, we have used the suffix **-tomy**, which always means to form an incision.

We can now fully understand the meaning of our first medical word:

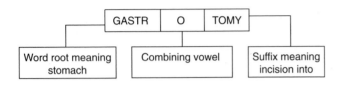

GASTR	O	TOMY
Word root meaning stomach	Combining vowel	Suffix meaning incision into

The meaning of gastrotomy is incision into the stomach. Gastrotomy is a name used by surgeons to describe an operation in which a cut is made into the wall of the stomach.

The combining form

In our first example the root **gastr** can be combined with the vowel **o** to make **gastro**. This word component is called a **combining form** of a word root, ie,

Word root	+	combining vowel	=	combining form
gastr	+	o	=	gastro

Most combining forms end in **o**, and we will be using many of them in the exercises that follow.

Now that we have learnt the meaning of our first root, we can use it again with a new word component:

Example 2   Epigastric

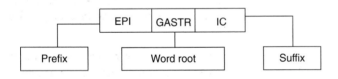

EPI	GASTR	IC
Prefix	Word root	Suffix

Here, we have split the word into its components, and we can see it begins with a prefix that appears before the root **gastr**.

The prefix

The prefix precedes the word root and changes its meaning. The prefix **epi-** means upon, and so it modifies the word to mean upon or above the stomach. Prefixes, like roots and suffixes, are also derived from Greek and Latin words.

The suffix **-ic**, meaning pertaining to, was also used in our second example, so we can now write the full meaning of epigastric:

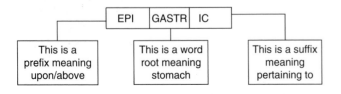

EPI	GASTR	IC
This is a prefix meaning upon/above	This is a word root meaning stomach	This is a suffix meaning pertaining to

The full meaning of epigastric is pertaining to above or upon the stomach.

> **Key Point**
>
> The components of medical words are:
> * prefixes
> * roots
> * suffixes
> * combining vowels
> * combining forms

The use of prefixes, combining forms and suffixes

There are certain simple rules that need to be applied when building and analyzing medical words. To practise using these rules, some new combining forms are introduced. Do not worry about remembering their meanings at the moment; we will study them in a later unit.

Rule 1: Joining a combining form to a suffix

If we add the suffixes **-logy**, meaning study of, and **-algia**, meaning condition of pain, to the combining form gastr/o, we can make two new words:

gastr/o	+	-logy	=	gastrology (study of the stomach)
gastr/o	+	-algia	=	gastralgia (condition of pain in the stomach)

Notice that in gastrology the combining vowel **o** has been left in place, whilst in gastralgia it has been dropped. The **o** has been dropped in gastralgia because **-algia** begins with **a**, which is a vowel. Gastralgia is used in preference to gastroalgia.

> **Key Point**
>
> When a combining form of a root is joined to a suffix, the combining vowel is left in place if the suffix begins with a letter other than a vowel.

Here are some more examples where the vowel is left in place because the suffix begins with a letter other than a vowel:

gastr/o	+	-tomy	=	gastrotomy (incision into the stomach)
gastr/o	+	-scope	=	gastroscope (instrument to view the stomach)

Here are some examples where the vowel is dropped:

gastr/o	+	-itis	=	gastritis (inflammation of the stomach)
gastr/o	+	-ectomy	=	gastrectomy (removal of the stomach)

 Word Exercise 1

Use Rule 1 to join the combining forms of word roots and suffixes to make medical words. The meanings of the words will be studied in following units. The first has been completed for you.

Combining form of word root		Suffix		Medical word
(a) gastr/o	+	-pathy	=	gastropathy
(b) gastr/o	+	-scopy	=	
(c) hepat/o	+	-itis	=	
(d) hepat/o	+	-megaly	=	
(e) hepat/o	+	-oma	=	

Rule 2: Joining the combining forms of two word roots

Some medical words contain two or more combining forms of roots, as in Example 3.

Example 3   Gastroenterology

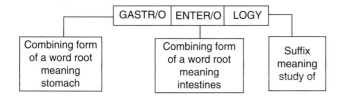

GASTR/O	ENTER/O	LOGY
Combining form of a word root meaning stomach	Combining form of a word root meaning intestines	Suffix meaning study of

The full meaning of gastroenterology is the study of the stomach and intestines. Notice that the vowel **o** between the two roots **gastr** and **enter** is left in place.

> **Key Point**
>
> When the combining forms of two roots are joined, the combining vowel of the first root is retained.

Here are some more examples:

pylor/o	+	gastr/o	+	ectomy	=	pylor**o**gastrectomy
duoden/o	+	enter/o	+	stomy	=	duoden**o**enterostomy

 Word Exercise 2

Use Rules 1 and 2 to join the combining forms of two roots with suffixes to make medical words. The meanings of the words will be studied in following units. The first has been completed for you.

Combining form of word root		Combining form of word root	Suffix		Medical word
(a) duoden/o	+	jejun/o	+ -stomy	=	duodenojeju-nostomy
(b) trache/o	+	bronch/o	+ -itis	=	
(c) gastr/o	+	enter/o	+ -stomy	=	
(d) laryng/o	+	pharyng/o	+ -ectomy	=	
(e) oste/o	+	arthro	+ -pathy	=	

> **Note.** There are a few exceptions to this rule which are hyphenated, eg, pharyngo-oral.

Rule 3: Joining a prefix to a root

When a prefix that ends in a vowel is added to a root that begins with a vowel or **h**, the vowel of the prefix is dropped.

Examine our second example, **epigastric**, again; notice the vowel **i** of **epi-** was retained because the root **gastr** begins with **g**, which is not a vowel.

Consider another example, which may be familiar to you: **antacid**, a drug used to neutralize stomach acid. This word is made from:

anti (prefix meaning against)	+	acid (root meaning acid)	=	antacid

The **i** is dropped because acid begins with the vowel **a**.

Here are some more examples; we will learn their meanings later.

Here, the vowel of the prefix is retained:

hemi-	+	col/o	+	-ectomy	=	hemicolectomy

Here the vowel of the prefix is dropped:

endo-	+ arter/i	+ -ectomy	=	endarterectomy		
anti-	+ helminth	+ -ic	=	anthelminthic (here **i** is dropped because helminth begins with **h**. Note: this is the only common example of this rule in use)		

> **Note.** Rule 3 is not a strict rule, and there are many exceptions to it, eg, periostitis.

Key Point

When a prefix that ends in a vowel is joined to a root, the vowel of the prefix is dropped if the root begins with a vowel or **h**.

📖 Word Exercise 3

Use the rules we have just described to join prefixes and combine forms of roots and suffixes to make medical words. The meanings of the words will be studied in following units. The first has been completed for you.

Prefix		Combining form of word root		Suffix		Medical word
(a) endo-	+	odont/o	+	-ic	=	endodontic
(b) prostho-	+	odont/o	+	-ist	=	
(c) para-	+	rect/o	+	-al	=	
(d) mono-	+	ocul/o	+	-ar	=	
(e) peri-	+	splen/o	+	-itis	=	

Reading and understanding medical words

Now that you have learnt the basic principle of building medical words, you should be able to deduce the meaning of an unfamiliar word from the meaning of its components. To illustrate this, we will use three examples.

Example 1   Cardiology

First

Split the word into its components: cardio/logy.

Then

Think of or look up the meaning of these components.

Finally

Read the meaning of the word beginning with the suffix, reading backwards:
eg, cardi/o[2], -logy[1]
1→study of
2→the heart
We read the full meaning of cardiology as the study of the heart.

Example 2   Pararectal

Here the prefix **para-** has modified the meaning of the root **rect/** to mean beside the rectum.

First

Split the word into its components: para/rect/al.

Then

Think of or look up the meaning of these components.

Finally

Read the meaning of the word beginning with the suffix, followed by the meaning of the modified root.
eg, pararect[2], al[1]
1→pertaining to
2→beside the rectum.
We read the full meaning of pararectal as pertaining to beside the rectum.

Example 3   Gastroenterology

First

Split the word into its components: gastro/entero/logy.

Then

Think of or look up the meaning of these components.

Finally

Read the meaning of the word starting with the suffix then back to the beginning of the word and across:
eg, gastr/o[2], enter/o[3], logy[1]
1→study of
2→the stomach and
3→intestines
Using this technique, we understand the meaning of gastroenterology to be the study of the stomach and intestines.

Key Point

When deducing the meanings of compound medical words, begin with the meaning of the suffix followed by those of the root(s) or modified root from left to right.

Once you have an understanding of these simple rules, you should be able to complete the exercises in Units 1–21. Each unit introduces different medical terms associated with a body system or medical specialty. The units can be completed in an order that complements your studies in anatomy, physiology and health care. Unit 22 provides additional word component exercises for all medical specialties studied in this self-teaching package.

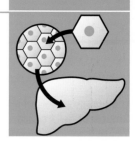

UNIT **1**
LEVELS OF ORGANIZATION

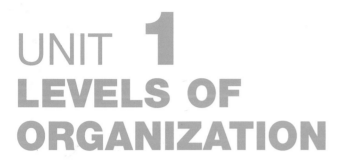

EXERCISE GUIDE

Use this list of word components and their meanings to complete the word exercises in this unit.

Prefixes

micro-	small

Roots / Combining forms

bio-	life/living
chem/(istry)	chemicals (study of)
chondr/o	cartilage
erythr/o	red
fibr/o	fibre (Am. fiber)
granul/o	granule
haem/o	blood
hem/o (Am.)	blood
leuc/o	white
leuk/o (Am.)	white
lymph/o	lymph
melan/o	pigment/melanin
oo	egg/ovum
oste/o	bone
path/o	disease
spermat/o	sperm

Suffixes

-blast	germ cell / cell that forms / an embryonic or immature cell
-genic	pertaining to formation / pertaining to originating in…
-genesis	formation of
-ic	pertaining to
-ical	pertaining to
-logist	a specialist who studies…
-logy	study of
-lysis	breakdown/disintegration
-pathy	disease of
-scope	an instrument used to view/examine
-scopist	a specialist who uses a viewing instrument
-scopy	technique of viewing/examining
-toxic	pertaining to being poisonous
-trophic	pertaining to nourishing

Levels of organization

The human body consists of basic units of life known as **cells**. Groups of cells similar in appearance, function and origin join together to form **tissues**. Different tissues then interact with each other to form **organs**. Finally, groups of organs interact to form body **systems**. Thus there are four levels of organization in the human body: cells, tissues, organs and systems. Let us begin by examining the first level of organization.

Cells

The cell is the basic unit of life, and the bodies of all plants and animals are built up of cells. Your body consists of millions of very small, specialized cells. It is interesting to note that all non-infectious disorders and diseases of the human body are really due to the abnormal behaviour of cells.

Body cells are all built on the same basic plan. Figure 1 represents a model cell.

Most cells have the same basic components as are shown in the model, but they are all specialized to carry out particular functions within the body. In your studies, you will come across many terms that relate to different types of cells. Now, we will examine our first word root which refers to cells:

▌Root

Cyt

(*From a Greek word* **kytos**, *meaning cell.*)

Combining forms　　Cyt/o, *also used as the suffix* -cyte

(*Remember from our introduction that combining forms are made by adding a combining vowel to the word root.*)

Here we have a word that contains the root **cyt**:

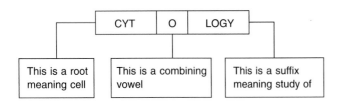

Reading from the suffix back, cytology means the study of cells.

(**Note.** When trying to understand medical words, first split the word into its components, then think of the meaning of each

component, and finally write the meaning, beginning with the suffix.)

Cytology is a very important topic in medicine as many diseases and disorders can be diagnosed by studying cells. Cells removed from patients are sent for cytological examination to a hospital cytology laboratory where they are examined with a microscope. (In the word cytological, *-ical* is a compound suffix meaning pertaining to or dealing with.)

The exercises that follow rely on the use of the Exercise Guide that appears at the beginning of this unit; use the guide to look up the meaning of path/o and -pathy, and then try Word Exercise 1.

📖 Word Exercise 1

(a) Name the components of the word and give their meanings:

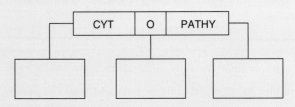

(b) Reading from the suffix back, the meaning of cytopathy is:

_____

The combining form **path/o** can be used at the beginning and in the middle of a compound word, as in the next two examples. Write the meaning of the words. Read the meaning of the word components in the order 1, 2, then 3.

(c) **path/o**[2]/logy[1]　　_____

(d) cyt/o[2]/**path/o**[3]/logy[1]　　_____

Using the Exercise Guide again, find the meaning of -logist, -lysis and toxic; then write the meaning of the words below. Remember to read the meaning from the suffix back to the beginning of each word as in (c) and (d):

(e) **cyt/o**/lysis　　_____

(f) **cyt/o**/tox/ic　　_____

(g) **cyt/o**/logist　　_____

In (g), **cyt/** was used at the beginning of a word. It can also be used in combination with other roots and at the end of words, as in lymph/o/**cyte**; its meaning remains the same. Here, **-cyte** is acting as a suffix, and it always means cell.

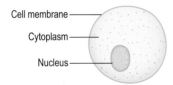

Figure 1　A cell.

Word Exercise 2

Here we have two more examples of the use of -**cyte** in a compound word:

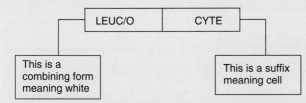

LEUC/O	CYTE

This is a combining form meaning white

This is a suffix meaning cell

The meaning of leucocyte is therefore white cell, a main type of blood cell (Am. leukocyte).

(a) Name the components of the following word, and find the meaning of erythr/o using your Exercise Guide.

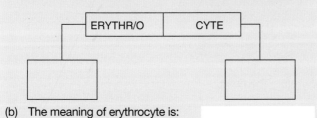

ERYTHR/O	CYTE

(b) The meaning of erythrocyte is: _____

Word Exercise 3

Figures 2 and 3 show two specialized cells, each one carrying out a different function.

Fig 2   This cell produces the pigment melanin that gives the dark colour to black or brown skin.

Fig 3   This cell produces white collagen fibres (Am. fibers) that give the skin strength.

Use your Exercise Guide to find the combining forms of melanin and fibre; then build words that mean:

(a) A cell containing melanin (melanin cell) _____

(b) A cell that produces fibres (fibre cell) _____

(c) Complete the table by looking up the combining forms of the following roots in your Exercise Guide and building words that name the cell types. The first one has been completed for you.

Root	Combining form	Name of cell
oste	osteo	osteocyte (bone cell)
lymph		
spermat		

Root	Combining form	Name of cell
oo		
granul		
chondr		

Now we will examine another root that refers to a special type of cell:

Root

Blast

(*A Greek word meaning bud or germ. Here blast/o means a cell that is forming something, a germ cell or an immature stage in cell development.*)

Combining forms   Blast/o, *also used as the suffix* -blast

Word Exercise 4

Without using your Exercise Guide, write the meaning of:

(a) oste/o/**blast** _____

(b) fibr/o/**blast** _____

Using your Exercise Guide, write the meaning of the word components in (c) in the order 1, 2, then 3.

(c) haem/o[2]/cyt/o[3]/blast[1] _____
    (Am. hem/o/cyt/o/blast)

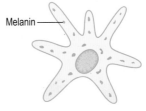

Melanin

Figure 2   A pigment cell.

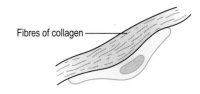

Fibres of collagen

Figure 3   A fibre cell (Am. fiber).

Tissues

As cells become specialized, they form groups of cells known as tissues. A definition of a tissue is a group of cells similar in appearance, function and origin. There are four basic types of tissue: epithelia, muscle, connective and nervous tissue; these form the second level of organization in the body. Figure 4 illustrates how cells associate to form a cuboidal epithelium in the kidney.

The study of tissues is known as histology, the combining form coming from a Greek word *histos* meaning web (web of cells). Histology is an important branch of biology and medicine because histological techniques are used to process and identify diseased tissues. The histology and cytology laboratories are usually sections of the pathology laboratory of a large hospital.

Root

Hist

(*From a Greek word* **histos**, *meaning web. Here hist/i/o means the tissues of the body.*)

Combining forms   Hist/i/o

Word Exercise 5

Using your Exercise Guide, find the meaning of:

(a) **hist/o**/chemistry

Without using your Exercise Guide, write the meaning of:

(b) **hist/o**[2]/**path/o**[3]/**logy**[1]

(c) **hist/o**/logist

(d) **hist/o**/lysis

Cells and tissues are very small and can only be examined using an instrument known as a microscope.

Word Exercise 6

Using your Exercise Guide, find the meaning of:

(a) **micro-**

(b) **micro/scope**

(c) **micro/scopy**

(d) **micro/scopist**

Note carefully the differences between **-scope**, **-scopy** and **-scopist**.

(e) **micro**[2]/**bio**[3]/**logy**[1]

Organs

Groups of different tissues interact to produce larger structures known as organs; these form the third level of

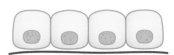

Figure 4   Cuboidal epithelium.

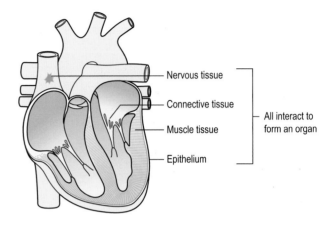

Figure 5   The heart.

organization. A familiar example is the heart (Fig. 5), which consists of muscle tissue, a covering of epithelium, nerve tissue and connective tissue. All these tissues interact so that the heart pumps blood.

Root

Organ

(*From a Greek word* **organon**, *meaning tool. Here organ/o means body organs.*)

Combining form   Organ/o

Word Exercise 7

Using your Exercise Guide, find the meaning of:

(a) **organ**/ic

(b) **organ/o**/genesis

(synonymous with organogeny)

(c) **organ/o**/genic

(d) **organ/o**/trophic

Systems

Groups of organs that interact for a common purpose form our fourth level of organization called the system; for example, the stomach, duodenum, colon, etc. interact to form the digestive system that processes our food. Units 2–17 introduce medical terms associated with the main body systems.

CASE HISTORY 1

The object of this exercise is to understand words associated with a patient's medical history.

To complete the exercise, do the following:

- Read through the passage on diagnosis of an AIDs-related infection; unfamiliar words are underlined, and you can find their meaning using the Word Help.

- Write the meaning of the medical terms shown in bold print on the lines that follow the Word Help.

Diagnosis of an AIDS-related infection

Mr A, a 34-year-old HIV-positive patient with symptoms of AIDs, was admitted to the unit following a chest X-ray that revealed a left upper lobe mass.

A CT scan confirmed the presence of a mass within the peripheral aspect of the left upper lobe, and a small left pleural effusion. CT-guided fine needle aspiration of the left upper lobe mass was performed, and the biopsy material was sent to the **histology** laboratory for analysis by the duty **pathologist**.

Cytological examination of direct smears using optical **microscopy** revealed a mucoid background, moderate cellularity, polymorphonuclear **leucocytes** (Am. leukocytes), **lymphocytes** and histiocytes. A significant number of oval yeast-like cells were observed that appeared to be budding. No malignant cells were observed.

A sample of the biopsy material was sent for culture and sensitivity testing to the **microbiology** laboratory. The report was positive for encapsulated fungal yeast forms morphologically compatible with **pathogenic** Cryptococcus species (Cryptococcus neoformans). Mr A's diagnosis was cryptococcosis, a condition seen mainly in AIDs patients and others with compromised immune systems.

Word Help

AIDs acquired immune deficiency syndrome

aspect part of a surface facing a designated direction

aspiration withdrawal by suction of a fluid

biopsy removal and examination of living tissue

budding performing asexual reproduction by producing buds that grow into new cells

cellularity state/condition of being made up of cells

compromised lacking the ability to mount an adequate immune response

Cryptococcus a yeast-like fungus that causes disease in humans

cryptococcosis abnormal condition of infection with Cryptococcus

CT computed tomography, a technique of using X-rays to image a slice or section through the body

culture and sensitivity testing growing microorganisms in the laboratory and testing them for sensitivity to antibiotics

effusion a fluid discharge into a part/escape of fluid into an enclosed space

encapsulated enclosed on a capsule or sheath

histiocytes the word means a tissue cell (actually a large cell found in connective tissue that helps defend against infection)

HIV-positive presence of antibodies to the human immunodeficiency virus in the blood; it indicates the virus has infected the body

lobe a division of an organ into smaller sections, here a lobe of the lung

malignant dangerous, life threatening

mass lump/collection of cohering cells

morphologically referring to the form and structure of an organism

mucoid resembling mucus

peripheral pertaining to the periphery, ie, the surface of an organ, outermost part, exteriority

pleural pertaining to the pleura/pleural membranes that surround the lungs

polymorphonuclear pertaining to or having nuclei of many shapes

Now, write the meaning of the following words from the Case History without using your dictionary lists:

(a) histology

(b) pathologist

(c) cytological

(d) microscopy

(e) leucocyte
    (Am. leukocyte)

(f) lymphocyte

(g) microbiology

(h) pathogenic

(Answers to the Case History exercise are given in the Answers to Word Exercises on page 333.)

Quick Reference

Combining forms relating to levels of organization:

Blast/o	immature cell/cell that forms…
Chondr/o	cartilage
Cyt/o	cell
Granul/o	granule
Hist/i/o	tissue
Lymph/o	lymph
Melan/o	pigment/melanin
Oo	egg/ovum
Organ/o	organ
Oste/o	bone
Path/o	disease
Spermat/o	sperm
System-	system/body systems

Abbreviations

Some common abbreviations related to cells and tissues are listed below. Note that some are not standard, and their meaning may vary from one healthcare setting to another. There is a more extensive list for reference on page 369.

Diff, diff	differential blood count (of cell types)
DNA	deoxyribonucleic acid
ECF	extracellular fluid
FBC	full blood count (of cells)
Histo	histology (lab)
HLA	human leucocyte antigen
ICF	intracelluar fluid
Lymphos	lymphocytes
NK	natural killer (cells)
PCV	packed cell volume
RBC	red blood (cell) count/red blood cell
WBC	white blood cell/white blood (cell) count

Associated words

Aerobic pertaining to requiring free oxygen

Anaerobic pertaining to living or occurring in the absence of free oxygen

Anatomy the science concerned with structure of the human body, especially that revealed by dissection and separation of its parts

Apoptosis condition of programmed cell death, the death of cells which occurs as a normal and controlled part of an organism's growth or development

Autolysis self-breakdown, the spontaneous breakdown/break-up of living tissues by enzymes produced in cells

Autopsy postmortem examination of a body to determine the cause of death

Corpuscle any small mass or body, an outdated term for a blood cell

Chromosome a structure in the nucleus containing a linear thread of DNA that carries genetic information

DNA deoxyribonucleic acid, a nucleic acid that forms the basic structure of genes

Fixation the process of preserving cells and tissues removed from the body to maintain their structure for examination in the laboratory; they are immersed in solutions such as formalin

Histocompatibility the ability of cells and tissues to be accepted and function in a new situation as in organ transplantation

Hyperplasia the condition of an increase in the number of normal cells in a tissue or organ

Hypertrophy the condition of an increase in size of cells and tissues

Meiosis a type of cell division in which a cell divides into four cells, each with half the number of chromosomes of the original cell; in humans, this process produces sperm and eggs in the reproductive organs

Mitosis the process by which a cell divides into two smaller cells that each contains the same number of chromosomes as the original cell; the human body grows by mitosis

Morphology the study of the form and structure of organisms

Multiple organ dysfunction syndrome a condition of altered function of vital organs that requires medical intervention to maintain life

Necrosis condition of death of cells due to disease, injury or failure of their blood supply

Organelle a specialized structure within a cell, eg, a mitochondrion

Pathologist a medical specialist who studies disease, especially the structural and functional changes in cells, tissues and organs; pathologists also perform autopsies to determine cause of death and confirm a diagnosis

Physiology the study of the functioning of the living organism and its parts

Tissue culture growing living cells extracted from the body in a medium conducive to their growth

Stem cell a cell taken from a person or other animal at an early stage of development that is capable of developing into cells of any type

Staining process of colouring cells and tissues to facilitate microscopic examination in the laboratory

NOW TRY THE WORD CHECK

WORD CHECK

This self-check exercise lists all the word components used in this unit. First, write down the meaning of as many word components as you can. Then check your answers using the Exercise Guide and Quick Reference box or the Glossary of Word Components (pp. 383–410).

Prefixes

micro-

Combining forms of word roots

bio-

blast/o

chem/o

chondr/o

cyt/o

erythr/o

fibr/o

granul/o

hist/i/o

leuc/o (Am. leuk/o)

lymph/o

melan/o

oo-

organ/o

oste/o

path/o

spermat/o

Suffixes

-blast

-cyte

-genic

-genesis

-ic

-ical

-logist

-logy

-lysis

-pathy

-scope

-scopist

-scopy

-toxic

-trophic

NOW TRY THE SELF-ASSESSMENT

SELF-ASSESSMENT

Test 1A

Prefixes, suffixes and combining forms of word roots

Match each meaning in Column C with a word component in Column A by inserting the appropriate number in Column B.

Column A	Column B	Column C
(a) chem/o		1. egg
(b) cyt/o		2. bone
(c) erythr/o		3. white
(d) granul/o		4. study of
(e) hist/i/o		5. pigment (black)
(f) leuc/o or leuk/o		6. sperm cells
(g) -logist		7. chemical
(h) -logy		8. tissue
(i) lymph/o		9. person who studies (specialist)
(j) -lysis		10. small
(k) melan/o		11. specialist who views/examines
(l) micro-		12. breakdown disintegration
(m) oo		13. poisonous/pertaining to poison
(n) oste/o		14. cell
(o) -pathy		15. visual examination
(p) -scope		16. disease
(q) -scopist		17. lymph
(r) -scopy		18. red
(s) spermat/o		19. granule
(t) -toxic		20. viewing instrument

Score

20

Test 1B

Write the meaning of:

(a) chondrolysis

(b) leucocytolysis

(c) histotoxic

(d) osteopathy

(e) lymphoblast

Score

5

Test 1C

This type of test may seem difficult at first but, as the terms become familiar, you will improve.

Build words that mean:

(a) small cell

(b) person who specializes in the study of disease

(c) person who specializes in the study of cell disease

(d) scientific study of cartilage

(e) pertaining to disease of cells

Score

5

Check answers to Self-Assessment Tests on page 359.

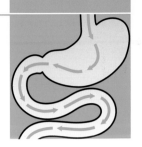

UNIT 2
THE DIGESTIVE SYSTEM

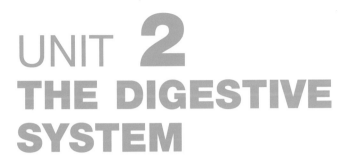

OBJECTIVES

Once you have completed Unit 2, you should be able to do the following:

- understand the meaning of medical words relating to the digestive system
- build medical words relating to the digestive system
- associate medical terms with their anatomical position
- understand common medical abbreviations relating to the digestive system

EXERCISE GUIDE

Use this list of word components and their meanings to complete the word exercises in this unit.

Prefixes

a-	without
endo-	inside/within
epi-	upon/above
mega-	large
para-	beside
peri-	around

Roots / Combining forms

an/o	anus

Suffixes

-aemia	condition of blood
-al	pertaining to
-algia	condition of pain
-clysis	infusion / injection into
-ectomy	removal of
-emia (Am.)	condition of blood

-gram	X-ray/tracing/recording
-graphy	technique of recording/making X-ray
-ia	condition of
-iasis	abnormal condition
-ic	pertaining to
-ist	specialist
-itis	inflammation of
-lith	stone
-lithiasis	abnormal condition of stones
-logist	specialist who studies…
-logy	study of
-lysis	breakdown/disintegration
-megaly	enlargement
-oma	tumour/swelling (Am. tumor)
-pathy	disease of
-scope	an instrument used to view/examine
-scopy	technique of viewing/examining
-stomy	formation of an opening into…
-tomy	incision into
-toxic	pertaining to poisoning
-uria	condition of the urine

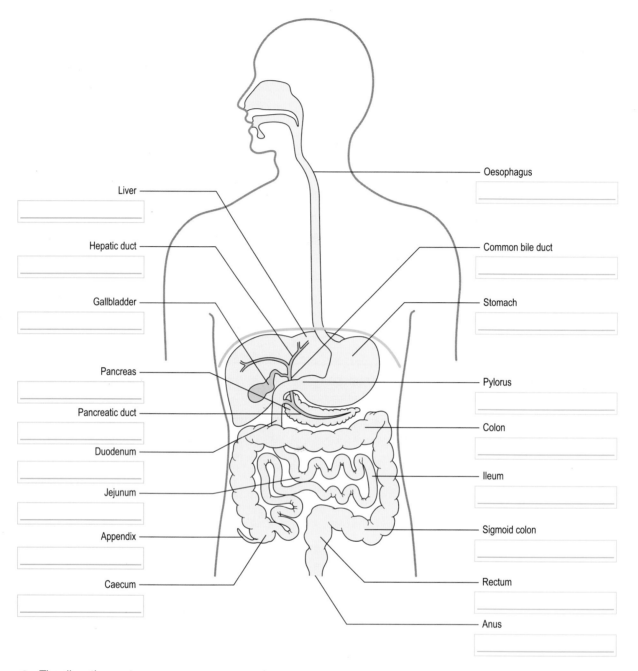

Figure 6   The digestive system.

 ANATOMY EXERCISE

When you have finished Word Exercises 1–12, look at the word components listed below. Complete Figure 6 by writing the appropriate combining form on each line. (You can check their meanings in the Quick Reference box on page 24.)

Appendic/o	Gastr/o	Pancreatic/o
Caec/o, Cec/o (Am.)	Hepatic/o	Pancreat/o
Cholecyst/o	Hepat/o	Proct/o
Choledoch/o	Ile/o	Pylor/o
Col/o	Jejun/o	Rect/o
Duoden/o	Oesophag/o, Esophag/o (Am.)	Sigmoid/o

The digestive system

The organs that compose the digestive system digest, absorb and process nutrients taken in as food. Materials not absorbed into the lining of the intestine form the faeces (Am. feces) and leave the body through the anus.

Our study of the digestive system begins at the point where food leaves the mouth and enters the gullet or oesophagus (Am. esophagus).

Use the Exercise Guide at the beginning of this unit to complete Word Exercises 1 to 12, unless you are asked to work without it.

The oesophagus and stomach

Food that enters the mouth is chewed, mixed with saliva and formed into a ball called a *bolus*. The bolus is forced to the back of the oral cavity and is swallowed into the oesophagus. Muscular contractions in the wall of the oesophagus help propel the food into the superior opening of the stomach. The stomach continually mixes the food, acts as a holding reservoir, and begins the digestion of protein by secreting a juice containing enzymes and hydrochloric acid from its lining. The strong hydrochloric acid (at pH 2) is secreted to activate the enzyme pepsin that digests protein; the stomach is well protected from self-digestion by the secretion of an alkaline mucus onto its lining.

▌Root

Oesophag

(*From a Greek word* **oisophagos**, *meaning oesophagus or gullet.*)

Combining forms   Oesophag/o
                     Esophag/o *(Am.)*

Word Exercise 1

Using your Exercise Guide, look up -*scope*, -*ectomy*, -*tomy* and -*itis*; then write the meaning of:

(a) **oesophag/o**/scope
     (Am. **esophag/o**/scope)

Remember that, to understand the meaning of these medical terms, we read the components from the suffix towards the beginning of the word.

(b) **oesophag**/ectomy
     (Am. **esophag**/ectomy)

(c) **oesophag/o**/tomy
     (Am. **esophag/o**/tomy)

(d) **oesophag**/itis
     (Am. **esophag**/itis)

Once you have learnt the suffixes in Word Exercise 1, it is easy to work out the meaning of other words with similar endings. Now we will use the same suffixes again with a different word root.

▌Root

Gastr

(*From a Greek word* **gaster**, *meaning stomach.*)

Combining form   Gastr/o

Word Exercise 2

Without using your Exercise Guide, write the meaning of:

(a) **gastr/o**/scope

(b) **gastr**/ectomy

(c) **gastr/o**/tomy

(d) **gastr**/itis

Using your Exercise Guide find the meaning of *epi-*, -*ic*, -*logist*, -*logy*, -*pathy* and -*scopy*, and then build words that mean:

(e) disease of the stomach

(f) study of the stomach

(g) pertaining to, upon or above the stomach

(h) a specialist who studies the stomach

(i) technique of viewing/ examining the stomach

Note. In the procedure nasogastric intubation, a naso**gastr**ic tube (nas/o meaning nose) passes through the nose to the stomach and can be used for suction, irrigation or feeding.

▌Root

Enter

(*From a Greek word* **enteron**, *meaning intestine or gut. Here enter/o means the intestines in general or the small intestine.*)

Combining form   Enter/o

Word Exercise 3

Without using your Exercise Guide, write the meaning of:

(a) **enter**/itis

(b) **enter/o**/pathy

(c) **enter/o**/tomy

Using your Exercise Guide find the meaning of:

(d) **enter/o**/stomy

(e) **enter/o**/lith

Here you need to note the difference between:

> **-ectomy**
> A surgical procedure in which a part is removed by cutting. (Synonymous with the words excision and resection.)
>
> **-stomy**
> A surgical procedure in which an opening is made into a cavity or a communication is formed between cavities. The word also refers to the name of the opening or stoma so created, eg, a colostomy is an opening into the colon or the procedure of forming the opening (from the Greek word *stoma* meaning mouth). This word component is also used in ana**stom**osis, an opening or communication formed between two parts (Fig. 7). Note: a stoma can be temporary or permanent.
>
> **-tomy**
> A surgical procedure in which an incision is made, as at the beginning of an operation, or the process of cutting.

Without using your Exercise Guide, build words that mean:

(f) study of the intestine

(g) a person who specializes in
     the study of the intestines

Now we can put the combining forms of two roots together to make a larger word. Although these words look complicated, it is now quite easy to understand their meaning. Read the word components as in (h) 1, 2 then 3.

Without using your Exercise Guide, write the meaning of:

(h) gastr/o^2/**enter/o**^{3}/logy^1

(i) gastr/o/**enter/o**/pathy

(j) gastr/o/**enter**/itis

(k) gastr/o/**enter/o**/scopy

> **Note.** When the combining forms of two roots are joined, the combining vowel of the first root is retained.

Between the stomach and the small intestine, there is an aperture surrounded by a sphincter muscle known as the **pylorus** (see Fig. 6). This acts as a valve that opens periodically to allow digested food to leave the stomach and enter the small intestine.

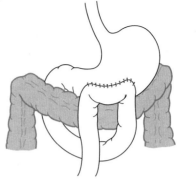 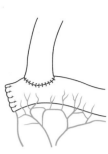

Stomach to intestine   Intestine to intestine
(side to side)   (side to end)

Figure 7   Surgical anastomoses.

Root

Pylor

*(From a Greek word **pylouros**, meaning gatekeeper. Here pylor/o means the pylorus, the opening of the stomach into the duodenum encircled by a sphincter muscle.)*

Combining form   Pylor/o

Word Exercise 4

Without using your Exercise Guide, write the meaning of:

(a) **pylor/o**/gastr/ectomy

(b) **pylor/o**/scopy

> **Note.** Bariatric surgery includes a variety of procedures performed on morbidly obese patients to enable them to lose weight. Weight loss is achieved by reducing the size of the stomach. Examples of these procedures include the following:
>
> **Laparoscopic adjustable gastric banding**
>
> In this procedure an inflatable silicone band (Lap Band) is placed around the top portion of the stomach using a laparoscope. When inflated, the band tightens and creates a small pouch at the top of the stomach that fills quickly and slows the passage of food to the lower part; this gives the sensation that the stomach is full and enables the patient to lose weight. The band is adjusted by introducing saline into a port with a special needle; the port is sutured to the abdominal wall just under the skin. The band can be loosened by withdrawing fluid from the port if necessary. See Figure 8(a).
>
> **Gastric bypass surgery (Roux-en-Y)**
>
> In this procedure a small pouch is created at the top of the stomach using staples. Food that enters the pouch is diverted by a surgical anastomosis (a gastrojejunostomy) into the jejunum, bypassing the duodenum and proximal jejunum; this reduces absorption of nutrients into the bloodstream. Roux-en-Y surgery

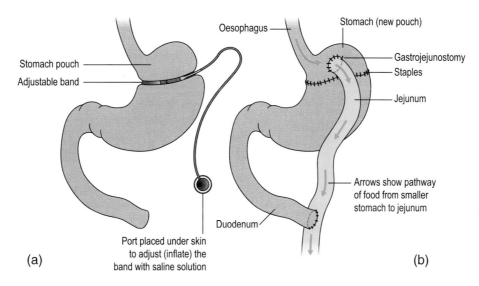

Figure 8 (a) Laparoscopic adjustable gastric banding, (b) Roux-en-Y gastric bypass procedure. (Adapted from Chabner D-E, Medical Terminology: A Short Course, 7th Edition, 2014, Saunders.)

is named after the surgeon who devised the procedure, Cesar Roux (1857–1934), and because the repositioned duodenum and jejunum form a Y-shape. See Figure 8(b).

The small intestine

Now we will examine the small intestine that consists of three parts: the **duodenum**, **jejunum** and **ileum**. The duodenum is concerned mainly with digestion of food, while the jejunum and ileum are specially adapted for the absorption of nutrients. Food is moved along the lumen (internal space) of the intestines and other parts of the alimentary canal by a process called **peristalsis** (from a Greek word *peristellein* meaning to clasp). This is brought about by a wave of contraction of smooth muscle in the wall of the intestine followed by a wave of relaxation.

Note. Although the root **enter** refers in general to intestines, it is sometimes used to mean the small intestine. However, there are also special roots that describe the different regions of the small intestine; we shall use these in the next three exercises.

▌Root

Duoden

(*From a Latin word* **duodeni**, *meaning twelve. Here duoden/o means the duodenum, the structure that forms the first 12 inches of the small intestine.*)

Combining form   Duoden/o

▌Root

Jejun

(*From a Latin word* **jejunus**, *meaning empty. Here jejun/o means the jejunum, the part of the intestine between the duodenum and ileum, approximately 2.4 m in length.*)

Combining form   Jejun/o

▌Root

Ile

(*From a Latin word* **ilia**, *meaning flank, guts or innards. Here ile/o means the ileum, the part that forms the lower three-fifths of the small intestine.*)

Combining form   Ile/o

📖 Word Exercise 5

Without using your Exercise Guide, write the meaning of words (a) to (c). Read the word components as in (a) 1, 2 then 3.

(a) **duoden/o²enter/o³/stomy¹**

(b) **jejun/o/jejun/o/stomy**

Using your Exercise Guide, find the meaning of:

(c) **duoden/o/jejun/al**

Without using your Exercise Guide, build words that mean:

(d) formation of an opening into the ileum

(e) inflammation of the ileum

(Exception to the 'rule' two vowels together)

A permanent opening or **ileostomy** is made when the whole of the large intestine has been removed. This acts as an artificial anus. The ileum opens directly on to the abdominal wall, and the liquid discharge from it is collected in a plastic **ileostomy bag** (Fig. 9).

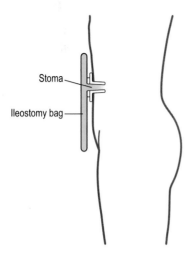

Figure 9   Ileostomy.

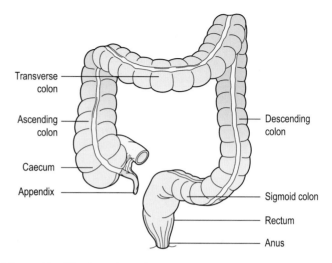

Figure 10   The large intestine.

After passing through the small intestine, any remaining material passes into the large intestine. A fold of mucous membrane called the ileocaecal valve or sphincter guards the opening from the ileum into the large intestine. This controls the movement of material from the ileum into the caecum (Am. cecum).

(Note: **small bowel** and **large bowel** are used colloquially to mean the small and large intestine.)

The large intestine

The large intestine has a wider diameter than the small intestine, and it is shorter. Its main function is to absorb water from the materials that remain after digestion and eject them from the body as faeces (Am. feces) during defaecation. The large intestine is made up of the **caecum** (Am. cecum), **appendix**, **colon**, **rectum** and **anus** (Fig. 10).

The next six roots refer to the large intestine:

 Root

Caec

(*From a Latin word* **caecus**, *meaning blind. Here caec/o means the caecum, the blindly ending pouch that is attached to the vermiform appendix and separated from the ileum by the ileocaecal valve.*)

Combining forms   Caec/o
                         Cec/o *(Am.)*

Root

Append

(*From a Latin word* **appendix**, *meaning appendage. Here appendic/o means the appendix, a blindly ending sac attached to the caecum.*)

Combining forms   Appendic/o
                     Append/o *(Am.)*

Root

Col

(*From a Greek word* **kolon**, *meaning colon, the part of the large intestine (large bowel) extending from the caecum to the rectum.*)

Combining forms   Col/o, colon/o

Word Exercise 6

Using your Exercise Guide, find the meaning of:

(a) mega/**colon**

Without using your Exercise Guide, write the meaning of:

(b) **appendic**/itis

(c) **col**/ectomy

(d) **col/o**/stomy
    (see Fig. 11)

A colostomy may be temporary or permanent and acts as an opening through which the effluent from the colon is discharged. The effluent is collected in a **colostomy bag**, which is attached to the surface of the abdomen.

Without using your Exercise Guide and beginning with the underlined root, build words that mean:

(e) formation of an opening into
    the caecum (Am. cecum)

(f) removal of the appendix

(g) formation of an opening
    (anastomosis) between the
    stomach and colon

(h) an instrument used to view
    the colon

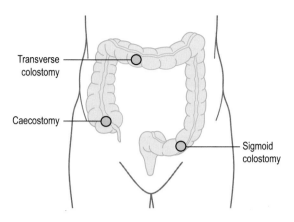

Transverse colostomy

Caecostomy

Sigmoid colostomy

Figure 11   Common sites of stomas of the large intestine (large bowel).

Root

Sigm

(*From a Greek word* **sigma**, *meaning the letter S. Here sigmoid/o means the sigmoid colon, the last part of the descending colon, which has an S shape.*)

Combining form   Sigmoid/o

Root

Rect

(*From a Latin word* **rectus**, *meaning straight. Here rect/o means the rectum, the last part of the large intestine, which is straight.*)

Combining form   Rect/o

Root

Proct

(*From a Greek word* **proktos**, *meaning anus. Here proct/o means the anus or rectum. The word anus is derived from Latin meaning a ring.*)

Combining form   Proct/o

Word Exercise 7

Using your Exercise Guide, find the meaning of:

(a) para/**rect**/al

(b) **an**o/rect/al

(c) peri/**proct**/itis

(d) **proct/o**/clysis

(e) **proct**/algia

Without using your Exercise Guide and beginning with the underlined root, build words that mean:

(f)   instrument to view <u>anus/ rectum</u> (use proct/o)

(g) formation of an opening between the <u>anus/rectum</u> and caecum (use proct/o)

(h) formation of an opening between the <u>caecum</u> (Am. cecum) and sigmoid colon

(i)   an instrument used to view the <u>sigmoid colon</u>

(j)   technique of examining or viewing the <u>sigmoid colon</u>

Sometimes the lining of the intestine develops enlarged pouches or sacs. Each is known as a **diverticulum** (plural **diverticula**). These can become inflamed as in **diverticul**itis and may have to be removed by **diverticul**ectomy.

The outer layer of the intestines and the lining of the cavity in which they lie consist of serous membranes. These membranes secrete a serum-like fluid called serous fluid that acts as a lubricant. A film of serous fluid allows organs to slide over each other as they move by peristalsis.

Root

Peritone

(*From Greek words* **peri**, *meaning around, and* **teinein**, *meaning to stretch. Here peritone/o means the peritoneum, the serous membrane lining the abdominal and pelvic cavities and covering all abdominal organs.*)

Combining forms   Periton/e/o

Word Exercise 8

Without using your Exercise Guide, write the meaning of:

(a) **periton**/itis

(b) **peritone/o**/scopy

Accessory organs of the digestive system

The pancreas

This large gland is found beneath the stomach (see Fig. 6). Its function is to produce **pancreatic juice** and pass it to the duodenum via the pancreatic duct. The juice neutralizes stomach acid and contains enzymes that digest all the main components of food. The pancreas also controls blood sugar levels by secreting the hormones **insulin** and **glucagon** directly into the blood.

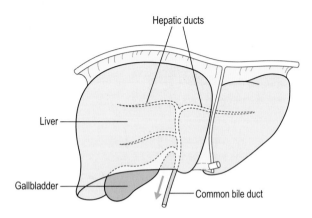

Figure 12   The liver and bile ducts.

Root

Pancreat

(*From a Greek word* **pankreas**, *meaning the pancreas.*)

Combining forms   Pancreat/o

A combining form **pancreatic/o** *is also derived from this root. It is used to mean the pancreatic duct. This duct transfers pancreatic juice containing digestive enzymes from the pancreas to the duodenum.*

The liver

The liver is the largest abdominal organ and is located just beneath the diaphragm (see Fig. 12). It processes nutrients received from the intestine, stores materials and excretes wastes in the form of **bile** into the intestine.

Root

Hepat

(*From a Greek word* **hepatos**, *meaning the liver.*)

Combining forms   Hepat/o

A combining form **hepatic/o** *is also derived from this root and is used to mean the hepatic bile duct.*

Word Exercise 9

Using your Exercise Guide, find the meaning of:

(a) **pancreat/o**/lysis

(b) **hepat/o**/megaly

(c) **hepat**/oma

(d) **hepat/o**/toxic

Without using your Exercise Guide, write the meaning of:

(e) **hepatic/o**/gastr/o/stomy

(f) **pancreatic/o**/duoden/al

Root

Chol

(*From a Greek word* **chole**, *meaning bile.*)

Combining form   Chol/e

Liver cells produce a yellowish-brown waste known as bile. This drains through small canals and hepatic ducts into a sac known as the gallbladder. Bile leaves the gallbladder through the common bile duct and enters the intestine. Although bile is a waste product, the bile salts it contains help to emulsify lipids (fats) in the intestine and neutralize acid entering from the stomach. The structures in which bile is transported are referred to as the **biliary** system (*bili-* meaning bile, *-ary* meaning pertaining to).

Word Exercise 10

Using your Exercise Guide, find the meaning of:

(a) a/**chol**/ia

(b) **chol/e**/lith

(c) **chol/e**/lith/iasis

(d) **chol**/aemia
    (Am. chol/emia)

(e) **chol**/uria

A word root commonly combined with **chol/e** is **cyst**, meaning bladder. **Cholecyst/o**, literally meaning a bladder of bile, is now used to mean the gallbladder.

Without using your Exercise Guide, write the meaning of:

(f) **cholecyst/o**/tomy

(g) **cholecyst**/ectomy

(h) **cholecyst/o**/lithiasis

A second word root often combined with **chol/e** is **angi**, meaning vessel. **Cholangi/o** means bile vessel or bile duct.

Using your Exercise Guide, find the meaning of:

(i) **cholangi/o**/gram

(j) **cholangi/o**/graphy

A third word root often combined with **chol/e** is **doch**, meaning to receive. **Choledoch/o** means the common bile duct, ie, that which receives the bile.

Without using your Exercise Guide, write the meaning of:

(k) **choledoch/o**/lith/iasis

(l) **choledoch/o**/lith/o/tomy

Here we need to distinguish between three suffixes that often cause some confusion:

-gram

This refers to a tracing. In practice in medicine, it usually refers to an X-ray picture, paper recording or to a trace on a screen.

-graphy

This refers to the technique or process of making a recording, eg, an X-ray or tracing. It can also refer to a written description.

-graph

This means a description or writing, but more often it is used in medicine for the name of an instrument that carries out a recording. It is also used to mean a recording or X-ray picture in the term radiograph.

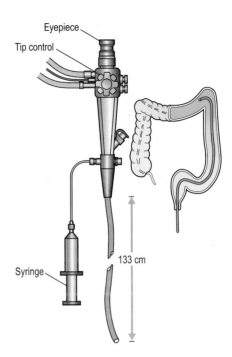

Figure 13   A fibreoptic endoscope used to view the colon.

Root

Lapar

(*From a Greek word* **lapara**, *meaning loin, the soft part between the ribs and hips. By common usage, it has come to mean the abdominal wall.*)

Combining form   Lapar/o

 Word Exercise 11

Without using your Exercise Guide, write the meaning of:

(a) **lapar/o**/scopy

(b) **lapar/o**/tomy

Laparotomy is an exploratory operation performed when the diagnosis of an abdominal problem is uncertain. With advances in diagnostic procedures such as computed tomography (CT) scanning, ultrasonography and laparoscopy, it has become less common.

Laparoscopy is performed using a laparoscope, a device consisting of a thin tube containing a lens system that can be passed through a small hole made with a *trocar* into the abdominal cavity. The trocar is a sharp pointed instrument that penetrates the abdominal wall and contains a cannula (tube) through which the laparoscope tube can pass. The laparoscope allows the internal organs (viscera) to be viewed and manipulated by a surgeon (a procedure commonly called 'keyhole' surgery).

Medical equipment and clinical procedures

The use of medical equipment and clinical procedures enables doctors to make a **diagnosis**; this means naming the patient's

disease and distinguishing it from others (from *dia-* meaning through and *-gnosis* meaning knowledge). The information also enables a **prognosis** or forecast of the probable course and determination of a disease to be made (from *pro-* meaning forward).

Endoscopes

In this unit, we have named several instruments used in the examination of the digestive system. Let us review their names:

Oesophagoscope   Sigmoidoscope
(Am. esophagoscope)
Gastroscope   Proctoscope
Colonoscope   Laparoscope

All of these instruments are used to view various parts of the digestive system. Now fibreoptic endoscopes have replaced many of the original viewing instruments. Endoscope means an instrument to view or examine within (**endo-** means within/inside); in practice, they are used to view the inside of tubular structures and cavities. The procedure of using an endoscope is known as **endoscopy**, and the person trained to use the equipment as an **endoscopist** (**-ist** meaning specialist).

Fibreoptic endoscopes utilize flexible tubes (Fig. 13) that can be inserted into body cavities or into small incisions made in the body wall. Each is provided with illumination and a system of lenses that enables the operator to view the inside of the body. The inclusion of electronic chips at the end of the fibreoptic tube allows the view to be transmitted to a video screen.

The endoscope can be adapted to view particular areas of the body. In the case of the digestive system, the fibreoptic tube can be passed into the mouth to examine the oesophagus, stomach and intestine; this procedure is known as oesophago-gastroduodenoscopy or OGD (Am. EGD). Alternatively, it can be passed into the anus to view the rectum and colon. Note that when an endoscope is adapted to examine the stomach, it may be referred to as a gastroscope.

When endoscopes are used to examine several different structures at the same time, for example, the mouth, oesophagus, voice box, nose and larynx, the term **pan**endoscopy is sometimes used (**pan-** meaning all).

Capsule endoscopy has recently been brought into use to examine parts of the intestines that cannot be reached with a fibreoptic endoscope. The procedure involves swallowing a pill-sized capsule that contains a camera, battery, light and transmitter. The camera can take several pictures every second for up to 8 hours and the images can be transmitted to a recorder worn around the patient's waist.

In addition to viewing cavities, endoscopes can be fitted with a variety of attachments, such as forceps and catheters, and they can then be used for special applications. One such procedure is:

ERCP or endoscopic, retrograde, cholangiopancreatography

Let's examine the words separately:

endoscopic	referring to an endoscope/endoscopy
retrograde	going backwards
chol	bile
angio	vessel
pancreato	pancreas
graphy	technique of making a tracing/X-ray recording

Analyzing the words making up ERCP helps us to understand the nature of the procedure.

A technique of making an X-ray (graphy) of the bile vessels and pancreas (chol/angi/o/pancreat/o) by passing a tube called a catheter backwards (retrograde) into them using an endoscope (endoscopic). Dye is injected through a catheter into the vessels to outline them on the X-ray, although this is not evident from the word analysis.

 Word Exercise 12

Match each description in Column C with a term in Column A by placing the appropriate number in Column B.

Column A	Column B	Column C
(a) capsule endoscopy		1. an instrument used to view the rectum or anus
(b) enteroscope		2. technique of taking images of the intestines using an internal camera
(c) endoscope		3. visual examination of the colon
(d) enteroscopy		4. an instrument used to view the intestines
(e) endoscopy		5. visual examination of all structures, eg, oesophagus, mouth, larynx and nose
(f) endoscopist		6. an instrument used to view body cavities
(g) colonoscopy		7. visual examination of the intestines
(h) proctoscope		8. a person who operates an endoscope
(i) sigmoidoscopy		9. visual examination of body cavities
(j) panendoscopy		10. visual examination of the sigmoid colon

Other procedures widely used to investigate the digestive system besides those mentioned in the word exercises include:

Abdominal ultrasonography The technique of using high-frequency sound waves to produce images of abdominal organs; it is especially useful for examining the gallbladder.

Computed tomography (CT) The technique of recording a series of X-rays showing abdominal structures in multiple cross-sectional views.

Faecal occult blood test (Am. fecal) A screening test for colon cancer; it uses guaiac, a chemical that changes colour when it reacts with any blood present in a stool sample.

Liver biopsy Sections of liver are removed using a needle to aid the diagnosis of cirrhosis, tumours (Am. tumors) and hepatitis.

Liver function tests A set of tests that detect the presence of enzymes and bilirubin in the blood. When the liver is damaged, it releases enzymes, and the levels of proteins produced by the liver drop. The tests aid diagnosis of hepatitis, cirrhosis and alcohol-related liver disease.

Magnetic resonance imaging The technique of using strong magnetic fields and radio waves to create detailed images in three planes; here it is used to image the abdominal organs.

X-ray imaging X-ray imaging is used in several ways to detect pathological changes in the digestive system, including X-ray imaging of the colon and rectum following injection of barium into the rectum (a barium enema). This procedure is known as a lower gastrointestinal series, and it produces a set of X-ray images of the rectum and colon. X-ray imaging of the oesophagus (Am. esophagus), stomach and small intestine following ingestion of barium by mouth (a barium meal or swallow) is known as an upper gastrointestinal series.

ANATOMY EXERCISE

Now complete the Anatomy Exercise on page 14.

 CASE HISTORY 2

The object of this exercise is to understand words associated with a patient's medical history. To complete the exercise:

- Read through the passage on gallstones; unfamiliar words are underlined, and you can find their meaning using the Word Help.

- Write the meaning of the medical terms shown in bold print on the lines that follow the Word Help.

Gallstones (cholelithiasis)

Miss B, a 35-year-old woman, presented to her general practitioner complaining of pain emanating from the **epigastric** and right hypochondrial regions radiating to the back. The pain lasted for about 3 hours following each meal and was accompanied by nausea and occasional vomiting. Her GP's initial diagnosis was **biliary** colic, and he prescribed the analgesic pethidine. The pain did not resolve, and she was admitted to the **gastroenterology** unit.

Initial ultrasound investigations revealed multiple stones (calculi) in the gallbladder and a dilated common bile duct. A date was set for an early elective **laparoscopic cholecystectomy**. Miss B was counselled on her perioperative drug regimen and was introduced to the concept of patient-controlled analgesia (PCA) using a syringe driver. Unfortunately, her elective procedure was delayed by an episode of acute **cholecystitis**.

Once recovered, Miss B was admitted again, but due to her excessive weight, laparoscopy was deemed inappropriate by the surgeon, and she was advised of the associative risks of an alternative procedure.

Vital signs on admission:

Pulse: 90/min	Oral temp: 37 °C	BP: 140/70
Height: 1.52 m	Weight: 85 kg	Smoker: 25/day
Moderate drinker	Medication: none	

An open cholecystectomy was performed, and the inflamed gallbladder was found to contain three gallstones, each approximately 15 mm in diameter. A bile sample was sent for culture and sensitivity testing, and a **nasogastric** tube was passed. Antibiotic prophylaxis (cefuroxime) was administered prior to her operation and continued for 48 hours. Miss B also received low-dose subcutaneous heparin injections as part of her thromboembolic prophylaxis.

The patient tolerated surgery well, PCA controlled her pain, and she was apyrexial. In the immediate postoperative period, she received an intravenous (IV) infusion of dextrose 4%, NaCl 0.18%, KCl 0.05% at a rate of 125 mL/hr.

On day four following her operation, the nasogastric tube and wound drains were removed, and IV fluid replacement ceased. Miss B left the unit on day six and was provided with diclofenac 50 mg analgesic tablets to be taken up to 3 times daily, when required. She agreed to an appointment with the dietician to discuss the desirability of reducing her weight.

Word Help

analgesic a pain-relieving drug

apyrexial absence of fever

calculi abnormal concretions composed of mineral salts and bile components

culture and sensitivity testing growing microorganisms in the laboratory and testing them for sensitivity to antibiotics

dietician/dietitian specialist who plans and advises on diet with the approval of medical staff

elective voluntary/not an emergency/at a planned date

GP general practitioner (family doctor)

heparin an anticoagulant drug that prevents blood clotting

hypochondrial the region to the side, just below the ribs

intravenous pertaining to within a vein

open refers to surgery via an incision (here into the abdomen)

perioperative around the time of an operation

postoperative pertaining to after/following an operation

prophylaxis preventative treatment

regimen a regulated scheme (eg, of taking drugs/medication)

subcutaneous pertaining to under the skin

syringe driver a motorized device that injects medication/drugs into the body

thromboembolic a thrombus or clot moving and blocking another blood vessel

ultrasound using sound waves to produce an image

Now write the meaning of the following words from the Case History without using your dictionary lists:

(a) cholelithiasis

(b) epigastric

(c) biliary

(d) gastroenterology

(e) laparoscopic

(f) cholecystectomy

(g) cholecystitis

(h) nasogastric

(Answers to the Case History exercise are given in the Answers to Word Exercises on page 335.)

Quick Reference

Combining forms relating to the digestive system:

An/o	anus
Appendic/o	appendix
Bil/i	bile
Caec/o	caecum
Cec/o (Am.)	cecum
Chol/e	bile
Cholangi/o	bile vessel/duct
Cholecyst/o	gallbladder
Choledoch/o	common bile duct
Col/o	colon
Colon/o	colon
Diverticul/o	diverticulum
Duoden/o	duodenum
Enter/o	intestine
Esophag/o (Am.)	esophagus
Gastr/o	stomach
Hepat/o	liver
Hepatic/o	hepatic duct
Ile/o	ileum
Jejun/o	jejunum
Lapar/o	flank / abdominal wall
Oesophag/o	oesophagus
Pancreatic/o	pancreatic duct
Pancreat/o	pancreas
Peritone/o	peritoneum
Proct/o	anus/rectum
Pylor/o	pyloric sphincter
Rect/o	rectum
Ser/o	serous/serum
Sigmoid/o	sigmoid colon

Abbreviations

Some common abbreviations related to the digestive system are listed below. Note that some are not standard, and their meaning may vary from one healthcare setting to another. There is a more extensive list for reference on page 369.

abdo	abdomen
BNO	bowels not open
BO	bowels open
CD	Crohn disease
DU	duodenal ulcer
GI	gastrointestinal
GU	gastric ulcer
IBD	inflammatory bowel disease
LLQ	left lower quadrant
LUQ	left upper quadrant
Pr/PR	per rectum
PU	peptic ulcer
RLQ	right lower quadrant
RUQ	right upper quadrant
UC	ulcerative colitis
UGI	upper gastrointestinal

Pathology notes

Anal fistula

An abnormal tube-like passageway in the skin near the anus that usually opens into the rectum. An anal fistula usually develops after an anal abscess that bursts, or when an abscess has not been completely treated. Anal fistulas can also be caused by conditions that affect the intestines, such as inflammatory bowel disease or diverticulitis.

Cancer

Stomach cancer has been linked to excessive alcohol consumption, use of chewing tobacco and eating smoked or preserved food. Most stomach cancers, usually adenocarcinomas, have already metastasized (spread) before they are found because patients treat themselves for the early warning signs of heartburn, belching and nausea. Later warning signs of stomach cancer include chronic indigestion, vomiting, anorexia, stomach pain and blood in the faeces. Surgical removal of the malignant tumours has been the most successful method of treating this condition.

Colorectal cancer is a malignancy, usually adenocarcinoma of the colon and rectum, that occurs most frequently after the age of 50; a low-fibre, high-fat diet and genetic predisposition are known risk factors. Early warning signs of this common type of cancer include changes in bowel habits, faecal blood (Am. fecal), rectal bleeding, abdominal pain, unexplained anaemia (Am. anemia) or weight loss and fatigue.

Colonic polyposis

A condition characterized by small growths on the lining of the colon or rectum. Polyps are usually less than 10 mm in size, although they can grow up to several centimetres. Sessile polyps appear as a bulge on the surface; pedunculated polyps have a stalk. Polyps are usually benign, but some become cancerous if left untreated. The cause of polyp formation is unknown, but familial polyposis is inherited, and unless the colon is removed the polyps will become malignant.

Gastrooesophageal reflux disease (GORD) (Am. Gastroesophageal reflux disease (GERD))

Backward flow (reflux) of hydrochloric acid from the stomach up into the oesophagus (Am. esophagus) causes sensations of burning and pressure behind the breastbone; these symptoms are commonly referred to as heartburn or acid indigestion. In their simplest form, GORD symptoms are mild and occur only infrequently. In these cases, avoiding problem foods or beverages, stopping smoking or losing weight may solve the problem. Additional treatment with over-the-counter antacids or nonprescription-strength acid-blocking medications called H_2-receptor antagonists may also be used. Over time if left untreated, serious pathological (precancerous) lesions may develop in the lining of the oesophagus; these changes are known as Barrett oesophagus.

Hepatitis

Hepatitis is a general term referring to inflammation of the liver. Hepatitis is characterized by jaundice (a yellowish discoloration of body tissues), liver enlargement, anorexia, abdominal discomfort, grey-white faeces (Am. feces) and dark urine. Various conditions can produce hepatitis, for example, excess alcohol, drugs, toxins and infection with bacteria, viruses or parasites. *Hepatitis A* results from infection by the hepatitis A virus, often acquired from contaminated food. It occurs commonly in young people and ranges in severity from mild to life threatening. Viral *Hepatitis B* is usually more severe; this is also called serum hepatitis because it is transmitted by contaminated blood serum. Hepatitis B causes severe illness that may lead to necrosis of the liver and death. It also predisposes victims to liver cancer. Hepatitis C is transmitted through blood, is common amongst IV drug users, and leads to chronic liver disease.

All these conditions may lead to a degenerative condition known as *cirrhosis*. The liver's ability to regenerate damaged tissue is well known, but it has its limits. When the toxic effects of alcohol accumulate faster than the liver can regenerate itself, damaged tissue is replaced with fibrous scar tissue instead of normal tissue. Cirrhosis is the name given to such degeneration.

Inflammatory bowel disease (IBD)

This is used to describe Crohn disease and ulcerative colitis:

Crohn disease (regional ileitis)

This is a chronic inflammation of the alimentary tract that usually occurs in young adults. The terminal ileum and rectum are most commonly affected, but the disease may be present anywhere from the mouth to the anus. The full thickness of the intestinal wall is inflamed in patches sometimes causing obstruction of the lumen of the intestine. The cause of Crohn disease is not clear, but an immunological abnormality may render the individual susceptible to infection by viruses or other organisms.

Ulcerative colitis

This is a chronic inflammatory disease of the inner lining (mucosa) of the colon and rectum that may ulcerate and become infected. It usually occurs in young adults and begins in the rectum and sigmoid colon. It can spread and involve part or the whole of the colon, and the cause is unknown. In severe cases surgical removal of the entire colon cures the condition.

Intussusception

A condition in which one part of the intestine telescopes into another; it causes severe colic and intestinal obstruction. The portion that has prolapsed in this way is called an intussusceptum.

Irritable bowel syndrome (IBS)

This is also called spastic colon and is a common chronic non-inflammatory condition that is often caused by stress. Diarrhoea (Am. diarrhea) or constipation with or without pain are the main symptoms.

Jaundice (icterus)

Jaundice is a term used to describe the yellowing of the skin and whites of the eyes when a bile pigment called bilirubin builds up in the tissues. It can be due to excessive destruction of red blood cells, malfunction of liver cells that prevents excretion of bilirubin, or posthepatic obstruction of bile flow by gallstones or a tumour.

Ulcers

An ulcer is an open wound or sore in the digestive system that is acted upon by the gastric juice. The two most common sites for ulcers are the stomach (gastric ulcers) and the upper part of the small intestine or duodenum (duodenal ulcers). Disintegration and death of tissue characterize ulcers as they erode the layers in the wall of the stomach or duodenum. Untreated ulcers cause persistent pain and may perforate the digestive tube, causing massive haemorrhage (Am. hemorrhage) and widespread inflammation of the abdominal cavity. Most experts now agree that hyperacidity is only partly to blame for most ulcers; the underlying cause is a spiral-shaped bacterium called *Helicobacter pylori*. The presence of this organism in the stomach lining impairs its ability to secrete mucus and opens the way for stomach acid to begin its destruction of the gastric tissue.

Volvulus

Twisting of a section of the intestine so as to occlude its lumen (internal space). Volvulus is a main cause of intestinal obstruction and constitutes a surgical emergency.

Associated words

Achalasia condition of failure of relaxation of a muscle sphincter causing dilation of the part above, eg, the oesophagus (Am. esophagus)

Adhesion a union between two surfaces that are normally separated

Anorexia nervosa a condition of complete loss of appetite and emaciation caused by psychological problems

Ascites accumulation of serous fluid in the abdominal cavity

Bariatrics a branch of medicine that deals with obesity

Borborygmi rumbling noises caused by movement of gas and fluid in the intestines (from a Greek word *borborizein*, to rumble in the bowels)

Bowel intestine

Brash also called water brash or heartburn, the reflux of dilute acid from the stomach into the pharynx giving a burning sensation

Bulimia condition of abnormal increase in the sensation of hunger; bulimia nervosa is a condition of 'binge eating' followed by controlled, self-induced vomiting

Cirrhosis condition of degeneration of the liver (the liver becomes yellow)

Coeliac pertaining to the abdomen (coeliac disease is a hypersensitivity to gluten that causes inflammation of the intestines and stomach) (Am. celiac)

Constipation difficult or delayed elimination of faeces (Am. feces)

Crepitus the noisy passing of flatus from the bowels

Deglutition the process of swallowing

Diarrhoea frequent loose, watery stools (Am. diarrhea)

Dysentery inflammation of the intestines, diarrhoea (Am. diarrhea) and abdominal cramps caused by bacteria, protozoa or parasitic worms

Emesis vomiting, the process of expelling the stomach contents through the mouth

Emulsification breaking up of fats (lipids) into small globules that are dispersed in water to form an emulsion; the globules form a large surface area for digestion of fat by enzymes

Enema introduction of fluid into the rectum or a solution introduced into the rectum to promote evacuation of faeces (Am. feces)

Enzyme a protein catalyst that speeds up a chemical reaction; enzymes are secreted by the mouth, stomach, pancreas and intestines to digest our food

Eructation belching, the process of expelling gas from the stomach through the mouth

Eventration protrusion of the bowels through the abdomen; removal of the abdominal viscera

Flatulence is the presence of large amounts of gas dilating the stomach and intestines (From a Latin word *flatus*, meaning a blowing)

Flatus gas in the stomach and intestines, usually applied to that passed rectally

Gut the intestine or bowel

Haematochezia a condition of passing blood in the faeces (Am. hematochezia, feces)

Hernia protrusion of any internal organ through the structures enclosing them, eg, protrusion of the intestine through the inguinal canal

Hiatus hernia protrusion of part of the stomach through the oesophageal opening in the diaphragm (Am. esophageal)

Hyperchlorhydria condition of secreting too much hydrochloric acid into the gastric juice

Hypochlorhydria condition of secreting too little hydrochloric acid into the gastric juice

Ileus an obstruction of the intestine usually applied to failure of peristalsis

Mastication the chewing of food

Melena black tarry stools caused by blood in the faeces (Am. feces)

Motion evacuation of the bowels, defaecation (Am. defecation)

Nausea a feeling of sickness making one vomit

Palpation examination of organs by touch or pressure of the hand

Paracentesis puncture of the abdomen to remove fluid (ascites), synonym, and not Synonym abdominocentesis

Postprandial occurring after a meal

Regurgitation return of material from the stomach to the mouth

Retch a strong involuntary effort to vomit

Steatorrhoea the flow of fat in the faeces due to poor digestion and absorption (Am. steatorrhea, feces)

Stool a motion or discharge from the bowel; faeces (Am. feces)

Tympanites swelling of the abdomen caused by gas in the intestines or peritoneal cavity

NOW TRY THE WORD CHECK

WORD CHECK

This self-check exercise lists all the word components used in this unit. First, write down the meaning of as many word components as you can. Then check your answers using the Exercise Guide and Quick Reference box or the Glossary of Word Components (pp. 383–410).

Prefixes

a-

endo-

epi-

mega-pan-

para-

peri-

retro-

Combining forms of word roots

an/o

angi/o

appendic/o

bil/i

caec/o (Am. cec/o)

chol/e

choledoch/o

col/o

colon/o

cyst/o

diverticul/o

duoden/o

enter/o

gastr/o

hepat/o

hepatic/o

ile/o

jejun/o

lapar/o

nas/o

oesophag/o (Am. esophag/o)

pancreat/o

pancreatic/o

peritone/o

proct/o

pylor/o

rect/o

ser/o

sigmoid/o

tox/o

Suffixes

-aemia (Am. -emia)

-al

-algia

-ary

-clysis

-ectomy

-grade

-gram

-graph

-graphy

-ia

-iasis

-ic

-ist

-itis

-lith

-lithiasis

-logist

-logy

-lysis

-megaly

-oma

-pathy

-scope

-scopy

-stomy

-tomy

-toxic

-uria

NOW TRY THE SELF-ASSESSMENT

SELF-ASSESSMENT

Test 2A

Next are some combining forms that refer to the anatomy of the digestive system. Indicate which part of the system they refer to by putting a number from the diagram (Fig. 14) next to each word. You can use a number more than once.

(a) pylor/o

(b) gastr/o

(c) proct/o

(d) hepat/o

(e) appendic/o

(f) choledoch/o

(g) col/o

(h) pancreat/o

(i) sigmoid/o

(j) oesophag/o
    (Am. esophag/o)

(k) cholecyst/o

(l) ile/o

(m) caec/o (Am. cec/o)

(n) duoden/o

(o) rect/o

Score [   ]
      15

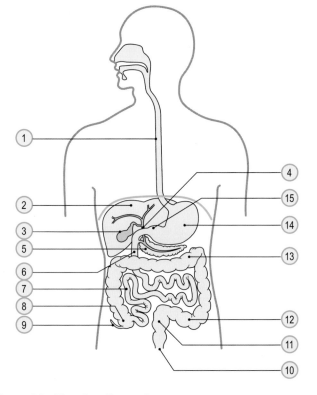

Figure 14   The digestive system.

Test 2B

Prefixes and suffixes

Match each meaning in Column C with a prefix or suffix in Column A by inserting the appropriate number in Column B.

Column A	Column B	Column C
(a) a-		1. enlargement
(b) -aemia (Am. -emia)		2. condition of pain
(c) -algia		3. study of
(d) -clysis		4. around
(e) -ectomy		5. injection/infusion
(f) endo-		6. X-ray/tracing
(g) -gram		7. inflammation
(h) -graph		8. condition of urine
(i) -graphy		9. within/inside
(j) -itis		10. beside/near
(k) -lithiasis		11. tumour (Am. tumor)
(l) -logy		12. abnormal condition of stones
(m) mega-		13. all
(n) -megaly		14. without
(o) -oma		15. technique of making an X-ray/ tracing/recording
(p) pan-		16. large
(q) para-		17. instrument that records

Column A	Column B	Column C
(r) peri-		18. incision into
(s) -tomy		19. removal of
(t) -uria		20. condition of blood

Score 20

Column A	Column B	Column C
(r) pylor/o		18. pancreas
(s) rect/o		19. liver
(t) sigmoid/o		20. appendix

Score 20

Test 2C

Combining forms of word roots

Match each meaning in Column C with a combining form of a word root in Column A by inserting the appropriate number in Column B.

Column A	Column B	Column C
(a) angi/o		1. pylorus
(b) appendic/o		2. sigmoid colon
(c) caec/o (Am. cec/o)		3. peritoneum
(d) chol/e		4. jejunum
(e) choledoch/o		5. intestine
(f) colon/o		6. vessel
(g) cyst/o		7. duodenum
(h) duoden/o		8. colon
(i) enter/o		9. rectum
(j) gastr/o		10. rectum/anus
(k) hepat/o		11. bladder
(l) jejun/o		12. stomach
(m) lapar/o		13. oesophagus
(n) oesophag/o (Am. esophag/o)		14. bile
(o) pancreat/o		15. abdomen/flank
(p) peritone/o		16. common bile duct
(q) proct/o		17. caecum

Test 2D

Write the meaning of:

(a) gastroenterocolitis

(b) hepatography

(c) ileorectal

(d) proctosigmoidoscopy

(e) pancreatomegaly

Score 5

Test 2E

Build words that mean:

(a) inflammation of the duodenum

(b) condition of pain in the stomach

(c) incision into the liver

(d) study of the anus/ rectum

(e) formation of an opening/ anastomosis between the ileum and anus

Score 5

Check answers to Self-Assessment Tests on page 359.

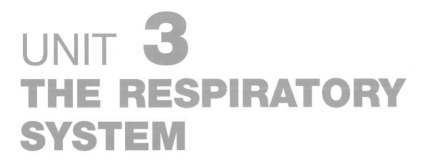

UNIT 3
THE RESPIRATORY SYSTEM

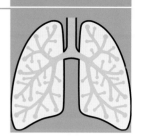

OBJECTIVES

Once you have completed Unit 3, you should be able to do the following:

- understand the meaning of medical words relating to the respiratory system
- build medical words relating to the respiratory system
- associate medical terms with their anatomical position
- understand common medical abbreviations relating to the respiratory system

EXERCISE GUIDE

Use this list of word components and their meanings to complete the word exercises in this unit.

Prefixes

a-	without
brady-	slow
dys-	difficult/painful
endo-	within
hyper-	above/excessive
hypo-	below/low
inter-	between
ortho-	straight
tachy-	fast

Roots / Combining forms

chondr/o	cartilage
esophag/o (Am.)	esophagus
gastr/o	stomach
haem/o	blood
hem/o (Am.)	blood
hepat/o	liver
myc/o	fungus
oesophag/o	oesophagus
radi/o	radiation/X-ray

Suffixes

-al	pertaining to
-algia	condition of pain
-ary	pertaining to
-centesis	surgical puncture to remove fluid
-desis	fixation/bind together by surgery / sticking together
-dynia	condition of pain
-eal	pertaining to
-ectasis	dilatation/stretching
-ectomy	removal of
-genic	pertaining to formation / originating in
-gram	X-ray/tracing/recording
-graphy	technique of recording/making X-ray
-ia	condition of
-ic	pertaining to
-itis	inflammation of
-logy	study of
-meter	measuring instrument
-metry	process of measuring
-osis	abnormal condition / disease of
-pathy	disease of
-plasty	surgical repair/reconstruction
-pexy	surgical fixation/fix in place
-plegia	condition of paralysis
-rrhaphy	stitching/suturing
-rrhea (Am.)	excessive discharge/flow
-rrhoea	excessive discharge/flow
-scope	an instrument used to view/examine
-scopy	technique of viewing/examining
-spasm	involuntary contraction
-stenosis	abnormal condition of narrowing
-stomy	formation of an opening into...
-tomy	incision into
-us	thing / a structure (indicates an anatomical part)

ANATOMY EXERCISE

When you have finished Word Exercises 1–16, look at the word components listed below. Complete Figure 15 by writing the appropriate combining form on each line; more than one component may relate to the same position. (You can check their meanings in the Quick Reference box on p. 40.)

Bronchiol/o	Nas/o	Pneumon/o
Bronch/o	Nasopharyng/o	Pulmon/o
Cost/o	Pharyng/o	Rhin/o
Laryng/o	Phren/o	Steth/o
Lob/o	Pleur/o	Trache/o

The respiratory system

Humans breathe air into paired lungs through the nose and mouth during inspiration. Whilst air is in the lungs, gaseous exchange takes place; in this process, oxygen enters the blood in exchange for carbon dioxide. During expiration, air containing less oxygen and more carbon dioxide leaves the body. The oxygen obtained through gaseous exchange is required by body cells for cellular respiration, a process that releases energy from food.

Our study of the respiratory system begins at the point where air enters the body, the nose.

Use the Exercise Guide at the beginning of this unit to complete Word Exercises 1 to 16, unless you are asked to work without it.

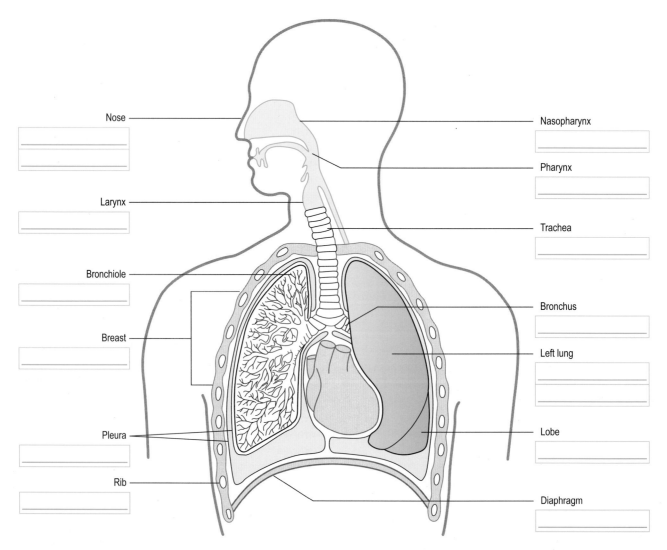

Figure 15   The respiratory system.

Root

Rhin

(*From a Greek word* **rhinos**, *meaning nose.*)

Combining form   Rhin/o

 Word Exercise 1

Using your Exercise Guide, find the meaning of:

(a) **rhin/o**/scope

(b) **rhin/o**/pathy

(c) **rhin**/algia

(d) **rhin**/itis

(e) **rhin/o**/rrhoea
    (Am. **rhin/o**/rrhea)

(f) **rhin/o**/plasty

(g) **rhino**scopy

Root

Nas

(*From a Latin word* **nasus**, *meaning nose.*)

Combining form   Nas/o

 Word Exercise 2

Using your Exercise Guide, find the meaning of:

(a) **nas/o**/gastr/ic tube

(b) **nas/o**-oesophag/eal tube
    (Am. **nas/o**-esophag/eal)

Root

Pharyng

(*From a Greek word* **pharynx**, *meaning throat. Here pharyng/o means the pharynx, the cone-shaped cavity at the back of the mouth lined with mucous membrane.*)

Combining form   Pharyng/o

 Word Exercise 3

Without using your Exercise Guide, write the meaning of:

(a) **pharyng**/algia

(b) **pharyng/o**/rrhoea (Am.
    pharyng/o/rrhea)

Without using your Exercise Guide and beginning with the underlined root, build words that mean:

(c) surgical repair of the
    pharynx

(d) inflammation of the phar-
    ynx and nose (use rhin/o)

(e) an instrument used to
    view the pharynx

Root

Laryng

(*From a Greek word* **larynx**, *meaning the voice box. Here laryng/o means the larynx, the organ that produces the voice.*)

Combining form   Laryng/o

 Word Exercise 4

Using your Exercise Guide, find the meaning of:

(a) **laryng/o**/logy

(b) **laryng/o**[2]/**pharyng**[3]/
    ectomy[1]

Without using your Exercise Guide and beginning with the underlined root, build words that mean:

(c) an instrument used
    to view the voice box

(d) technique of viewing
    the larynx

(e) the study of the larynx
    and nose (use rhin/o)

When swallowing, food is prevented from falling into the larynx by the **epiglottis**, a thin flap of cartilage lying above the glottis and behind the tongue. When the epiglottis moves, it covers the opening into the larynx and sound-producing glottis. **Epiglott/o** is the combining form derived from epiglottis; inflammation of the epiglottis may produce **epiglott**itis, and tumours may be removed by an **epiglott**ectomy.

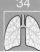
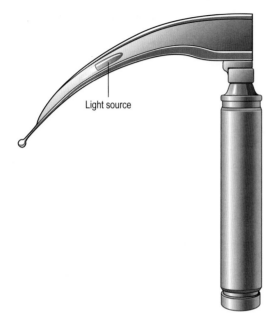

Figure 16   A laryngoscope.

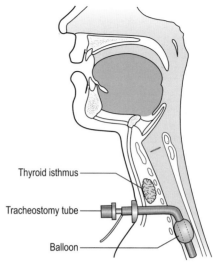

Figure 18   Tracheostomy.

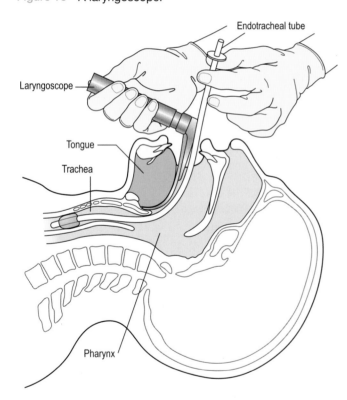

Figure 17   Endotracheal intubation using a laryngoscope. (Adapted from Chabner D-E, The Language of Medicine, 10th Edition, 2013, Saunders.)

▌Root

Trache

(*From Greek* **tracheia**, *meaning rough. Here trache/o means the trachea or windpipe, a structure containing rings of cartilage that give it a rough appearance.*)

Combining form   Trache/o

 Word Exercise 5

Using your Exercise Guide, find the meaning of:

(a) **trache/o**/tomy

(b) endo/**trache**/al

(c) **trache/o**/stomy

(An operation performed to maintain the airway or the name of the opening so created; see Fig. 18.)

Bronch

(*From a Greek word* **bronchos**, *meaning windpipe. Here bronch/o means the bronchi, two large air passages formed by division of the trachea that enter the lungs.*)

Combining forms   Bronch/i/o

 Word Exercise 6

Using your Exercise Guide, find the meanings of -ectasis, -gram, -graphy and -plegia; then build words that mean:

(a) condition of paralysis of the bronchi

(b) an X-ray picture of the bronchi

(c) technique of making an X-ray of the bronchi

(d) dilation of the bronchi

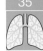

Using your Exercise Guide, find the meaning of:

(e) **bronch**/us (Plural bronchi)

(f) **bronch/o**/rrhaphy

(g) **bronch/o**/myc/osis

(h) **bronch/o**/genic

(i) **bronch/o**/spasm

(j) trache/o/**bronchi**/al

Without using your Exercise Guide, write the meaning of:

(k) **bronch/o**/scope

(l) **bronch/o**/rrhoea (Am. bronch/o/rrhea)

(m) laryng/o/trache/o/**bronch**/itis

(n) **bronch**/oesophag/o/stomy (Am. **bronch**/esophag/o/stomy)

Note. The combining form **bronchiol/o** is used when referring to the very small subdivisions of the bronchi known as **bronchioles**, eg, **bronchiol**itis for inflammation of the bronchioles.

The smallest bronchioles end in microscopic air sacs known as **alveoli** (from Latin *alveus*, meaning hollow cavity). Alveoli form a large surface area of the lungs across which the gases oxygen and carbon dioxide are exchanged and therefore play an essential role in maintaining life. The combining form is **alveol/o**, but few terms are in use, eg, **alveol**itis.

At the alveolar surface, oxygen diffuses into the blood from the cavities of the alveoli; carbon dioxide diffuses in the opposite direction and is lost from the body in expired air. Disorders of the respiratory and cardiovascular systems can affect gaseous exchange and therefore the concentration of these gases in the blood. **Hypoxia** is a condition of deficiency of oxygen in the tissues (*hypo-* meaning below/low, *-oxia* meaning condition of oxygen). **Hypercapnia** is a condition of too much carbon dioxide in the blood (*hyper-* meaning above/excessive, *-capnia* meaning a condition of carbon dioxide).

Poor oxygenation also results in the presence of large amounts of unoxygenated haemoglobin (Am. hemoglobin) in the blood. This produces **cyanosis**, an abnormal condition in which unoxygenated haemoglobin gives a blue tinge to the skin, lips and nail beds (*cyan/o* meaning blue, *-osis* meaning abnormal condition).

Root

Pneumon

(*A Greek word, meaning lung.*)

Combining form   Pneumon/o

Word Exercise 7

Without using your Exercise Guide, write the meaning of:

(a) **pneumon/o**/tomy

(b) **pneumon/o**/rrhaphy

(c) **pneumon**/osis

Without using your Exercise Guide, build words that mean:

(d) removal of a lung

(e) disease of a lung

Using your Exercise Guide, find the meaning of:

(f) **pneumon/o**/centesis

(g) **pneumon/o**/pexy

Note. Pneumonia means a condition of the lungs. It refers to an inflammation of the lungs with exudation caused by infection. (The exudate is a fluid that has escaped from capillaries lining the lungs.)

Root

Pneum

(*From a Greek word* **pneuma**, *meaning air. In the following examples, pneum/o and pneumat/o mean gas or air, but they can be used to mean the lungs or breathing.*)

Combining forms   Pneum/a/o, Pneumat/o

At this point, we need to introduce the word **pneumothorax**. The components of this word refer to air and thorax (chest), but the meaning of the word is not obvious. It means air or gas in the pleural cavity, ie, the space between the wall of the thorax and the lungs. A pneumothorax is formed by puncture of the chest wall; a stab wound or incision made as part of a surgical procedure can cause this. A pneumothorax causes the lung to collapse and can be life-threatening.

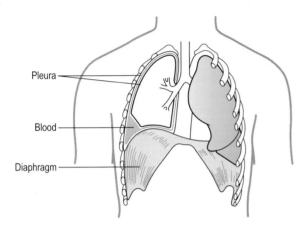

Pleura

Blood

Diaphragm

Figure 19   Haemothorax (Am. hemothorax).

Word Exercise 8

Using your Exercise Guide, find the meaning of:

(a) **pneum/o**/haem/o/thorax (Am. **pneum/o**/hem/o/thorax; see Fig. 19)

(b) **pneum/o**/radi/o/graphy (This term does not refer specifically to the respiratory system. It is a technique used to enhance the contrast of X-rays of body cavities by injecting air into them.)

A combining form, **-pnoea** (Am. -pnea), is derived from the Greek word **pnoia** meaning breathing or from **pnein** meaning to breathe.

Using your Exercise Guide, find the meaning of:

(c)   a/**pnoea** (Am. a/**pnea**)

(d) dys/**pnoea** (Am. dys/**pnea**)

(e) hyper/**pnoea** (Am. hyper/**pnea**)

(f) hypo/**pnoea** (Am. hypo/**pnea**)

(g) tachy/**pnoea** (Am. tachy/**pnea**)

(h)   brady/**pnoea** (Am. brady/**pnea**)

Note. The word ortho**pnoea** (Am. ortho**pnea**) means a condition of difficult breathing except in the upright (straight) position, eg, sitting up in bed.

Root

Lob

(*From a Greek word* **lobos**, *meaning lobe, a rounded section of an organ. In the lungs, lobes are formed by fissures or septa that divide the right lung into three lobes and the left lung into two. Note that other organs in the body are lobar.*)

Combining form   Lob/o

Word Exercise 9

Without using your Exercise Guide, build words that mean:

(a) incision into a lobe

(b) removal of a lobe

Root

Pulmon

(*From a Latin word* **pulmonis**, *meaning lung.*)

Combining form   Pulmon/o

Word Exercise 10

Using your Exercise Guide, find the meaning of:

(a) **pulmon**/ic

(b) **pulmon**/ary

Root

Pleur

(*From a Greek word* **pleura**, *meaning rib. Here pleur/o means pleura, the shiny membranes covering the lungs and internal surfaces of the thorax. The space in between these membranes is known as the pleural cavity.*)

Combining form   Pleur/o

Word Exercise 11

Without using your Exercise Guide, write the meaning of:

(a) **pleur**/itis (also called pleurisy)

(b) **pleur/o**/centesis

Without using your Exercise Guide, build a word that means:

(c) technique of making an X-ray/recording of the pleura (pleural cavity)

Using your Exercise Guide, find the meaning of:

(d) **pleur/o**/dynia

(e) **pleur/o**/desis

Note. Mesothelioma is a malignant tumour (Am. tumor) that arises in the pleura and is caused by exposure to asbestos.

Root

Phren

(*A Greek word, meaning midriff. Here phren/o means the dia-phragm, the muscular septum separating the thorax and abdomen that acts as the main respiratory muscle.*)

Combining form   Phren/o

Word Exercise 12

Using your Exercise Guide, find the meaning of:

(a) **phren/o**/gastr/ic

(b) **phren/o**/hepat/ic

(c) **phren/o**/plegia

Root

Thorac

(*From a Greek word **thorax**, meaning chest.*)

Combining form   Thorac/o; -thorax *is used as a suffix*

Word Exercise 13

Without using your Exercise Guide, build words that mean:

(a) disease of the thorax

(b) incision into the chest

Without using your Exercise Guide, write the meaning of:

(c) **thorac/o**/centesis

(d) **thorac/o**/scope

Using your Exercise Guide, find the meaning of:

(e) **thorac/o**/stenosis

Root

Cost

(*From a Latin word costa, meaning rib, one of the 12 pairs of curved bones that form part of the thorax.*)

Combining form   Cost/o

Word Exercise 14

Using your Exercise Guide, find the meaning of:

(a) inter/**cost**/al

(b) **cost/o**/genic

(c) **cost/o**/chondr/itis

Medical equipment and clinical procedures

In this unit, we have named several instruments used to examine the respiratory system. Some of those mentioned may be modified fibreoptic endoscopes. Here is a review of their names:

Rhinoscope   Pharyngoscope   Laryngoscope
Bronchoscope   Thoracoscope

The nose and pharynx can be superficially examined using a source of illumination with a tongue depressor and a Thudi-chum nasal speculum (Figs 20 and 21), named after physician Johann Ludwig Wilhelm Thudichum (1829–1901). Both of these items are usually disposable to prevent cross-infection during examination. Figure 20 shows a stainless-steel tongue depressor that can be sterilized and reused.

Note. The word **speculum** refers to an instrument used to hold the walls of a cavity apart so that its interior can be examined visually.

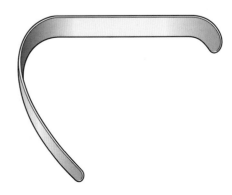

Figure 20   A tongue depressor.

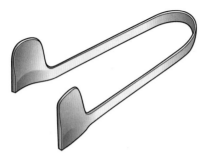

Figure 21   Thudichum nasal speculum.

Other instruments used to investigate the respiratory system include:

Mediastinoscope

This is a type of endoscope used to examine the mediastinum, the space in the chest cavity between the lungs. Mediastinoscopy is used to check whether cancer cells have spread from the lungs to the front part of the mediastinum and for the presence of infection.

Spirograph

Spir/o is from a Latin word *spirare*, meaning to breathe, the spirograph is an instrument that records the breathing movements of the lungs.

Spirometer

The spirometer is an instrument that measures breathing. The technique for using this instrument is known as spirometry (synonymous with pneumatometry). The spirometer is used for **pulmonary function tests** (PFTs) by recording the volumes of inhaled and exhaled air over a period of time. Many different values can be recorded, for example, **forced vital capacity** (FVC) and **peak expiratory flow rate** (PEF or PEFR).

Stethoscope

From a Greek word *stethos*, meaning breast, the stethoscope is an instrument used for listening to sounds from the chest (auscultation of the heart and lungs). See Figure 29.

> Here, we need to distinguish between the suffixes:
>
> **-meter**
> an instrument that measures
>
> **-metry**
> the technique of measuring, ie, using a measuring instrument

Now review the names and uses of all instruments and clinical procedures mentioned in this unit, and then try Exercises 15 and 16.

 Word Exercise 15

Match each description in Column C with a term in Column A by placing the appropriate number in Column B.

Column A	Column B	Column C
(a) bronchoscope		1. a person who may use a nasal speculum
(b) laryngoscopy		2. an instrument used to examine the vocal cords
(c) rhinoscope		3. an instrument used to examine the bronchi
(d) pharyngoscope		4. visual examination of the vocal cords
(e) bronchoscopy		5. a device used to allow air through the tracheal wall
(f) rhinologist		6. an instrument used to view the back of the mouth
(g) tracheostomy tube		7. visual examination of the bronchi
(h) laryngoscope		8. an instrument used to view nasal cavities

 Word Exercise 16

Match each description in Column C with a term in Column A by placing the appropriate number in Column B.

Column A	Column B	Column C
(a) thoraco-scope		1. an instrument used to open the nostrils
(b) stethoscope		2. technique of making an X-ray/recording of the pleura (pleural cavity)
(c) spirometer		3. technique of recording breathing movements

Column A	Column B	Column C
(d) spirography		4. technique of measuring lung capacity
(e) nasal speculum		5. an instrument used to view the thorax
(f) nasogastric tube		6. an instrument that measures lung capacity
(g) pleurography		7. an instrument used to examine/listen to the breast
(h) spirometry		8. a tube inserted into the stomach via the nose

Other procedures widely used to investigate the respiratory system besides those mentioned in the Word Exercises include:

Chest X-ray (CXR) Radiographic imaging of the thoracic cavity

Computed tomography (CT) The technique of recording a series of X-rays showing thoracic structures in multiple cross-sectional views

Lung biopsy A lung needle biopsy is a method of removing a piece of lung tissue for microscopic examination. If performed through the chest wall, it is called a transthoracic lung biopsy or percutaneous lung biopsy.

Magnetic resonance imaging The technique of using strong magnetic fields and radio waves to create detailed images in three planes; here, it is used to image the chest.

Mantoux test A test for latent tuberculosis; it is performed by injecting tuberculin, a purified protein derivative, into the skin. If a hard red bump develops within 48 to 72 hours, the test is positive, and the patient may have an active tuberculosis infection. The test is also known as the tuberculin skin test (TST).

Positron emission tomography This is the technique of scanning the lungs following the administration of radioactive glucose into the bloodstream. The images produced indicate the extent of uptake of glucose by lung tissue and are used to identify malignant tumours (Am. tumor).

Sputum test The patient expels sputum by coughing, or it is taken via an endotracheal tube. The specimen is then analyzed for the presence of pathogenic microorganisms in the laboratory.

ANATOMY EXERCISE

Now complete the Anatomy Exercise on page 32.

CASE HISTORY 3

The object of this exercise is to understand words associated with a patient's medical history.

To complete the exercise, do the following:

- Read through the passage on chronic obstructive pulmonary disease; unfamiliar words are underlined, and you can find their meaning using the Word Help.

- Write the meaning of the medical terms shown in bold print on the lines that follow the Word Help.

Chronic obstructive pulmonary disease

Mr C is 56 years of age and has a long history of chronic obstructive **pulmonary** disease (COPD). He began smoking at the age of 14 and until 6 years ago smoked approximately 25 to 30 cigarettes per day, but now he only smokes two or three per week. Five years ago, he developed a squamous cell carcinoma and had a right upper **lobectomy**.

Mr C has had two acute exacerbations of bronchitis in the past year. His wife says that over the last few days he has become increasingly out of breath and has difficulty in walking, speaking and eating. He was seen in casualty with increasing **dyspnoea (Am. dyspnea)**, **cyanosis** and a productive, purulent sputum.

Vital signs on admission

Pulse 100/min	Oral temp 38°C	BP 150/95

Medication

Home oxygen therapy	salbutamol 5 mg nebulized prednisolone 30 mg/day

Blood gas analysis

paCO₂ 8.90 kPa (4.5–6.1)	Standard bicarbonate 29.2 (22–28)	PEFR 180 L/min
paO₂ 4.5 kPa (12–15)	Blood pH 7.05 (7.32–7.42)	

On examination, he had a degree of **bronchospasm** and was showing signs of **hypoxia** and **hypercapnia**. His serious condition required his immediate transfer to the intensive therapy unit (ITU) for mechanical ventilatory support. An arterial catheter for blood gas sampling was inserted via the left radial artery, and he was sedated. He was given a muscle relaxant intravenously to enable endotracheal intubation and commencement of intermittent positive pressure ventilation (IPPV).

Mr C was initially diagnosed as having basal **pneumonia** in the right lung complicating his COPD. He was administered one intravenous dose of 500 mg of ampicillin, followed by 500 mg amoxicillin each 8 hours.

Word Help

acute symptoms and signs of short duration

carcinoma a malignant growth of epidermal cells / a cancer

catheter a tube inserted into the body

chronic lasting or lingering for a long time

endotracheal pertaining to within the trachea

exacerbations acute increased severity of symptoms

intravenous pertaining to within a vein

intubation insertion of a tube into a hollow organ, in this case the trachea

productive producing, eg, producing mucus/sputum

purulent resembling pus / infected

sedated state of reduced activity, usually as a result of medication

sputum material expelled from the respiratory passages by coughing or clearing the throat

squamous pertaining to scale-like / from a squamous epithelium

Epiglott/o	epiglottis
Laryng/o	larynx
Lob/o	lobe
Nas/o	nose
Nasopharyng/o	nasopharynx
Pharyng/o	pharynx
Phren/o	diaphragm
Pleur/o	pleura
Pneum/o	gas/air/lung
Pneumon/o	lung/air
-pnoea	breathing
-pnea (Am.)	breathing
Pulmon/o	lung
Rhin/o	nose
Spir/o	to breathe
Steth/o	breast
Thorac/o	thorax
Trache/o	trachea

Now write the meaning of the following words from the Case History without using your dictionary lists:

(a) pulmonary

(b) lobectomy

(c) dyspnoea (Am. dyspnea)

(d) cyanosis

(e) bronchospasm

(f) hypoxia

(g) hypercapnia

(h) pneumonia

(Answers to the Case History exercise are given in the Answers to Word Exercises on page 336.)

Quick Reference

Combining forms relating to the respiratory system:

Alveol/o	alveolus
Bronch/o	bronchus
Bronchiol/o	bronchiole
Chondr/o	cartilage
Cost/o	rib

Abbreviations

Some common abbreviations related to the respiratory system are listed below. Note that some are not standard, and their meaning may vary from one healthcare setting to another. There is a more extensive list for reference on page 369.

BRO	bronchoscopy
COAD	chronic obstructive airway disease
COPD	chronic obstructive pulmonary disease
CPR	cardiopulmonary resuscitation
CXR	chest X-ray
ET	endotracheal; endotracheal tube
FVC	forced vital capacity
LLL	left lower lobe (of lung)
PE	pulmonary embolism
PEF/PEFR	peak expiratory flow rate
PFTs	pulmonary function tests
RDS	respiratory distress syndrome
RSV	respiratory syncytial virus
RUL	right upper lobe (of lung)
SOB	shortage of breath
URI	upper respiratory infection
URTI	upper respiratory tract infection
VC	vital capacity

Pathology notes

Asthma

Asthma is an obstructive lung disorder characterized by recurring inflammation of mucous membranes and spasms of smooth muscles in the walls of bronchial air passages. The inflammation and contraction of smooth muscle narrow the airways and make breathing difficult. Initial onset of asthma can occur in children or adults. Stress, heavy exercise, infection or exposure to allergens or other irritants such as dusts, vapours (Am. vapors), or fumes can trigger acute episodes of asthma, so-called asthma

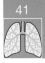

attacks. Many patients with asthma have a family history of allergies. Dyspnoea (Am. dyspnea) is the major symptom, but hyperventilation, headaches, numbness and nausea can occur. One way to treat asthma is by using inhaled or systemic bronchodilators that reduce muscle spasms and open the airways. Other types of treatment use nonsteroidal leukotriene modifiers that reduce the inflammation associated with asthma.

Atelectasis

A condition in which there is collapse of lung tissue with a consequent reduction in gaseous exchange. It may be due to failure of the alveoli to expand in the newborn (congenital atelectasis) or to resorption of air from the alveoli (collapse).

Chronic obstructive pulmonary disease (COPD)

This is a broad term used to describe conditions of progressive, irreversible obstruction of expiratory airflow. Patients with COPD have a productive cough, difficulty in breathing (mainly emptying their lungs) and develop visibly hyperinflated chests. The major disorders observed in people with this condition are bronchitis, emphysema and asthma.

Cor pulmonale

Failure of the right side of the heart to pump sufficient blood to the lungs; it results from chronic respiratory disease.

Emphysema

In this condition the walls of the alveoli lose their elasticity and remain filled with air on expiration. As emphysema progresses, large numbers of alveoli are damaged, and they become permanently dilated due to loss of interstitial connective tissue. These changes result in a hyperinflated chest known as a 'barrel chest'. Emphysema is associated with long-term exposure to cigarette smoke or air pollution, and victims often suffer the effects of hypoxia.

Lung cancer

Lung cancer is a malignancy of pulmonary tissue that not only destroys the vital gas exchange tissues of the lungs but also, like other cancers, may invade other parts of the body (metastasis). Lung cancer most often develops in damaged or diseased lungs. The most common predisposing condition associated with lung cancer is cigarette smoking (accounting for about 75% of cases). Other factors include exposure to second-hand cigarette smoke, asbestos, chromium, coal products, petroleum products, rust and ionizing radiation (as in radon gas).

Lung cancer may be arrested if detected early in routine chest X-ray films or other diagnostic procedures such as bronchoscopy. Depending on the size, location and exact type of malignancy involved, several strategies are available for treatment. Chemotherapy can cause a cure or remission in selected cases, as can radiation therapy. Photodynamic therapy (PDT) is also used to treat cancer of the lining of the bronchial tubes. Surgery

is the most effective treatment known, but less than half of those diagnosed are good candidates for surgery because of extensive metastatic spread.

Pertussis (whooping cough)

A highly contagious bacterial infection of the upper respiratory tract (pharynx, larynx and trachea) caused by *Bordatella pertussis*.

Pneumoconiosis

A condition caused by the presence of dust in the lungs characterized by inflammation, infection and bronchitis. Different forms of this condition are named according to the type of dust particle inhaled: anthracosis from coal dust; asbestosis from the mineral asbestos; silicosis from silica, a constituent of sandstone, glass and other rocks; byssinosis from cotton or linen dust.

Pulmonary embolism

A pulmonary embolism is a sudden obstruction of a pulmonary vessel by an embolus. Emboli can form from blood clots, fat, air and infective material. An embolus in a pulmonary vessel obstructs circulation of blood through the lungs.

Pulmonary oedema (Am. edema)

Pulmonary oedema is a condition in which there is an abnormal accumulation of fluid in the intercellular spaces and alveoli of the lungs; it is due to changes in hydrostatic forces in the capillaries or to an increase in capillary permeability. The condition is characterized by severe dyspnoea (Am. dyspnea); it may develop slowly, as in the patient with renal failure, or suddenly in the patient with left ventricular failure.

Restrictive pulmonary disease

Restrictive pulmonary diseases involve restriction of the alveoli, or reduced compliance, leading to decreased lung inflation. The hallmark of these disorders, regardless of their cause, is a decrease in lung volume, inspiratory reserve volume and vital capacity. Factors that restrict breathing can originate within the lung or the environment. Causes of restrictive lung disorders include *alveolar fibrosis* (scarring) secondary to occupational exposure to asbestos, toxic fumes, coal dust or other contaminants and immunological disease.

Tuberculosis (TB)

An infectious communicable disease caused by one of two forms of mycobacterium. Humans are the main host for *Mycobacterium tuberculosis* spread either by droplet infection or dust contaminated with infected sputum. *Mycobacterium bovi* (bovine TB) is transmitted from cows to humans via consumption of unpasteurized milk causing initial infection in the alimentary canal. Tuberculosis can affect any organ but, in humans, the main focus is in the lungs and pleurae, where it is marked by formation of tubercles and necrotic tissue. Immunization with attenuated BCG (Bacille-Calmette-Guérin) mycobacterium protects susceptible individuals who are identified by skin testing.

Associated words

Asphyxia condition of lack of oxygen and buildup of carbon dioxide in the blood; causes include drowning, a blocked airway and electrocution

Aspiration the entry of fluids or solids into the airway

Auscultation listening to the sounds given out by the internal organs, such as the lungs, with a stethoscope

Catarrh inflammation of mucous membranes, usually applied to the upper respiratory system

Coryza acute viral infection of the upper respiratory tract; the common cold

Cough a sudden, noisy expulsion of air from the lungs

Croup an acute respiratory syndrome in infants obstructing the larynx caused by allergy, infection or foreign body; characterized by a harsh cough and stridor

Effusion escape of fluid into a part; effused material, eg, pleural effusion, escape of fluid into the pleural cavity

Expectoration secretions coughed up from the air passages; sputum

Exudate a slow discharge of fluid and cell debris from blood capillaries that accumulates in tissues

Haemoptysis the coughing up of blood from the lungs or bronchi (Am. hemoptysis)

Hiccup repeated spasmodic inspiration associated with sudden closure of the glottis and contraction of the diaphragm

Hypoxaemia condition of below normal levels of oxygen in the blood (Am. hypoxemia)

Infiltrate a collection of fluid or other material within the lung seen on a radiographic image

Mediastinum the region between the lungs in the chest cavity that contains the trachea, oesophagus, heart and bronchi (Am. esophagus)

Midriff the diaphragm

Nares the nostrils

Oximeter a device that measures the oxygen saturation of the blood

Paroxysmal pertaining to a sudden occurrence such as a worsening of symptoms; a seizure or spasm

Percussion a method of diagnosis by tapping with the fingers or a light hammer upon any part of the body

Pleural rub a grating sound produced by the pleural surfaces rubbing against each other

Rale a crackling or rattling sound produced on inspiration when there is fluid in the alveoli (plural rales)

Rhonchus a loud rale (a crackling sound caused by air passing through bronchi obstructed by secretions) (plural rhonchi)

Sputum material expelled from the respiratory passages by coughing or clearing the throat

Stridor a high-pitched sound made on inspiration associated with an obstructed airway

Wheeze a whistling sound heard on expiration associated with constricted bronchi

NOW TRY THE WORD CHECK

WORD CHECK

This self-check exercise lists all the word components used in this unit. First, write down the meaning of as many word components as you can. Then, check your answers using the Exercise Guide and Quick Reference box or the Glossary of Word Components (pp. 383–410).

Prefixes

a-	
brady-	
dys-	
endo-	
hyper-	
hypo-	
inter-	
ortho-	
tachy-	

Combining forms of word roots

alveol/o	
bronch/o	
bronchiol/o	
chondr/o	
cost/o	
cyan/o	
epiglott/o	
gastr/o	
haem/o (Am. hem/o)	
hepat/o	
laryng/o	
lob/o	
myc/o	
nas/o	
oesophag/o (Am. esophag/o)	
pharyng/o	
phren/o	
pleur/o	
pneum/o	

pneumon/o	
-pnoea (Am. -pnea)	
pulmon/o	
radi/o	
rhin/o	
spir/o	
sten/o	
thorac/o	
trache/o	

Suffixes

-al	
-algia	
-ary	
-capnia	
-centesis	
-desis	
-dynia	
-ectasis	
-ectomy	
-genic	
-gram	
-graphy	
-ia	

-ic	
-itis	
-logy	
-meter	
-metry	
-osis	
-oxia	
-pathy	
-pexy	
-plasty	
-plegia	
-rrhaphy	
-rrhoea (Am. rrhea)	
-scope	
-scopy	
-spasm	
-stomy	
-tomy	
-us	

NOW TRY THE SELF-ASSESSMENT

SELF-ASSESSMENT

Test 3A

Below are some combining forms that refer to the anatomy of the respiratory system. Indicate which part of the system they refer to by putting a number from the diagram (Fig. 22) next to each word. The numbers may be used more than once.

(a) bronch/o

(b) nasopharyng/o

(c) phren/o

(d) lob/o

(e) pleur/o

(f) pneum/o

(g) trache/o

(h) laryng/o

(i) pharyng/o

(j) rhin/o

Score

10

Test 3B

Prefixes and suffixes

Match each meaning in Column C with a prefix or suffix in Column A by inserting the appropriate number in Column B.

Column A	Column B	Column C
(a) -centesis		1. measuring instrument
(b) -desis		2. pertaining to originating in/formation
(c) -dynia		3. opening into/connection between two parts
(d) dys-		4. between
(e) -ectomy		5. abnormal condition/disease of
(f) -genic		6. fixation (by surgery)
(g) hyper-		7. condition of pain
(h) hypo-		8. removal of
(i) inter-		9. excessive flow/discharge
(j) -meter		10. fast
(k) -metry		11. above/above normal
(l) -osis		12. difficult/painful
(m) -pexy		13. surgical repair
(n) -plasty		14. puncture
(o) -plegia		15. condition of paralysis
(p) -rrhaphy		16. to bind together
(q) -rrhoea (Am. rrhea)		17. incision into
(r) -stomy		18. below/below normal
(s) -tachy		19. technique of measuring
(t) -tomy		20. suturing/stitching

Score

20

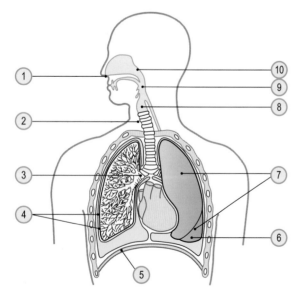

Figure 22   The respiratory system.

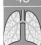

Test 3C

Combining forms of word roots

Match each meaning in Column C with a combining form of a word root in Column A by inserting the appropriate number in Column B.

Column A	Column B	Column C
(a) bronch/o		1. larynx
(b) cost/o		2. diaphragm
(c) enter/o		3. bronchus
(d) epiglott/o		4. thorax
(e) gastr/o		5. intestine
(f) hepat/o		6. pleural membranes
(g) laryng/o		7. stomach
(h) lob/o		8. trachea
(i) myc/o		9. breathing (wind)
(j) nas/o		10. nose (i)
(k) pharyng/o		11. nose (ii)
(l) phren/o		12. fungus
(m) pleur/o		13. lobe
(n) pneum/o		14. pharynx
(o) pneumon/o		15. liver
(p) -pnoea (Am. -pnea)		16. gas/air/wind
(q) rhin/o		17. lung
(r) sten/o		18. epiglottis
(s) thorac/o		19. rib
(t) trache/o		20. narrowing

Score

20

Test 3D

Write the meaning of:

(a) bronchogenic

(b) tracheostenosis

(c) pulmonologist

(d) phrenodynia

(e) laryngoplegia

Score

5

Test 3E

Build words that mean:

(a) surgical repair of the bronchus

(b) technique of visually examining bronchi

(c) suturing of the trachea

(d) study of the nose (use rhin/o)

(e) pertaining to the ribs and diaphragm

Score

5

Check answers to Self-Assessment Tests on pages 359–360.

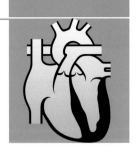

UNIT 4
THE CARDIOVASCULAR SYSTEM

OBJECTIVES

Once you have completed Unit 4, you should be able to do the following:

- understand the meaning of medical words relating to the cardiovascular system
- build medical words relating to the cardiovascular system
- associate medical terms with their anatomical position
- understand common medical abbreviations relating to the cardiovascular system

EXERCISE GUIDE

Use this list of word components and their meanings to complete the word exercises in this unit.

Prefixes

a-	without
brady-	slow
dextro-	right
endo-	within/inside
pan-	all
peri-	around
tachy-	fast

Roots / Combining forms

dynam/o	force
ech/o	echo/reflected sound
electr/o	electrical
lith/o	stone
man/o	pressure
my/o	muscle
necr/o	dead / death of
phon/o	sound/voice

Suffixes

-ac	pertaining to
-algia	condition of pain
-ar	pertaining to
-centesis	surgical puncture to remove fluid
-clysis	infusion/injection/irrigation
-ectasis	dilatation/stretching
-ectomy	removal of

-genesis	capable of causing / pertaining to formation
-gram	X-ray/tracing/recording
-graph	usually an instrument that records
-graphy	technique of recording/making X-ray
-ia	condition of
-ic	pertaining to
-itis	inflammation of
-logy	study of
-lysis	breakdown/disintegration
-megaly	enlargement
-meter	measuring instrument
-metry	process of measuring
-oma	tumour/swelling (Am. tumor)
-osis	abnormal condition/disease of
-ous	pertaining to/of the nature of
-pathy	disease of
-plasty	surgical repair/reconstruction
-pexy	surgical fixation / fix in place
-plegia	condition of paralysis
-poiesis	formation
-rrhaphy	stitching/suturing
-sclerosis	abnormal condition of hardening
-scope	an instrument used to view/examine
-spasm	involuntary contraction of muscle
-stasis	stopping/controlling/cessation of movement
-stenosis	abnormal condition of narrowing
-tome	cutting instrument
-tomy	incision into
-um	thing / a structure / anatomical part
-us	thing / a structure / anatomical part

ANATOMY EXERCISE

When you have finished Word Exercises 1–16, look at the word components listed below. Complete Figure 23 by writing the appropriate combining form on each line; more than one component may relate to the same position. (You can check their meanings in the Quick Reference box on p. 57.)

Aort/o	Pericardi/o	Venacav/o
Arteri/o	Phleb/o	Ven/o
Cardi/o	Valv/o	
Myocardi/o	Valvul/o	

The cardiovascular system

In order to remain alive, cells within the body need a continuous supply of oxygen and nutrients for their metabolism. Any metabolic wastes excreted by these cells must be transported to the excretory organs where they can be removed from the body. The cardiovascular system provides a transport system for supply and removal of materials to and from the tissue cells; it consists of the heart and blood vessels.

The heart

The heart is a four-chambered muscular pump that continuously pushes blood into arteries. The right and left atria (singular atrium) form the top chambers and the right and left ventricles the lower chambers.

The atria receive blood from veins and push it into the ventricles. The right ventricle then forces blood through the pulmonary arteries to the lungs where it is oxygenated. Simultaneously, the left ventricle forces blood into the systemic circulation through the aorta.

The heart muscle (**myocardium**) that forms the walls of the chambers is stimulated to contract rhythmically by a special patch of tissue called the sino-atrial (SA) node or 'pacemaker'. For this reason the normal rhythm of the heart is called the sinus rhythm. Although the SA node gives the heart the ability to contract by itself, its rate of contraction is determined by nerve impulses from centres in the brain.

The heart muscle receives a supply of fully oxygenated blood from branches of the aorta known as the **coronary arteries**. If a coronary artery becomes blocked, the muscle it supplies dies, triggering a heart attack. Another common cause of death is **heart failure**, defined as the inability of the heart to maintain a flow of blood sufficient to meet the body's needs; the term is most often applied to the heart muscle of either the left or right

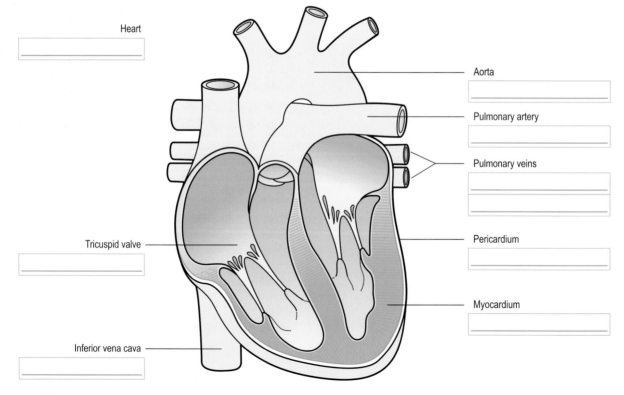

Figure 23   The heart.

ventricle. If both ventricles are affected, it is known as **biventricular** heart failure (bi- means two).

The term **atrial** means pertaining to an atrium, and **ventricular** means pertaining to a ventricle (-*al* and -*ar* both mean pertaining to).

Use the Exercise Guide at the beginning of this unit to complete Word Exercises 1 to 16, unless you are asked to work without it.

 Root

Card

(*From a Greek word* **kardia**, *meaning heart.*)

Combining forms   Card/i/o

 Word Exercise 1

Using your Exercise Guide, find the meaning of:

(a) **cardi**/ac

(b) **cardi**/algia

(c) **cardi/o**/scope

(d) **cardi/o**/graph

(e) **cardi/o**/gram

(f) tachy/**card**/ia

Using your Exercise Guide find the meaning of -logy, -megaly, -pathy and -plasty, and then build words using cardi/o that mean:

(g) enlargement of the heart

(h) surgical repair of the heart

(i) disease of the heart

(j) study of the heart

Using your Exercise Guide, find the meaning of:

(k) my/o/**cardi**/um

(l) **cardi/o**²/my/o³/pathy¹

(m) **cardi/o**/rrhaphy

(n) electro/**cardi/o**/graph

(o) endo/**card**/itis

(p) pan/**card**/itis

(q) brady/**card**/ia

(r) dextro/**card**/ia

(s) phon/o/**cardi/o**/graphy

(t) echo/**cardi/o**/graphy

(u) electro/**cardi/o**/gram

To make an electrocardiogram (ECG; Fig. 24), electrodes are attached to the skin at various sites on the body. The heart muscle generates electrical impulses that can be detected at the surface of the body, amplified and converted into a trace on a screen or paper. The P wave appears when the atria are stimulated, the QRS complex when the impulse passes to the ventricles, and the T wave is generated when the ventricles contract. Abnormal electrical activity and changes in heart rate (**arrhythmia** or **dysrrhythmia**) seen in coronary heart disease can be detected from the ECG.

The heart is continuously supplied with blood through coronary arteries (see Fig. 25). Narrowing of these vessels results in **ischaemia** (**Am.** ischemia), a deficient blood supply (*isch*- meaning to check) that produces the chest pain known as **angina pectoris**. If the flow of blood to the heart muscle is interrupted, the muscle dies; this is a **myocardial infarction** or heart attack. Heart muscle deprived of oxygen produces a rapid, uncoordinated, quivering contraction known as **fibrillation**. Applying an electric shock with an instrument known as a **defibrillator** can sometimes terminate the fibrillation and allow the normal sinus rhythm to be reestablished by the sino-atrial node (pacemaker).

Around the heart, there is a double membranous sac known as the **pericardium** (*peri*-, prefix meaning around). Between the membranes is the pericardial cavity containing a small

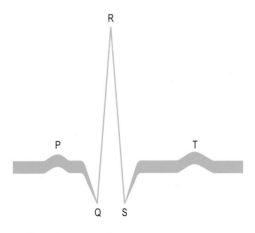

Figure 24   The electrocardiogram.

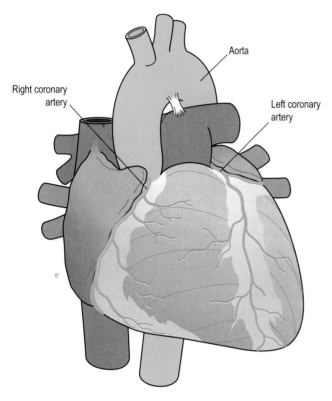

Right coronary artery

Aorta

Left coronary artery

Figure 25 The heart showing the main coronary arteries.

amount of fluid. The combining forms of pericardium are **pericard/o** and **pericardi/o**. The inner surface of the heart is lined with endothelial cells that form a membrane called the **endocardium**.

Word Exercise 2

Without using your Exercise Guide, build a word that means:

(a) inflammation of the pericardium

Using your Exercise Guide, find the meaning of:

(b) cardi/o/**pericardi/o**/pexy

(c) **pericardi/o**/centesis

(d) **pericardi**/ectomy

Root

Valv

(*From Latin **valva**, meaning fold. Here valv/o means a valve, a fold or flap in a tube or passage that permits flow of fluid in one direction only.*)

Combining form   Valv/o

Valves control blood flow through the heart. Between the right atrium and the right ventricle there is a **tricuspid valve** (with three flaps or cusps) that allows blood to flow from the right atrium to the right ventricle but not in the opposite direction. Similarly, there is a valve on the left side of the heart that allows blood to flow from the left atrium to the left ventricle. This is known as the **bicuspid valve** or the **mitral valve** (with two flaps or cusps).

The **aortic semilunar valve** in the aorta and the **pulmonary semilunar valve** in the pulmonary artery prevent backflow of blood into the ventricles.

Word Exercise 3

Without using your Exercise Guide, build words that mean:

(a) surgical repair of a heart valve

(b) removal of a heart valve

Valvul/o is a New Latin combining form also derived from *valva*; using your Exercise Guide, find the meaning of:

(c) cardio/**valvul/o**/tome

Note. -tome comes from *tomon,* meaning cutter. Using your Exercise Guide, find the meaning of:

(d) **valvul**/ar

(e) **valv/o**/tomy

The blood vessels

Blood circulates through a closed system of blood vessels throughout the body. It flows away from the heart in arteries that divide into smaller arterioles and then into capillaries. Blood flows back to the heart through venules and then into larger vessels known as veins. The system that supplies blood to the tissues is known as the **arterial system** and that which takes it away the **venous system**. Now, we will look at some of the terms concerned with blood vessels.

Root

Vas

(*A Latin word, meaning **vessel**. Here vas/o means a blood vessel of any type.*)

Combining forms   Vas/o

Vascul/o, *also derived from vas, means a small blood vessel of any type.*

Word Exercise 4

Using your Exercise Guide, find the meaning of:

(a) **vas/o**/spasm

Blood vessels can widen (**vaso**dilatation) and they can narrow (**vaso**constriction) because of the activity of smooth muscle in their walls. If a vessel widens, then the blood pressure within it falls. Some drugs are designed to stimulate this action (ie, reducing blood pressure) and are known as **vasodilators** and antihypertensives.

(b) a/**vascul**/ar

Without using your Exercise Guide, build words using vascul/o that mean:

(c) inflammation of blood vessels

(d) disease of blood vessels

Root

Angi

*(From a Greek word **angeion**, meaning vessel. Here angi/o means a blood vessel of any type.)*

Combining form   Angi/o

Word Exercise 5

Without using your Exercise Guide, write the meaning of:

(a) **angi/o**/gram

(b) **angi/o**/cardi/o/gram

(c) **angi/o**/cardi/o/graphy

Angiography is the technique of making X-rays or images of blood vessels. Both arteries and veins can be made visible on radiographic film following the injection of a contrast medium. This results in an X-ray film on which the injected vessels cast a shadow showing their size, shape and location.

Digital subtraction angiography (DSA) is very similar, except, instead of having an X-ray film, the X-rays are detected electronically, and a computer builds an image of the blood vessels on a monitor.

One problem in visualizing blood vessels is that overlying tissues cast an image on the picture. To eliminate these unwanted images, an X-ray is taken before and after dye is injected. A computer then subtracts the first image from the second, removing the interfering image. The picture produced by DSA is superior to a film-based angiogram.

Without using your Exercise Guide, build words that mean:

(d) study of blood vessels

(e) surgical repair of blood vessels

A common surgical repair is a balloon angioplasty. In this procedure a catheter containing an inflatable balloon is inserted into a narrowed vessel (see Fig. 26). When the balloon is inflated and moved along the lining, any fatty plaques are displaced, and the flow of blood through the vessel is restored. An expandable slotted tube called a **stent** can be left in position to serve as a permanent scaffold that maintains a wide lumen (space within the vessel); this reduces the chance of the vessel narrowing again (a process called restenosis).

Using your Exercise Guide, find the meaning of:

(f) **angi**/oma

(g) **angi**/ectasis

(h) **angi/o**/poiesis

(i) **angi/o**/sclerosis

The above roots refer generally to blood vessels. Now we will look at roots that refer to specific types of vessel.

Root

Aort

*(From Greek **aorte**, meaning great vessel. Here aort/o means the aorta, the largest artery in the body. The aorta leaves the left ventricle of the heart and divides into smaller arteries that supply all body systems with oxygenated blood.)*

Combining form   Aort/o

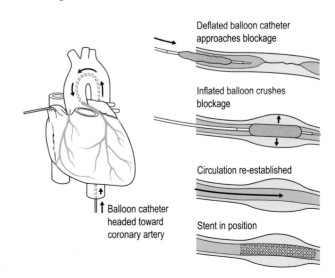

Figure 26   Balloon angioplasty.

Word Exercise 6

Without using your Exercise Guide, build words that mean:

(a) disease of the aorta

(b) technique of X-raying the aorta

Root

Arter

(*From a Greek word* **arteria**, *meaning artery. The function of arteries is to move blood away from the heart. Arteries divide into smaller arterioles and then into capillaries that exchange materials with the tissue cells.*)

Combining forms   Arter/i/o

Word Exercise 7

Without using your Exercise Guide, build words using arteri/o that mean:

(a) suturing of an artery

(b) condition of hardening of arteries

Using your Exercise Guide, find the meaning of:

(c) end/**arter**/ectomy

(In this procedure, fatty deposits are removed from the lining of the artery.)

(d) **arteri/o**/necr/osis

(e) **arteri/o**/stenosis

Root

Vena cav

(*From Latin* **vena cavum**, *meaning hollow vein. Here venacav/o means the venae cavae, the great veins of the body that drain blood into the heart.*)

Combining form   Venacav/o

Venae cavae are the great veins of the body; the **superior vena cava** drains blood from the head and upper body; the **inferior vena cava** drains blood from the lower parts of the body. They pass their blood into the right atrium of the heart.

Word Exercise 8

Without using your Exercise Guide, write the meaning of:

(a) **venacav/o**/gram

(b) **venacav/o**/graphy

Root

Ven

(*From a Latin word* **vena**, *meaning vein. The function of veins is to transfer blood back to the heart. Capillaries are drained by small vessels called venules; these join and form larger veins. Unlike arteries, veins contain valves that prevent the backflow of blood.*)

Combining form   Ven/o

Word Exercise 9

Using your Exercise Guide, find the meaning of:

(a) **ven**/ectasis

(b) **ven/o**/clysis

(c) **ven**/ous

Without using your Exercise Guide, build words that mean:

(d) X-ray picture of a vein (after injection of opaque dye)

(e) technique of making an X-ray of a vein or the venous system

Root

Phleb

(*From a Greek word* **phlebos**, *meaning vein.*)

Combining form   Phleb/o

Word Exercise 10

Without using your Exercise Guide, write the meaning of:

(a) **phleb**/arteri/ectasis

(b) **phleb/o**/clysis

(c) **phleb/o**/tomy

Using your Exercise Guide, find the meaning of:

(d) **phleb/o**/stasis

(e) **phleb/o**/man/o/meter

(f) **phleb/o**/lith

Root

Thromb

(*From a Greek word* **thrombos**, *meaning a clot. Blood clots are formed mainly of platelets, fibrin and blood cells; they can block blood vessels, restricting or stopping the flow of blood.*)

Combining form   Thromb/o

 Word Exercise 11

Without using your Exercise Guide, write the meaning of:

(a) **thromb/o**/poiesis

(b) **thromb/o**/phleb/itis

(c) **thromb/o**/end/arter/ ectomy

Without using your Exercise Guide, build words that mean:

(d) abnormal condition of having a clot

(e) removal of a clot

Using your Exercise Guide, find the meaning of:

(f) **thromb/o**/genesis

(g) **thromb/o**/lysis

The sudden blocking of an artery by a clot is referred to as an **embolism**. Thrombi, as well as other foreign materials such as fat, air and infective material, can cause emboli. The combining form **embol/o** is used when referring to an **embolus**, eg, as in **embol**ectomy.

The development of enzymes that can dissolve blood clots in situ has led to the development of **thrombolytic therapies**. For example, the drug streptokinase, extracted from bacteria, can be injected into the coronary vessels to lyse a clot and thereby restore blood in the coronary system. Thrombolytic drugs such as streptokinase and the tissue plasminogen activators (tPAs) alteplase and anistreplase have all been shown to reduce mortality when given by the intravenous route following a heart attack.

Root

Ather

(*From a Greek word* **athere**, *meaning porridge or meal. Here ather/o means atheroma, a fatty plaque that forms on the inner walls of blood vessels.*)

Combining form   Ather/o

The term **ather**oma means a porridge-like tumour and is used to indicate the presence of fatty plaques in the lining of arteries. Atheroma is a common disorder of blood vessels, and the presence of such deposits is often related to aspects of one's lifestyle such as smoking, lack of exercise and diets rich in certain types of fat. Atheroma in coronary arteries increases the chance of their becoming blocked, thus predisposing the heart to myocardial infarction.

Word Exercise 12

Without using your Exercise Guide, write the meaning of:

(a) **ather/o**/genesis

(b) **ather/o**/embolus

Atherosclerosis is a common form of arteriosclerosis that results from the presence of atheroma and calcification in vessel walls. Contributing factors to the development of this condition include advanced age, diabetes, high-fat and high-cholesterol diets, hypertension and smoking.

Root

Aneurysm

(*From Greek* **aneurysma**, *meaning a dilatation. Here aneurysm/o means an aneurysm, a dilated vessel, usually an artery. An aneurysm is caused by a localized fault in a vessel wall through a defect, disease or injury; it appears as a pulsating swelling that can rupture.*)

Combining form   Aneurysm/o

Word Exercise 13

Without using your Exercise Guide, write the meaning of:

(a) **aneurysm/o**/plasty (see Fig. 27)

(b) **aneurysm/o**/rrhaphy

Root

Sphygm

(*From a Greek word* **sphygmos**, *meaning pulsation. Here sphygm/o means the pulse, the rhythmical throbbing that can be felt wherever an artery is near the surface of the body. The pulsation is due to the heart forcing blood into the arterial*

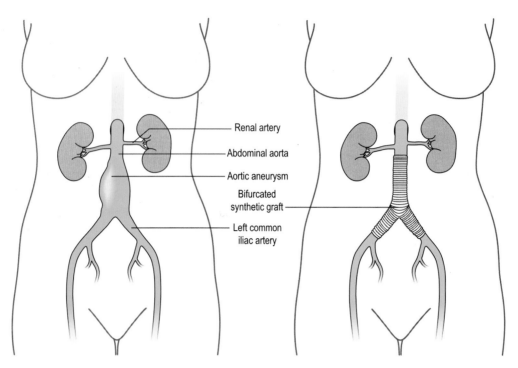

Figure 27   An abdominal aortic aneurysm (AAA) and its repair with a synthetic graft (aneurysmoplasty). (Adapted from Chabner D-E, The Language of Medicine, 10th Edition, 2013, Saunders.)

system at ventricular systole (contraction). Pulse rate is therefore a measure of heart rate.)

Combining form   Sphygm/o

 Word Exercise 14

Using your Exercise Guide, find the meaning of:

(a) **sphygm/o**/dynam/o/
    meter

(b) **sphygm/o**/man/o/meter

(c) **sphygm/o**/metry

Without using your Exercise Guide, write the meaning of:

(d) **sphygm/o**/graph

(e) **sphygm/o**/gram (refers
    to movements created
    by the arterial pulse)

(f) **sphygm/o**/cardi/o/graph

Note. Man/o comes from Greek *manos*, meaning rare. Manometers were first used for measuring rarefied air, ie, gases. The combining form **man/o** is now used to mean pressure.

A sphygmomanometer is an instrument that uses a manometer to measure the pressure of the pulse that is blood pressure (BP). Two pressures are measured: the **systolic** pressure when the ventricles of the heart are forcing blood into the circulation, and the **diastolic** pressure, which is the pressure within the vessels when the heart is dilating and refilling. The ideal blood pressure in adults should be close to $^{120}/_{80}$ mm Hg; the first number is the systolic pressure, and the second is the diastolic pressure (Hg = mercury).

The sphygmomanometer can be used to detect **hypertension**, ie, a persistently high arterial blood pressure, or **hypotension**, an abnormally low blood pressure. Both of these conditions have a variety of causes. Figure 28 shows a clinical mercury sphygmomanometer that is used to measure blood pressure by the Korotkoff or auscultatory method. The procedure requires the use of a **stethoscope** (see Fig. 29) to listen to sounds made by blood flowing through the brachial artery in the arm. As mercury is toxic, mercury-free models are being introduced in many countries. (Named after Nikolai Sergeyevich Korotkov (1874–1920), a Russian surgeon, the sounds heard in the arm are called Korotkoff sounds.)

Figure 30 shows a digital sphygmomanometer that provides a blood pressure reading without listening to blood flow sounds and is easy to operate without training; these are often used for routine blood pressure measurement and screening.

Note. In medicine, the suffix -scope usually refers to an instrument used for visual examination. However, it is used in stethoscope to mean an instrument to examine

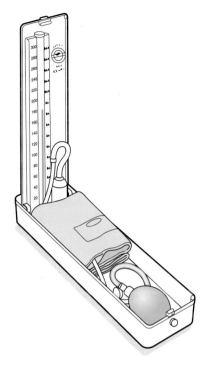

Figure 28　A mercury sphygmomanometer.

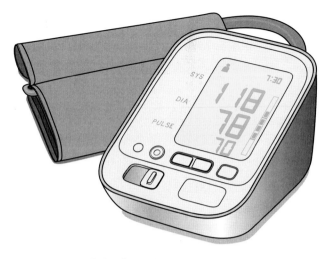

Figure 30　A digital sphygmomanometer.

> **man/o**
> means pressure. In sphygmo**mano**meter, it refers to the pressure of the pulse, ie, arterial blood pressure.
>
> **dynam/o**
> means power. In sphygmo**dynamo**meter, it refers to the force of the pulse (volume and pressure).

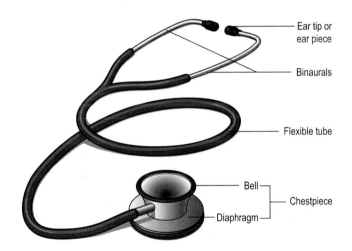

- Ear tip or ear piece
- Binaurals
- Flexible tube
- Bell
- Chestpiece
- Diaphragm

Figure 29　A stethoscope.

> **Note.** Words ending in **-graph** usually refer to a recording instrument, and those ending in **-scope** to a viewing instrument. Remember, there are exceptions: for example, a radiograph is an X-ray picture, and the stethoscope is used for listening to sounds.

Review the names of all instruments and clinical procedures mentioned in this unit, and then complete Exercises 15 and 16.

> the breast (from **steth/o-** breast). We can use it in this way because -scope comes from the Greek word *skopein* that means to examine. In practice, a stethoscope is used for listening to body sounds (auscultation).

Medical equipment and clinical procedures

In this unit, we have named several instruments that are used to examine the cardiovascular system. The following combining forms have been introduced with them. Review their meanings before completing the next two exercises:

Word Exercise 15

Match each description in Column C with a term in Column A by placing the appropriate number in Column B.

Column A	Column B	Column C
(a) cardioscope		1. an instrument that measures arterial blood pressure (the pressure of the pulse)
(b) cardiograph		2. an instrument used to cut a heart valve

Column A	Column B	Column C
(c) electrocardio-graph		3. technique of X-raying the blood vessels and heart after injection of radio-opaque dye
(d) cardioval-votome		4. an instrument that records the heart (beat)
(e) angiocardio-graphy		5. an instrument that records the electrical activity of the heart
(f) sphygmoma-nometer		6. an instrument used to view the heart

 Word Exercise 16

Match each description in Column C with a term in Column A by placing an appropriate number in Column B.

Column A	Column B	Column C
(a) echocardio-graphy		1. a recording of heart sounds
(b) sphygmocar-diograph		2. pertaining to the force of the pulse
(c) stethoscope		3. a tracing or recording of the electrical activity of the heart
(d) phonocardio-gram		4. an instrument that measures the pressure within a vein
(e) electrocardio-gram		5. an instrument that records the pulse and heart beat
(f) phleboma-nometer		6. technique of recording the heart using reflected ultrasound
(g) sphygmo-dynamic		7. an instrument used to listen to sounds within the chest

Other procedures used to investigate the cardiovascular system besides those mentioned in the word exercises include:

Cardiac catheterization In this procedure a thin flexible tube is guided into the heart via a vein or artery. A contrast medium that is visible on X-ray images is administered through the tube whilst images are taken of the heart and blood vessels.

Cardiac CT (computed tomography) Contrast material visible on X-rays is injected via a small peripheral vein whilst multiple cross-sectional images are made of the heart and coronary vessels.

Doppler echocardiography A form of echocardiography that uses ultrasound technology to determine the speed and direction of blood flow through the heart and blood vessels. It is particularly useful in assessing leakage and narrowing of the heart valves, and for assessing holes between the chambers of the heart.

Exercise tolerance test or stress test A test that determines the heart's response to physical exertion. The patient's vital signs and electrocardiogram are monitored whilst exercising on a treadmill or exercise bike.

Holter monitoring A portable electrocardiograph is worn during a 24-hour period to record cardiac arrhythmias and correlate them with symptoms in the patient.

Phonocardiography The technique of recording heart sounds using a phonocardiograph during the cardiac cycle. The procedure enables the detection of subaudible sounds and murmurs that are not detectable with a stethoscope.

Positron emission tomography (PET) Images made using this procedure show blood flow through the heart, the activity of the myocardium and the presence of heart disease by tracing the uptake of radioactive glucose administered to the patient.

Troponin test This measures the levels of a group of proteins, troponin-I and troponin-T, that are released into the blood stream following injury to the myocardium. Levels are raised when heart muscle has been damaged by lack of oxygen (myocardial infarction).

ANATOMY EXERCISE

Now complete the Anatomy Exercise on page 48.

 CASE HISTORY 4

The object of this exercise is to understand words associated with a patient's medical history.

To complete the exercise:

- Read through the passage on cardiac failure; unfamiliar words are underlined, and you can find their meaning using the Word Help.

- Write the meaning of the medical terms shown in bold print on the lines that follow the Word Help.

Cardiac failure

Mr D, a 65-year-old male builder, was referred by his <u>GP</u> to the **Cardiology** Unit. He had been healthy until 8 months previous, but since then he has developed fatigue, exertion <u>dyspnoea</u> (Am. dyspnea) and <u>paroxysmal nocturnal</u> dyspnoea. He also described discomfort in his chest and felt his heart was 'thumping'.

On the morning of admission, he had become unwell and was pale, cold and sweating and seemed confused. Initial examination revealed tender, smooth hepatic enlargement and the presence of <u>ascites</u>. His <u>jugular</u> **venous** pulse was raised and <u>pitting oedema</u> (Am. edema) was present in his ankles. <u>Auscultation</u> revealed a left ventricular third sound with **tachycardia** (a gallop rhythm), and <u>crepitations</u> were heard at the lung bases. Mr D was connected to a 12-lead **electrocardiograph** to monitor his heart rate and rhythm. A <u>posteroanterior</u> chest X-ray revealed **cardiomegaly** and pulmonary oedema, and he was diagnosed as having acute **biventricular** heart failure.

Mr D was treated with furosemide (frusemide), a <u>diuretic</u>, to promote renal excretion of fluid. The loss of fluid provided symptomatic and <u>haemodynamic</u> (Am. hemodynamic) benefits, relieving his dyspnoea and reducing ventricular filling pressure. **Cardiac** output was improved by **vasodilator** therapy with <u>ACE inhibitors</u> in combination with positive <u>inotropic</u> agents.

Word Help

ACE inhibitor angiotensin-converting enzyme (drug used to reduce blood pressure)

ascites free fluid in the abdominal cavity

auscultation a method of listening to body sounds for diagnostic purposes

crepitations rattling or crackling sounds

diuretic an agent that increases the flow of urine

dyspnoea (Am. dyspnea) difficult/laboured breathing

GP general practitioner (family doctor)

haemodynamic (Am. hemodynamic) pertaining to the force of blood

inotropic pertaining to affecting the contraction of (heart) muscle increasing or decreasing the force of contraction

jugular pertaining to the neck/throat

nocturnal pertaining to during the night

oedema (Am. edema) accumulation of fluid in a tissue

paroxysmal intensification of symptoms/an attack

posteroanterior from the back/posterior to the front

pitting when pressure on a tissue leaves a mark

Now write the meaning of the following words from the Case History without using your dictionary lists:

(a) cardiology

(b) venous

(c) tachycardia

(d) electrocardiograph

(e) cardiomegaly

(f) biventricular

(g) cardiac

(h) vasodilator

(Answers to the Case History exercise are given in the Answers to Word Exercises on page 338.)

Quick Reference

Combining forms relating to the cardiovascular system:

Aneurysm/o	aneurysm
Angi/o	vessel
Aort/o	aorta
Arteri/o	artery
Ather/o	atheroma
Atri/o	atrium
Cardi/o	heart
Embol/o	embolism
My/o	muscle
Myocardi/o	myocardium
Pericardi/o	pericardium
Phleb/o	vein
Sphygm/o	pulse
Steth/o	breast
Thromb/o	thrombus/clot
Valv/o	valve
Valvul/o	valve
Vas/o	vessel
Vascul/o	vessel
Venacav/o	vena cava
Ven/o	vein
Ventricul/o	ventricle

Abbreviations

Some common abbreviations related to the cardiovascular system are listed below. Note that some are not standard, and their meaning may vary from one healthcare setting to another. There is a more extensive list for reference on page 369.

AAA	abdominal aortic aneurysm
AF	atrial fibrillation
AMI	acute myocardial infarction

BBB	bundle branch block
CABG	coronary artery bypass grafting
CAD	coronary artery disease
CCU	coronary care unit
CHF	congestive heart failure
CPR	cardiopulmonary resuscitation
CT	coronary thrombosis
DVT	deep vein thrombosis
ECG	electrocardiogram
IV	intravenous
MI	myocardial infarction / mitral insufficiency
MS	mitral stenosis
NSR	normal sinus rhythm
PAD	peripheral artery disease
VF	ventricular fibrillation

Pathology notes

Arrhythmia

Arrhythmia is an irregular heartbeat; the heart may beat too fast (tachycardia), too slowly (bradycardia), too early (premature contraction) or too irregularly (fibrillation). Arrhythmias occur when electrical impulses that coordinate the beating of the heart are not working correctly. The condition can be treated with drugs, artificial pacemakers, cardioversion (defibrillation) or catheter ablation. In the latter procedure a series of catheters called ablators (thin, flexible wires) are put into a blood vessel in the arm, groin or neck and are guided into the heart. A radio frequency alternating current (350–500 kHz) passed down the catheter and destroys the dysfunctional heart tissue causing the arrhythmia. Heating of heart tissue using radio frequency energy in this way can be used to treat atrial flutter, atrial fibrillation and supraventricular tachycardia (SVT).

Congestive heart failure (CHF)

CHF is a result of an inadequate pumping action of the heart. Congestion develops when the heart is unable to pump all of the blood it receives, and fluid accumulates in the lungs and peripheral tissues. The clinical presentation depends on how quickly heart failure develops and whether it involves the right or left sides of the heart or both.

In patients with *left ventricular failure*, the left ventricle fails to pump blood effectively, and as a result, blood backs up in the lungs. As a result, fluid accumulates in the lungs, and patients develop a sensation of breathlessness and have difficulty in breathing, particularly at night (paroxysmal nocturnal dyspnoea (Am. dyspnea)). Often such failure results from coronary artery disease and valve disorders.

In patients with *right ventricular failure*, the right ventricle fails to empty, and the right atrium and venae cavae become congested with blood followed by congestion throughout the venous system. The organs first affected are the liver, spleen and kidneys. Oedema (Am. edema) of the limbs and ascites (excess fluid in the peritoneal cavity) usually follow.

Symptoms include shortness of breath, pedal (foot) oedema and abdominal pain.

Coronary artery disease (CAD)

Coronary artery disease is one of the leading causes of death; it results from conditions that reduce the flow of blood to the myocardium (heart muscle). If a coronary artery is occluded, blood cannot reach the heart muscle cells it normally supplies and, deprived of oxygen, the cells soon die or are damaged. The death of heart muscle is termed a myocardial infarction (MI) or heart attack. The principal causes are atherosclerosis and the formation of clots in coronary arteries.

Coronary heart disease (CHD)

When symptoms of coronary artery disease appear and begin to affect the patient, the term coronary heart disease or CHD is used. Coronary heart disease, also called *ischaemic heart disease*, is due to the effects of atheroma causing narrowing or occlusion of one or more branches of the coronary arteries (Am. ischemic). Narrowing of coronary arteries leads to *angina pectoris* and occlusion to a *myocardial infarction* (heart attack).

Hypertension

This is a term used to describe a persistently higher than normal blood pressure for a particular age group. Arteriosclerosis contributes to increasing blood pressure with age, but it is not the only factor. Hypertension is described as essential, primary or idiopathic when the cause is unknown and as secondary hypertension when it results from other diseases. High blood pressure is of concern because it can damage the heart, brain and kidneys if it remains uncontrolled.

Myocardial infarction (heart attack)

An infarct is an area of tissue that has died because of lack of a supply of oxygenated blood. The failure of blood supply to cardiac muscle is called a myocardial infarction (MI). The most common cause is an atheromatous plaque complicated by thrombosis. Myocardial infarction is usually accompanied by severe chest pain which, unlike angina pectoris, continues when the individual is at rest. Myocardial infarction is often fatal, but recovery is possible if the amount of heart tissue damage is small.

Patent ductus arteriosus

This is a heart defect in which the ductus arteriosus fails to close at birth. Before birth the duct allows blood to pass between the pulmonary artery and aorta bypassing the pulmonary circulation. Shortly after birth when the pulmonary circulation is established, the duct should close completely; failure to do so results in congestion of the lungs and eventual cardiac failure.

Peripheral vascular disease (synonym peripheral arterial disease)

In this condition, arteries in the neck, groin or upper leg narrow or become blocked by atherosclerosis. Often the femoral artery and popliteal artery behind the knee are involved and blood flow to the lower leg and foot is reduced. An early sign of discomfort is intermittent claudication (pain, tension and weakness upon walking and absence of discomfort on resting). Treatment is exercise, avoidance of smoking, which causes vessels to constrict, and control of other risk factors such as diabetes. Surgical treatment includes endarterectomy and bypass grafting.

Rheumatic heart disease

Rheumatic heart disease is an autoimmune disease caused by *Streptococcus pyogenes* (beta-haemolytic group A) that occurs most often in children (Am. hemolytic). The antibodies developed to combat the infection damage the heart. A few weeks after an improperly treated streptococcal infection, the cardiac valves and other tissues in the body may become inflamed, a condition called *rheumatic fever.* If severe, the inflammation can result in stenosis (narrowing) and other deformities of the valves, and damage to the chordae tendinae or myocardium.

Tetralogy of Fallot

This is a congenital defect that results in cardiac function inadequate for a growing child. Four abnormalities are present: stenosis of the pulmonary artery, malposition of the aorta, a ventricular septal defect (a hole between the two ventricles) and right ventricular hypertrophy.

Varicose veins

Varicose veins are enlarged veins in which blood tends to pool rather than continue on toward the heart. The condition commonly occurs in superficial veins in areas seen externally as varicosities. The great saphenous vein, the largest superficial vein in the leg often becomes varicose in people who stand for long periods. The force of gravity slows the return of venous blood to the heart in such cases, causing blood-engorged veins to dilate. As the veins dilate, the distance between the flaps of venous valves widens, eventually making them incompetent (leaky and inefficient). Incompetence of valves causes even more pooling in affected veins, a positive feedback mechanism. Haemorrhoids (Am. hemorrhoids), also called *piles*, are varicose veins in the anal canal.

Associated words

Ablation destruction of tissue, eg, cardiac catheter ablation
Angina pectoris sudden chest pain that radiates to the arms due to insufficient oxygenated blood reaching the myocardium
Auricle an obsolete term for the atrium
Bruit an abnormal sound (murmur) from the heart heard on auscultation
Cardiac arrest the sudden stopping of heart action often leading to death
Cardioversion the restoration of the normal rhythm of the heart by electrical shock
Claudication limping, accompanied by severe pain in the legs on walking that disappears with rest; a sign of occlusive arterial disease

Clubbing broadening and thickening of the tips of the fingers and toes due to poor circulation, a sign of heart disease
Coarctation process of narrowing or contraction, eg, coarctation of the aorta
Fibrillation rapid, random, ineffectual and irregular contractions of the heart
Flutter rapid abnormal heart rhythm, eg, an atrial flutter
Heart block failure of proper conduction of impulses through the heart conducting system
Infarction process of forming an infarct, an area of dead tissue
Murmur an extra abnormal sound heard on auscultation, eg, presystolic murmur
Occlusion closure, eg, of a vessel such as a coronary artery
Pacemaker an electronic device that keeps the heart beating at a proper rate and overcomes arrhythmias
Palpitation rapid and forceful contraction of the heart sensed by the patient
Patent open
Petechia a small pinpoint spot due to haemorrhage under the skin (plural petechiae, Am. hemorrhage)
Stent a device to keep a tube or vessel open; it consists of a mesh of stainless steel, plastic or other material
Stricture narrowing or local contraction
Syncope a simple faint due to temporary interruption in cerebral blood flow
Tamponade compression, eg, cardiac tamponade, the compression of the heart caused by accumulation of fluid in the pericardium
Thrill a vibration felt on palpation, eg, of the chest
Vegetations collections of microorganisms, clotting proteins and platelets that stick to an inflamed or infected endocardium

NOW TRY THE WORD CHECK

WORD CHECK

This self-check exercise lists all word components used in this unit. First, write down the meaning of as many word components as you can. Then, check your answers using the Exercise Guide and Quick Reference box or the Glossary of Word Components (pp. 383–410).

Prefixes

a-	
bi-	
brady-	
dextro-	
endo-	
hyper-	
hypo-	

pan-

peri-

tachy-

Combining forms of word roots

aneurysm/o

angi/o

aort/o

arteri/o

ather/o

atri/o

cardi/o

ech/o

electr/o

embol/o

dynam/o

isch/o

man/o

my/o

necr/o

pericardi/o

phleb/o

phon/o

sphygm/o

sten/o

steth/o

thromb/o

valv/o

valvul/o

vas/o

vascul/o

venacav/o

ven/o

ventricul/o

Suffixes

-algia

-ar

-centesis

-clysis

-ectasis

-ectomy

-genesis

-gram

-graph

-graphy

-ia

-ic

-itis

-ium

-lith

-logy

-lysis

-megaly

-meter

-metry

-oma

-osis

-ous

-pathy

-pexy

-plasty

-poiesis

-rrhage

-rrhaphy

-sclerosis

-scope

-stasis

-tome

-tomy

-um

NOW TRY THE SELF-ASSESSMENT

SELF-ASSESSMENT

Test 4A

Below are some combining forms that refer to the anatomy of the cardiovascular system. Indicate which part of the system they refer to by putting a number from the diagram (Fig. 31) next to each word.

(a) aort/o

(b) venacav/o

(c) endocardi/o

(d) valv/o

(e) pericardi/o

(f) myocardi/o

Score

6

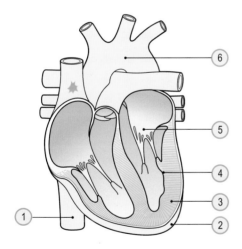

Figure 31　The heart.

Test 4B

Prefixes and suffixes

Match each meaning in Column C with a prefix or suffix in Column A by inserting the appropriate number in Column B.

Column A	Column B	Column C
(a) a-		1. formation (i)
(b) -ac		2. formation (ii)
(c) bi-		3. infusion/injection
(d) brady-		4. two
(e) -clysis		5. fast
(f) dextro-		6. pertaining to
(g) -ectasis		7. without
(h) endo-		8. dilatation
(i) -genesis		9. fixation
(j) -megaly		10. right
(k) pan-		11. around
(l) peri-		12. stopping/cessation
(m) -pexy		13. abnormal condition of narrowing
(n) -poiesis		14. condition of hardening
(o) -rrhaphy		15. slow
(p) -sclerosis		16. thing/structure/anatomical part
(q) -stasis		17. stitching/suturing
(r) -stenosis		18. all
(s) tachy-		19. enlargement
(t) -um		20. inside

Score

20

Test 4C

Combining forms of word roots

Match each meaning in Column C with a combining form of a word root in Column A by inserting the appropriate number in Column B.

Column A	Column B	Column C
(a) aneurysm/o		1. echo / reflected sound
(b) angi/o		2. artery
(c) aort/o		3. death/corpse
(d) arteri/o		4. sound
(e) ather/o		5. valve
(f) cardi/o		6. aorta
(g) dynam/o		7. porridge (yellow plaque on wall of blood vessel)
(h) ech/o		8. heart
(i) man/o		9. vessel (i)
(j) my/o		10. vessel (ii)
(k) necr/o		11. force
(l) phleb/o		12. aneurysm (swelling)
(m) phon/o		13. pressure/rare
(n) sphygm/o		14. muscle
(o) sten/o		15. vein (i)
(p) steth/o		16. vein (ii)
(q) thromb/o		17. clot
(r) valv/o		18. narrowing
(s) vas/o		19. pulse
(t) ven/o		20. breast

Score

20

Test 4D

Write the meaning of:

(a) cardiovalvulitis

(b) aortorrhaphy

(c) angioscope

(d) phlebostenosis

(e) thromboendarteritis

Score

5

Test 4E

Build words that mean:

(a) condition of hardening of veins (use phleb/o)

(b) puncture of the heart

(c) disease of an artery

(d) removal of a vein

(e) study of the blood vessels and heart (use angi/o)

Score

5

Check answers to Self-Assessment Tests on page 360.

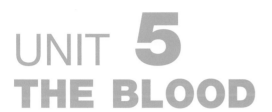

UNIT 5
THE BLOOD

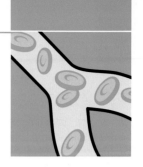

Once you have completed Unit 5, you should be able to do the following:

- understand the meaning of medical words relating to the blood
- build medical words relating to blood
- associate medical terms with the components of blood
- understand common medical abbreviations relating to the blood

EXERCISE GUIDE

Use this list of word components and their meanings to complete the word exercises in this unit.

Prefixes

a-	without
an-	without/not
ellipto-	shaped like an ellipse
hyper-	above / abnormal increase
hypo-	below / abnormal decrease
iso-	equal/same
macro-	large
micro-	small
normo-	normal/rule
peri-	around
poikil/o	varied/irregular
poly-	many

Roots / Combining forms

cyt/o, -cyte	cell
dynam/o	force/movement
fibr/o	fibre (Am. fiber)
path/o	disease
pericardi/o	pericardium
septic/o	sepsis/infection/putrefaction

Suffixes

-aemia	condition of blood
-apheresis	removal
-blast	germ cell/cell, cell that forms
-chromia	condition of colour/haemoglobin (Am. color)
-crit	separate / device for measuring cells
-cytosis	abnormal condition of cells (too many)
-emia (Am.)	condition of blood
-genesis	capable of causing / pertaining to formation of
-globin	protein
-ia	condition of
-ic	pertaining to
-ium	structure/anatomical part
-logy	study of
-lysis	breakdown/disintegration
-meter	measuring instrument
-oma	tumour/swelling (Am. tumor)
-osis	abnormal condition/disease of
-penia	condition of lack of / deficiency
-poiesis	formation
-ptysis	spitting up
-rrhage	bursting forth (of blood/bleeding)
-stasis	stopping/controlling / cessation of movement
-toxic	pertaining to poisoning
-um	thing / structure / anatomical part
-uria	condition of urine

ANATOMY EXERCISE

When you have finished Word Exercises 1 to 8, look at the word components listed below. Complete Figure 32 by writing the appropriate combining form on each line. (You can check their meanings in the Quick Reference box on p. 70.)

Bas/o	Leucocyt/o	Plasma-
Eosin/o	(Am. Leukocyt/o)	Thrombocyt/o
Erythrocyt/o	Lymphocyt/o	
Haem/o	Monocyt/o	
(Am. Hem/o)	Neutr/o	

The blood

Blood is a complex fluid classified as a connective tissue because it contains cells, plus an intercellular matrix known as plasma. In Figure 32 we can see the main components of whole blood.

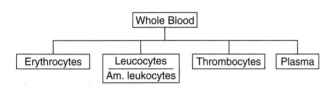

The blood cells carry out a variety of functions: erythrocytes (red blood cells) transport gases, whilst leucocytes (white blood cells) defend the body against invasion by microorganisms and foreign antigens. Thrombocytes, or platelets, are in fact fragments of larger cells concerned with the formation of blood clots following injury.

The plasma carries nutrients, wastes, hormones, antibodies and blood-clotting proteins. The study of blood is very important in medicine for the diagnosis of disease.

Use the Exercise Guide at the beginning of the unit to complete Word Exercises 1 to 7, unless you are asked to work without it.

Root

Haem

(*From a Greek word* **haima**, *meaning blood.*)

Combining forms Haem/o, haemat/o, -aem- *(Am. Hem/o, hemat/o, -em-)*

Word Exercise 1

Using your Exercise Guide, find the meaning of:

(a) **haemat/o**/logy
(Am. **hemat/o**/logy)

(b) **haem/o**[2]/path/o[3]/logy[1]
(Am. **hem/o**/path/o/logy)

(c) **haem/o**/dynam/ics
(Am. **hem/o**/dynam/ics)

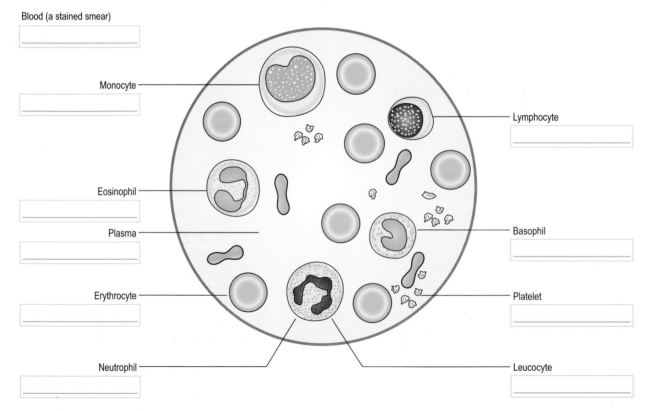

Blood (a stained smear)

Monocyte

Eosinophil

Plasma

Erythrocyte

Neutrophil

Lymphocyte

Basophil

Platelet

Leucocyte

Figure 32   **Blood.**

(d) **haem/o**/poiesis (Am. **hem/o**/poiesis)

(e) **haem/o**/stasis (Am. **hem/o**/stasis)

(f) **haem/o**/pericardi/um (Fig. 33) (Am. **hem/o**/pericardi/um)

(g) **haem/o**/ptysis (Am. **hem/o**/ptysis)

Using your Exercise Guide, look up the meaning of -lysis, -oma, -rrhage and -uria; then build words that mean:

(h) Swelling containing blood (use haemat/o, Am. hemat/o)

(i) Breakdown/disintegration of blood

(j) Condition of blood in the urine (use haemat/o, Am. hemat/o)

(k) Bursting forth of blood

Using your Exercise Guide, find the meaning of:

(l) poly/cyt/**haem**/ia (Am. poly/cyt/**hem**/ia)

(m) an/**aem**/ia (Am. an/**em**/ia)

(n) septic/**aem**/ia (Am. septic/**em**/ia)

Haemoglobin is a red pigment (globular protein) found inside red blood cells; it functions to transport oxygen and carbon dioxide. The presence of haemoglobin in the blood is of great importance to the efficiency of gaseous transport, and several types of investigation are performed to estimate its concentration.

Two of the medical terms that follow use the combining form **haemoglobin/o** meaning haemoglobin.

Using your Exercise Guide, find the meaning of:

(o) **haemoglobin/o**/meter (Am. **hemoglobin/o**/meter)

Without using your Exercise Guide, write the meaning of:

(p) **haem/o**/globin (Am. **hem/o**/globin)

(q) **haemoglobin**/uria (Am. **hemoglobin**/uria)

The amount of haemoglobin within red blood cells can be estimated, and abnormal levels are found in some patients. Terms describing these conditions have been formed from the suffix **-chromia** (from Greek *chroma*, meaning colour, Am. color). Here, the colour refers to the red pigment haemoglobin.

Using your Exercise Guide, find the meaning of:

(r) hypo/**chrom**/ia

(s) hyper/**chrom**/ia

(t) normo/**chrom**/ic

Another common term relating to the colour of haemoglobin is **cyanosis**. **Cyan/o** means blue. In the absence of oxygen, haemoglobin develops a bluish tinge. Nailbeds, lips and skin show signs of cyanosis (ie, look blue) when oxygenation of the blood is deficient. Tissues deprived of oxygen can also be described as **an/ox/ic**, meaning pertaining to without oxygen.

Now, we will examine word roots that refer to the different types of blood cells. All of these cells are suspended in the liquid matrix of the blood known as plasma.

Root

Erythr

(*From a Greek word* **erythros**, *meaning red. Here erythr/o means red or erythrocyte.*)

Combining form   Erythr/o

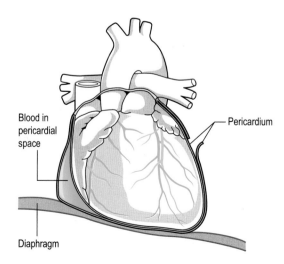

Blood in pericardial space

Pericardium

Diaphragm

Figure 33   Haemopericardium (Am. hemopericardium).

Word Exercise 2

Using your Exercise Guide, find the meaning of:

(a) **erythr/o**/penia

(b) **erythr/o**/genesis

(c) **erythr/o**/blast

(This refers to the cell which eventually forms the mature erythrocyte.)

Without using your Exercise Guide, write the meaning of:

(d) **erythr/o**/poiesis

(e) **erythr/o**/cyt/o/lysis

(f) **erythr/o**/cyt/haem/ ia (Am. **erythr/o/** cyt/hem/ia)

This last condition is synonymous with **erythrocyto- sis**, meaning an abnormal condition of red cells, ie, too many red cells. This condition is usually a physiological response to low levels of oxygen circulating in the blood. Besides changes in number, individual erythrocytes can suffer from various abnormalities, some of which are listed next.

Using your Exercise Guide, find the meaning of:

(g) micro/**cytosis**

(Note. Cytosis is used in (g) to (k) to mean too many red blood cells of a particular type.)

(h) macro/**cytosis**

(i) ellipto/**cytosis**

(j) an/iso/**cytosis**

(k) poikilo/**cytosis**

(l) normo/**cyt**/ic

Root

Reticul

(*From a Latin word* **reticulum,** *meaning a small net. Here reticul/o means reticulocyte, a very young erythrocyte lacking a nucleus; its cytoplasm gives it a net-like appearance when stained with basic dyes.*)

Combining form   Reticul/o

Word Exercise 3

Without using your Exercise Guide, build words that mean:

(a) an immature reticulo- cyte

(b) condition of too many reticulocytes

(c) condition of deficiency of reticulocytes

Root

Leuc

(*From a Greek word* **leukos**, *meaning white. Here leuc/o means white or leucocyte.*)

*Combining form*s   Leuc/o, leuk/o
(Leuc/o *is more commonly used in the UK,* leuk/o *in America.*)

Word Exercise 4

Without using your Exercise Guide, build words that mean:

(a) condition of deficiency of white cells

(b) the formation of white blood cells

Without using your Exercise Guide, write the meaning of:

(c) **leuc/o**/cyto/genesis (Am. **leuk/o**/cyto/ genesis)

(d) **leuk**/aem/ia (Am. **leuk**/em/ia. This is a malignant condition, ie, a type of cancer.)

(e) **leuc/o**/cytosis (Am. **leuk/o**/cytosis. (An excess of white cells seen during infection.)

(f) **leuc/o**/cyt/oma (Am. **leuk/o**/cyt/oma)

(g) **leuc/o**/blast (Am. **leuk/o**/blast)

(h) **leuc/o**/blast/osis (Am. **leuk/o**/blast/osis)

Using your Exercise Guide, find the meaning of:

(i) **leuc/o**/toxic (Am.
leuk/o/toxic)

Leucocyte is a general term meaning white cell, but there are many types of white cell. Some leucocytes contain granules and are known as **granulocytes**; those without granules are called **agranulocytes** (*a-* meaning without, *granul/o-* granule and *-cyte* cell).

Among the most common granulocytes are polymorpho-nuclear granulocytes or polymorphs. These all have nuclei that show many shapes (*poly-* many, *morph/o* shape and *nuclear* means nucleus). There are three types of polymorph:

Neutrophils

From *neuter*, meaning neither, and *philein*, meaning to love. These cells stain well with (love) **neutral** dyes. Neutrophils engulf microorganisms that have entered the blood and destroy them. These cells are sometimes referred to as phagocytes (*phag/o* means to eat, ie, cells that eat). The process of engulfing particles is known as phagocytosis.

Basophils

These cells stain well with basic (alkaline) dyes.

Eosinophils

These cells stain well with acid dyes like eosin, a red dye.

Among the agranular leucocytes are lymphocytes and large monocytes (*mono* means single). The latter can leave the blood and wander to sites of infection. Lymphocytes will be studied in Unit 6.

Note. The condition **pancytopenia** refers to an abnormal depression of all the cellular components of the blood (*pan-* meaning all, *cyt/o-* cell and *-penia* condition of deficiency).

Root

Myel

(*From a Greek word* **myelos**, *meaning marrow. Here myel/o means bone marrow, the substance that fills the medullary cavity and spaces of bone; it contains the blood-forming tissue that produces blood cells. Myel/o also means myelocyte, a precursor cell of the polymorphonuclear series of granulocytes found in the bone marrow.*)

Combining form   Myel/o

Word Exercise 5

Without using your Exercise Guide, write the meaning of:

(a) **myel/o**/cyte

(b) **myel/o**/fibr/osis

Without using your Exercise Guide, build words that mean:

(c) a germ cell of the marrow

(d) a tumour (Am. tumor) of myeloid tissue

Word Exercise 6

We have already used the combining form **thromb/o** meaning clot; here, it is combined with **-cyte** to make **thrombocyte**. Thrombocytes or **platelets** are fragments of cells that circulate in the blood. They play a major role in the clotting of blood.

Without using your Exercise Guide, write the meaning of:

(a) **thrombocyt/o**/penia

(b) **thrombocyt/o**/poiesis

(c) **thrombocyt/o**/lysis

(d) **thrombocyt/o**/pathy

Counting blood cells

The numbers and proportions of blood cells found in whole blood are important in the diagnosis of disease. The percentage volume of erythrocytes is known as the **haematocrit** (Am. hematocrit) (from Greek *krinein*, meaning to separate/judge/discern). The word haematocrit is also used for a device that measures the volume of erythrocytes in a blood sample. Similarly, a **thrombocytocrit** is a device that measures the volume of platelets in a given quantity of blood.

The number of blood cells can be counted using a device known as a **haemocytometer**. The simplest type of counter consists of a specially designed microscope slide that holds a precise volume of blood and a grid for the manual counting of cells. Today, the process of counting cells is performed automatically in a Coulter counter. A doctor may request particular types of cell count to aid diagnosis, for example:

Full blood count

A count of the number of red cells, white cells and platelets in a sample of blood. Reference intervals for the number of cells in a sample from a healthy person are:

Red blood cells (erythrocytes) $4.5–6.5 \times 10^{12}$/L in men, $3.8–5.3 \times 10^{12}$/L in women
White cells (leucocytes) $4.0–11.0 \times 10^{9}$/L
Platelets (thrombocytes) $150–400 \times 10^{9}$/L

Differential count

A count of the proportions of different types of cells in stained smears. Examples of reference intervals for the number of cells in a sample from a healthy person are:

Neutrophils (30–75%) $2.5–7.5 \times 10^{9}$/L
Basophils (< 1%) $< 0.1 \times 10^{9}$/L
Eosinophils (1–6%) $0.04–0.4 \times 10^{9}$/L

Techniques have been developed to take blood from a donor, remove wanted or unwanted components from it and return the cells in fresh or frozen plasma back into the body. When plasma is removed, the technique is known as **plasmapheresis**. Plasma refers to the liquid matrix of the blood in which cells are suspended and nutrients and wastes dissolved. Apheresis is from the Greek *aphairesis*, meaning a taking away.

 Word Exercise 7

Without using your Exercise Guide, write the meaning of:

(a) erythrocyt/**apheresis**

(b) thrombocyt/**apheresis**

(c) leuc/**apheresis**

Medical equipment and clinical procedures

Review the names of all instruments and clinical procedures mentioned in this unit and then complete Exercise 8.

 Word Exercise 8

Match each description in Column C with a term in Column A by placing the appropriate number in Column B.

Column A	Column B	Column C
(a) plasma-pheresis		1. a count of numbers of different blood cells/litre of blood
(b) differential count		2. an instrument that estimates the percentage volume of red cells in blood or the actual value (as a percentage of the volume) of red cells in blood
(c) haematocrit		3. an estimate of proportions/numbers of white cells in a stained smear
(d) haemoglobi-nometer		4. continuous removal of plasma from blood and retransfusion of cells
(e) complete blood count		5. an instrument that measures amount of haemoglobin in a sample

Other procedures used to investigate and treat blood disorders beside those mentioned in the word exercises include:

Blood transfusion A blood transfusion is a process that involves taking whole blood or cells from one person (the donor) and giving it to someone else (the recipient). You may need a blood transfusion for a number of reasons, including to replace blood lost during major surgery, childbirth or a severe accident. An organization called a blood bank collects, processes and stores transfused blood for such emergencies.

Before a recipient receives a transfusion, compatibility testing between donor and recipient blood must be carried out. The first step before a transfusion is given is to type and screen the recipient's blood. Typing of a recipient's blood determines its ABO and Rh status; then, the sample is screened for any antibodies in the recipient that may react with the donor blood. The ABO system classifies blood as type A, B, AB or O, and the Rh system as Rhesus-positive (Rh+) or Rhesus-negative (Rh–); A+, for example, means the patient has A type blood and it is Rhesus +. The blood bank scientist also checks the patient's medical history to see if they have previously identified any serological anomalies.

Bone marrow biopsy In this procedure a core of bone marrow is removed from the body using a thick, hollow needle pushed into a hipbone. Liquid bone marrow can also be removed by aspiration with a narrower syringe. The samples are then subjected to microscopic examination in the laboratory.

Erythrocyte sedimentation rate A sample of venous blood is mixed with an anticoagulant and left in an upright tube. The erythrocytes gradually fall to the bottom of the tube as sediment; the clear plasma is left at the top. The rate at which the cells move is measured in mm/h. The rate increases with the presence of inflammatory disease such as rheumatoid arthritis and polymyositis; it is also raised when infection and or malignant disease are present.

Prothrombin time (PT) This is a test of the ability of the blood to clot. Prothrombin time is used to determine how well anticoagulant therapy is working and aids the diagnosis of bleeding disorders.

ANATOMY EXERCISE

Now, complete the Anatomy Exercise on page 64.

 CASE HISTORY 5

The object of this exercise is to understand words associated with a patient's medical history.

To complete the exercise, do the following:

- Read through the passage on aplastic anaemia (Am. anemia); unfamiliar words are underlined, and you can find their meaning using the Word Help.

- Write the meaning of the medical terms shown in bold print on the lines that follow the Word Help.

Aplastic anaemia (Am. aplastic anemia)

Mr E, a 44-year-old chemistry teacher and former industrial chemist, had been unwell for many weeks before seeking advice from his GP. He complained of headache, breathlessness, fatigue and palpitation; the previous day he had become concerned about his condition following a severe epistaxis and **haemoptysis** (Am. hemoptysis). On examination, he appeared to have a lower respiratory tract infection and oral thrush. Initial blood investigation revealed a **pancytopenia**, and he was referred to the Haematology (Am. Hematology) Department.

Mr E looked pale and was troubled by ulcerative lesions in his mouth and pharynx. There was no lymphadenopathy or hepatosplenomegaly. A bone marrow trephine biopsy and smear confirmed a hypocellularity with the virtual absence of reticulocytes; no **leukaemic** or neoplastic cells were observed. Detailed haematological (Am. hematological) examination revealed a **normochromic**, **normocytic** anaemia with **granulocytopenia** and **thrombocytopenia**.

Mr E was diagnosed with a severe, secondary aplastic **anaemia** (Am. anemia) and was advised of its serious prognosis. He resigned from his post as a teacher, and a programme of supportive care aimed at treating his respiratory tract infection was established. He is currently being assessed for bone marrow transplantation by his HLA-identical brother.

Word Help

aplastic pertaining to without growth/unable to form new cells

epistaxis a nose bleed

GP general practitioner (family doctor)

haematological pertaining to study of blood (Am. hematological)

hepatosplenomegaly enlargement of the liver and spleen

HLA human leucocyte (Am. leukocyte) antigen, important for cross-matching of donor and recipient

hypocellularity condition of below normal number of cells

lesion pathological change in a tissue

lymphadenopathy disease of lymph nodes

neoplastic pertaining to new, abnormal growth of cells (cancer cells)

oral thrush fungal infection in the mouth (with *Candida albicans*)

palpitation unusual awareness of one's heartbeat

prognosis a forecast of the probable course and outcome of a disease

reticulocyte an immature erythrocyte

secondary here refers to a second type of aplastic anaemia caused by direct damage of the bone marrow by chemicals, radiation or infection

smear spreading material across a slide for microscopic examination

trephine biopsy using a trephine (device that removes a circular disc of bone) to take a sample of bone marrow

ulcerative having the form of an ulcer

Now write the meaning of the following words from the Case History without using your dictionary lists:

(a) haemoptysis (Am. hemoptysis)

(b) pancytopenia

(c) leukaemic (Am. leukemic)

(d) normochromic

(e) normocytic

(f) granulocytopenia

(g) thrombocytopenia

(h) anaemia
  (Am. anemia)

(Answers to the Case History exercise are given in the Answers to Word Exercises on page 339.)

Quick Reference

Combining forms relating to the blood:

Basophil/o	basophil
Cyt/o,-cyte	cell
Eosinophil/o	eosinophil
Erythr/o	red
Erythrocyt/o	erythrocyte/red cell
Fibr/o	fibre (Am. fiber)
Globin/o	protein
Granul/o	granule
Haem/o	blood
Hem/o (Am.)	blood
Leuc/o	white
Leucocyt/o	leucocyte/white cell
Leuk/o (Am.)	white
Leukocyt/o (Am.)	leukocyte/white cell
Lymphocyt/o	lymph cell
Monocyt/o	monocyte
Morph/o	shape/form
Myel/o	bone marrow/myelocyte
Neutrophil/o	neutrophil
Phag/o	eating/consuming
Plasma	plasma, the liquid part of the blood
Reticul/o	immature erythrocyte
Thromb/o	clot
Thrombocyt/o	thrombocyte/platelet

Abbreviations

Some common abbreviations related to the blood are listed below. Note that some are not standard, and their meaning may vary from one healthcare setting to another. There is a more extensive list for reference on page 369.

ALL	acute lymphocytic leukaemia (Am. leukemia)
AML	acute myeloid leukaemia (Am. leukemia)
CBC	complete blood count
CLL	chronic lymphocytic leukaemia (Am. leukemia)
CML	chronic myeloid leukaemia (Am. leukemia)
diff	differential blood count (of cell types)
ESR	erythrocyte sedimentation rate
FBC	full blood count
Hb, Hgb	haemoglobin (Am. hemoglobin)
H/ct, h.ct	haematocrit (Am. hematocrit)
HDL	high density lipoprotein
INR	international normalized ratio (prothrombin time)
LDL	low density lipoprotein

MCH	mean corpuscular haemoglobin (Am. hemoglobin)
MCHC	mean corpuscular haemoglobin concentration (Am. hemoglobin)
PCV	packed cell volume
PT	prothrombin time
RBC	red blood (cell) count/red blood cell
TIBC	total iron-binding capacity
WBC	white blood cell count

Pathology notes

Anaemia (Am. anemia)

The term anaemia is used to describe different disease conditions caused by an inability of the blood to carry sufficient oxygen to the body cells. The condition can result from inadequate numbers of red blood cells or a deficiency of haemoglobin (Am. hemoglobin) within them. Signs and symptoms are related to the inability of the blood to supply body cells with sufficient oxygen. All types of anaemia lead to a feeling of fatigue and intolerance to cold conditions. There are many types, for example:

Acute blood loss anaemia loss of red blood cells due to haemorrhage (Am. hemorrhage), often associated with trauma, extensive surgery or another situation involving a sudden loss of blood

Aplastic anaemia characterized by an abnormally low number of red blood cells. Although idiopathic forms of this disease occur, most cases result from destruction of bone marrow by drugs, toxic chemicals or radiation. As many different cells in the bone marrow are affected, aplastic anaemia is usually accompanied by a decreased number of white blood cells and platelets. Bone marrow transplants have been successful in treating some cases.

Folate deficiency anaemia similar to pernicious anaemia because it also causes a decrease in the red blood cell count resulting from a vitamin deficiency. In this condition, it is folic acid (vitamin B_9) that is deficient. Folic acid deficiencies are common among alcoholics and other malnourished individuals.

Haemolytic anaemia a condition in which red blood cells are destroyed and removed from the bloodstream before their normal lifespan is over. Intrinsic haemolytic anaemia, an inherited condition, develops when the red blood cells produced by the body are defective; for example, sickle-cell anaemia. Extrinsic haemolytic anaemia develops when the spleen traps and destroys healthy red blood cells; this can also be due to autoimmune disease, infection or a side-effect of medication.

Iron deficiency anaemia the most common type of anaemia. It is caused by inadequate absorption of dietary iron or excessive loss from the body. Iron (Fe) is a critical component of the haemoglobin molecule and, without it, the body cannot manufacture enough haemoglobin. Red blood cells seen in this type of anaemia are classed as hypochromic, meaning they have an abnormally low haemoglobin content.

Pernicious anaemia characterized by insufficient production of red blood cells due to a lack of vitamin B_{12}. Vitamin B_{12} is absorbed from the diet and used in the formation of new red blood cells in the bone marrow. In many cases, the condition results from the failure of the stomach lining to produce intrinsic factor, a substance that allows vitamin B_{12} to be absorbed. Pernicious anaemia can be fatal if not successfully treated; one method of treatment involves intramuscular injections of vitamin B_{12}.

Sickle-cell anaemia characterized by the manufacture of an abnormal haemoglobin (Hb^S) that causes red blood cells to assume a sickle-shape when deoxygenated. The sickle cells easily rupture, increase the viscosity of blood and stick to the walls of small blood vessels, restricting blood supply to tissues. The condition originated in Africa and is more common in black people.

Thalassaemia (Am. thalassemia) an inherited condition caused by the presence of autosomal recessive genes seen most commonly in populations living around the Mediterranean Sea and Southeast Asia. Reduced or absent synthesis of globin chains of haemoglobin (Am. hemoglobin) characterizes the condition. How an individual is affected depends on the genes they have inherited; they can be asymptomatic or have mild to severe anaemia (Am. anemia).

Granulocytopenia (neutropenia)

Granulocytopenia is a general term used to indicate an abnormal reduction in the number of circulating granulocytes (polymorphonuclear leucocytes, Am. leukocytes) and is commonly called neutropenia because 40–75% of granulocytes are neutrophils. A reduction in the number of circulating granulocytes occurs when production does not keep pace with the normal removal of cells or when the life span of the cells is reduced. Extreme shortage or absence of granulocytes is called agranulocytosis. Cytotoxic drugs, irradiation damage, disease of bone marrow and severe microbial infections may cause inadequate formation of granulocytes.

Haemophilia (Am. hemophilia)

Haemophilia is an inherited disorder caused by a gene linked to the X-chromosome. It affects one in every 5000 males worldwide but is rare in females. The condition results from a failure to produce one or more plasma proteins responsible for blood clotting and is characterized by a relative inability to form blood clots. Sufferers experience severe episodes of prolonged bleeding often without signs of trauma. Minor blood vessel injuries common in ordinary life can be life-threatening as they result in excessive loss of blood. There is also recurrent bleeding into joints causing pain and damage to articular cartilage. The most common form is called haemophilia A caused by absence of Factor VIII, a clotting protein; this affects more than 300,000 people around the world.

Leukaemia (Am. leukemia)

The term leukaemia applies to a group of malignant diseases characterized by proliferation of white blood cell precursors in the bone marrow. The leukaemic cells may eventually leave the bone marrow and infiltrate the lymph nodes, liver, spleen, central nervous system and other parts of the body. Approximately 5% of all deaths are due to leukaemia. Continuous production and accumulation of immature leucocytes (Am. leukocytes) characterize acute leukaemia. Overproduction of these cells leads to crowding out of normal bone marrow cells and platelets, and it results in bleeding problems. In chronic leukaemia, there is an accumulation of mature leucocytes in the blood that do not die at the end of their normal span.

The main types of leukaemia include the following: acute lymphoblastic or lymphocytic leukaemia (ALL), acute myeloid or myelogenous leukaemia (AML), chronic lymphoblastic or lymphocytic leukaemia (CLL), chronic myeloid or myelogenous leukaemia (CML) and hairy cell leukaemia.

Polycythaemia (Am. polycythemia)

In this condition, there are an abnormally large number of erythrocytes in the blood. This increases blood viscosity, slows the rate of flow and increases the risk of intravascular clotting, ischaemia (Am. ischemia) and infarction. *Polycythaemia rubra vera* is a primary condition of unknown cause in which there is an abnormal excessive production of erythrocyte precursors.

Purpura

A condition in which multiple pinpoint haemorrhages (Am. hemorrhages) accumulate under the skin and mucous membranes. The lesions appear as purple spots and are due to bleeding caused by a reduction in the number of platelets (thrombocytopenia). Autoimmune thrombocytopenic purpura is a condition in which the patient makes antibody to their platelets, which are then destroyed.

Thrombocytopenia

A condition characterized by bleeding from many small blood vessels throughout the body, most visibly in the skin and mucous membranes. If the number of thrombocytes falls to 20×10^9/L or less (normal range is $150–400 \times 10^9$/L), catastrophic bleeding may occur. Although a number of different mechanisms can result in thrombocytopenia, the usual cause is bone marrow destruction by drugs, immune system disease, chemicals, radiation or cancer.

Associated words

Agglutination the clumping together of the recipient's red blood cells when incompatible bloods are mixed
Albumin a protein found in blood plasma

Antibody a chemical that circulates in the blood destroying specific foreign substances that have entered the body

Antigen any substance that enters the body and stimulates antibody production or a response associated with sensitized T-cells

Coagulation blood clotting

Cross-matching a test of the compatibility of donor blood to be transfused into a patient

Diapedesis the condition of blood cells passing through capillary walls, particularly white blood cells

Differentiation the changes that occur in cells as they grow and specialize to perform different functions, ie, become different or specialized

Donor an individual from whom tissue is removed and collected for transfer to another

Dyscrasia an abnormality of component parts such as blood or bone marrow

Exsanguination condition of extensive blood loss due to internal or external haemorrhage (Am. hemorrhage)

Extravasation the escape of fluid into surrounding tissue, as in a bruise

Globulin a protein that forms a constituent of blood as in immunoglobulin

Haemochromatosis a condition caused by too much iron being deposited in the body (Am. hemochromatosis)

Haemosiderosis a condition in which iron accumulates in tissues and organs, due to excessive breakdown of red blood cells (Am. hemosiderosis)

Hypovolaemia a condition of severe reduction in the volume of circulating blood due to external loss of blood or increased permeability of blood vessels (Am. hypovolemia)

Immunoglobulin a protein with antibody activity, eg, IgG or IgM

Mononucleosis a condition caused by infection with Epstein-Barr virus (EBV) characterized by an increase in the number of atypical mononuclear leucocytes. It is transmitted orally by kissing and is known by the common name glandular fever.

Morphology having a particular form, shape, or structure; the study of form and structure of cells and organisms

Palliative a treatment that relieves symptoms but does not cure

Perfusion the passage of fluid or blood through a tissue or organ, particularly blood through the lungs

Pernicious highly destructive, fatal

Recipient an individual receiving a blood transfusion or organ transplant

Relapse deterioration in condition after apparent improvement or recovery

Remission period when a disease subsides and there are no signs or symptoms

Sanguineous pertaining to containing blood

Serum the fluid part of the blood that remains after clotting

Undifferentiated like a primitive cell without any development to a more specialized type

NOW TRY THE WORD CHECK

WORD CHECK

This self-check exercise lists all the word components used in this unit. First, write down the meaning of as many word components as you can. Then, check your answers using the Exercise Guide and Quick Reference box or the Glossary of Word Components (pp. 383–410).

Prefixes

a-	
an-	
baso-	
ellipto-	
eosino-	
hyper-	
hypo-	
iso-	
macro-	
micro-	
neutro-	
normo-	
pan-	
peri-	
poikil/o	
poly-	

Combining forms of word roots

cardi/o	
cyan/o	
cyt/o	
dynam/o	
erythr/o	
fibr/o	
globin/o	
granul/o	
haem/o (Am. hem/o)	
leuc/o (Am. leuk/o)	
monocyt/o	

morph/o

myel/o

norm/o

ox/y

path/o

phag/o

plasma-

reticul/o

septic/o

thromb/o

thrombocyt/o

Suffixes

-aemia (Am.
-emia)

-apheresis

-blast

-chromia

-crit

-cytosis

-genesis

-ic

-ium

-logy

-lysis

-meter

-oma

-osis

-penia

-phil

-poiesis

-rrhage

-stasis

-toxic

-um

-uria

NOW TRY THE SELF-ASSESSMENT

SELF-ASSESSMENT

Test 5A

Next are some combining forms that relate to the components of blood. Indicate which part of the blood they refer to by putting a number from the diagram (Fig. 34) next to each word. You may use a number more than once.

(a) plasma

(b) erythr/o

(c) lymph/o

(d) neutr/o

(e) thrombocyt/o

Score

5

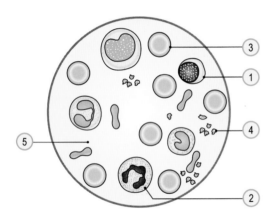

Figure 34   Blood.

Test 5B

Prefixes, suffixes and combining forms of word roots

Match each meaning in Column C with a word component in Column A by inserting the appropriate number in Column B.

Column A	Column B	Column C
(a) -aemia (Am. -emia)		1. condition of urine
(b) an-		2. disintegration/ breakdown

Column A	Column B	Column C
(c) baso-		3. red
(d) -blast		4. measuring instrument
(e) -chromia		5. abnormal condition of
(f) ellipt/o		6. basic/alkaline
(g) eosin/o		7. white
(h) erythr/o		8. clot
(i) granul/o		9. equal/same
(j) iso-		10. condition of blood
(k) leuc/o (Am. leuk/o)		11. disease
(l) -lysis		12. granule
(m) macro-		13. germ cell
(n) -meter		14. cessation of flow
(o) micro-		15. affinity for / loving
(p) neutr/o		16. condition of deficiency / lack of
(q) -osis		17. not/without
(r) -pathy		18. small
(s) -penia		19. condition of colour / haemoglobin (Am. hemoglobin)
(t) -phil		20. oval/elliptoid
(u) septic/o		21. large
(v) -stasis		22. eosin (acid dye)
(w) thromb/o		23. neutral
(x) -uria		24. decay/sepsis/ infection

Score

24

Test 5C

Write the meaning of:

(a) leucocyturia (Am. leukocyturia)

(b) myelocytosis

(c) reticulocytopenia

(d) thrombocythaemia (Am. thrombo-cythemia)

(e) phagocytolysis

Score

5

Test 5D

Build words that mean:

(a) any disease of blood (use haem/o, Am. hem/o)

(b) condition of too many platelets in the blood

(c) a physician who specializes in the study of blood (use haemat/o, Am. hemat/o)

(d) pertaining to the poison-ing of blood

(e) condition of deficiency in the number of neutrophils

Score

5

Check answers to Self-Assessment Tests on pages 360–361.

Test your recall of the meanings of word components in Units 1–5 by completing the appropriate self-assessment tests in Unit 22 on pages 324–325.

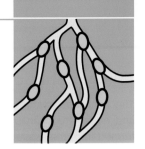

UNIT 6
THE LYMPHATIC SYSTEM AND IMMUNOLOGY

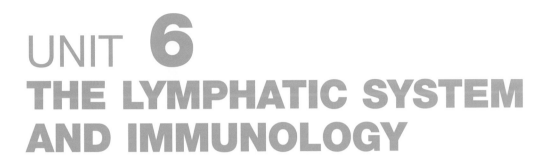

EXERCISE GUIDE

Use this list of word components and their meanings to complete the word exercises in this unit.

Prefixes

auto-	self

Roots / Combining forms

aden/o	gland
angi/o	vessel
cyt/o, -cyte	cell
helc/o	ulcer
hepat/o	liver
path/o	disease
pharyng/o	pharynx
port/o	portal vein

Suffixes

-aemia	condition of blood
-cele	swelling/protrusion/hernia
-cytosis	abnormal increase in cells
-eal	pertaining to
-ectasis	dilatation/stretching
-ectomy	removal of
-emia (Am.)	condition of blood
-genesis	pertaining to formation
-genic	pertaining to formation / originating in
-globulin	protein
-gram	X-ray/tracing/recording
-graphy	technique of recording/making X-ray
-ic	pertaining to
-itis	inflammation of
-ity	state/condition
-logy	study of
-lysis	breakdown/disintegration
-malacia	condition of softening
-megaly	enlargement
-oma	tumour/swelling (Am. tumor)
-osis	abnormal condition / disease of
-pathy	disease of
-pexy	surgical fixation/fix in place
-poiesis	formation
-rrhagia	condition of bursting forth
-rrhea (Am.)	excessive discharge/flow
-rrhoea	excessive discharge/flow
-tic	pertaining to
-tome	cutting instrument

The lymphatic system

The lymphatic system consists of capillaries, vessels, ducts and nodes that transport a fluid known as lymph. Lymph is formed from the tissue fluid that surrounds all tissue cells. The system performs three important functions: (1) transportation of lymphocytes that defend the body against infection and foreign antigens, (2) transportation of lipids and (3) the drainage of excess fluid from the tissues.

We'll begin by examining the terms associated with the cells and components of the system. Use the Exercise Guide at the beginning of this unit to complete Word Exercises 1–8, unless you are asked to work without it.

Root

Lymph

(From Latin **lympha***, meaning water. Here lymph/o means lymph or lymphatic tissue.)*

Combining forms   Lymph/a/o

 Word Exercise 1

Using your Exercise Guide, find the meaning of:

(a) **lymph/o**/cyt/osis

(b) **lymph/o**/rrhagia

(c) **lymph**[2]/angi/o[3]/graphy[1]

(d) **lymph**/angi/o/gram

(e) **lymph**/angi/ectasis

(f) **lymph**/oma

Note. The next four words use the combining form lymphaden/o meaning lymph gland. The structures referred to by this combining form are no longer called glands because, unlike true glands, they do not produce secretions. Lymphaden/o is now used to mean lymph node. A node is a mass of lymphoid tissue containing cells that defend the body against noxious agents such as microorganisms and toxins.

(g) **lymphaden**/ectomy

(h) **lymphaden/o**/pathy

(i) **lymphaden**/itis

Lymph nodes consist of lymphatic channels held in place by fibrous connective tissue that forms a capsule. The nodes

contain **lymphocytes** (lymph cells, *-cyte* meaning cell) and special cells called **macrophages** (large eaters) which, like neutrophils, can engulf foreign substances and microorganisms by phagocytosis. Lymph nodes often trap and destroy malignant cells as well as microorganisms. During infection, lymphocytes multiply rapidly in germinal centres (Am. centers), causing the nodes to swell; they may become inflamed and sore. Lymphocytes and macrophages leave the nodes in lymph (a clear fluid) that eventually drains through ducts into blood vessels near the heart. These cells then circulate in the blood and form a proportion of the white blood cell population. See Figure 36 on p. 80.

If disease in the lymphatic system is suspected, a **nodal biopsy** (nod- meaning node and *-al* meaning pertaining to) may be performed; in this procedure a node is removed for examination by a histopathologist (*hist/o* meaning tissue, *path/o* disease and *-logist* a specialist who studies).

The macrophages that line the lymph organs are part of a large system of cells known as the **reticuloendothelial system** or macrophage system. Cells that form this network have a common ancestry and carry out phagocytosis (Fig. 37) in the liver, bone marrow, lymph nodes, spleen, nervous system, blood and connective tissues. Macrophages found in connective tissues are known as **histiocytes** (ie, tissue cells). If there is an increase in the number of histiocytes without infection, this is known as a **histiocytosis**.

Distinct patches of lymphatic tissue have been given specific names; the familiar ones mentioned here include the spleen, tonsils, adenoids and thymus.

Root

Splen

(A Greek word, meaning spleen. The spleen has four main functions: destruction of old blood cells, blood storage, blood filtration and participation in the immune response.)

Combining form   Splen/o

 Word Exercise 2

Using your Exercise Guide, find the meaning of:

(a) **splen/o**/megaly

(b) **splen/o**/hepat/o/megaly

(c) **splen/o**/pexy

(d) **splen/o**/cele

(e) **splen/o**/malacia

(f) **splen/o**/lysis

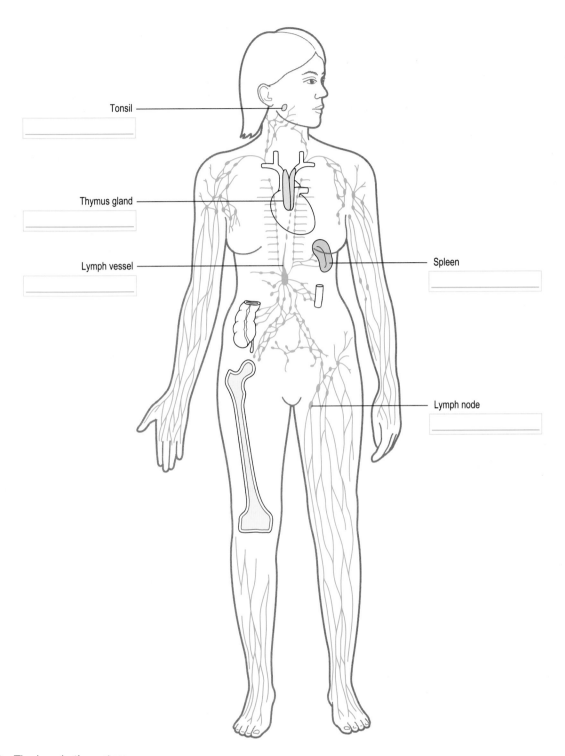

Tonsil

Thymus gland

Lymph vessel

Spleen

Lymph node

Figure 35   The lymphatic system.

Without using your Exercise Guide, write the meaning of:

(g) **splen/o**/graphy

(h) **splen/o**/port/o/gram

(**Port/o** refers to the portal vein that drains blood from the intestines, stomach, pancreas and spleen into the liver.)

 ANATOMY EXERCISE

When you have finished Word Exercises 1–8, look at the word components listed next. Complete Figure 35 by placing the appropriate combining form on each line. (You can check their meanings in the Quick Reference box on p. 84.)

| Lymphaden/o | Splen/o | Tonsill/o |
| Lymphangi/o | Thym/o | |

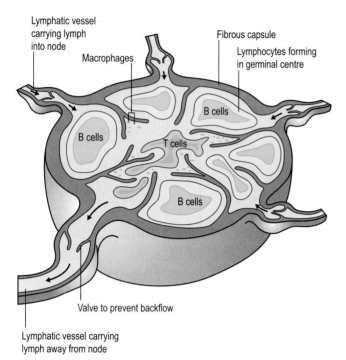

Figure 36   A lymph node. (Adapted from Chabner D-E, The Language of Medicine, 10th Edition, 2013, Saunders.)

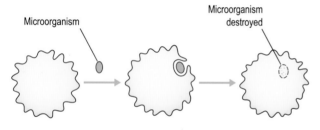

Figure 37   Phagocytosis.

Root

Tonsill

(*From Latin* **tonsillae**, *meaning tonsils. These form a ring of lymphoid tissue at the back of the mouth and nasopharynx. They are important in the formation of antibodies and lymphocytes.*)

Combining form   Tonsill/o

 Word Exercise 3

Without using your Exercise Guide, build words that mean:

(a) inflammation of the tonsils

(b) removal of the tonsils

Using your Exercise Guide, find the meaning of:

(c) **tonsill/o**/pharyng/eal

(d) **tonsill/o**/tome

Note. An adenoid is a pharyngeal tonsil; the term **adenoids** is used for enlarged pharyngeal tonsils that obstruct the passage of air or interfere with hearing when they block the entrance to the auditory tube. Removal of the adenoids is known as an **adenoid**ectomy.

Root

Thym

(*From a Greek word* **thymos**, *meaning soul or emotion. Here, thym/o means the thymus gland that lies high in the chest above the aorta. It controls the development of the immune system in early life.*)

Combining forms   Thym/o, thymic/o

Word Exercise 4

Without using your Exercise Guide, build words using thym/o that mean:

(a) a cell of the thymus

(b) disease of the thymus

(c) protrusion/swelling of the thymus

Using your Exercise Guide, find the meaning of:

(d) **thym**/elc/osis (Look up helc)

(e) **thymic/o**/lympha/tic

Immunology

Immunology is the scientific study of immunity and related disciplines such as immunotherapy and immunochemistry. Immunological research has intensified because of the spread of the immunodeficiency virus (HIV) that causes AIDS. Many pharmaceutical companies are actively engaged in the search for vaccines and new treatments based on our increased knowledge of the immune process.

Immunity is the condition of being immune to infectious disease and antigenic substances that might damage the body. It is brought about by the production of antibodies and cells that destroy invading pathogens before they can do us harm. During our lifetime, we naturally acquire immunity to common disease-producing organisms, such as viruses that cause colds and influenza. We can also artificially acquire immunity to more serious diseases by vaccination.

Understanding the meaning of the following terms will help you understand the basis of the immune process.

Antigen

An antigen is any foreign substance that enters the body and stimulates antibody production or a response associated with sensitized T-cells. Note that antigens will be present on the surface of any foreign cell that enters the body, and these will provoke a response from the immune system.

Antibody

An antibody is a chemical that circulates in the blood destroying or precipitating specific foreign substances (antigens) that have entered the body. (*Anti-* means against, *-body* is an Anglo-Saxon word, in this case referring to a foreign body.)

Root

Immun

(*From Latin* **immunis**, *meaning exempt from public burden. Here, immun/o means immunity, the condition of being immune (exempt) from disease.*)

Combining form   Immun/o

📖 Word Exercise 5

Using your Exercise Guide, look up the meaning of -logy and path/o, and then build words that mean:

(a) the study of immunity

(b) branch of medicine
concerned with the study
of immune reactions
associated with disease

Using your Exercise Guide, find the meaning of:

(c) **immun/o/genesis**

(d) auto/**immun**/ity

(e) **immun/o**/globulin

Two basic types of cell bring about immunity:

T-cells (thymic cells)

T-cells are types of lymphocytes formed in the bone marrow of the embryo that move to the thymus to be processed into T-cells (hence the name T-cell). The T-cells then move to other parts of the lymphatic system where they are responsible for the **cell-mediated response**. Once sensitized to a specific antigen, these cells multiply rapidly, producing various cell types, all of which play a role in the immune response. One type of cell that forms is the cytotoxic (killer) T-cell; this attacks and kills infectious microorganisms containing the specific antigen. These cells are particularly effective against slowly growing bacteria and fungi, cancer cells and skin grafts.

B-cells

B-cells are types of lymphocytes named for historical reasons after the site where they were first seen in birds, in the bursa of Fabricius. In humans, B-cells first differentiate in the fetal liver and transform into large **plasma cells** when confronted with specific antigens. Once sensitized by an antigen, the plasma cell multiplies to form a large clone of similar cells (**plasmacytosis**). Each cell in the clone secretes the same antibody to the sensitizing antigen; this is known as the **humoral response**. Some antibodies activate a protein in the blood known as **complement**, which aids the antibody in destroying the antigen. (Note. Plasmacytosis means an excess of plasma cells in the blood.)

T-cells and B-cells are produced in lymph nodes in large numbers in response to infection. See Figure 36.

Root

Ser

(*From a Latin word* **serum**, *meaning whey. Here, ser/o means serum, the clear portion of any liquid separated from its more solid elements. Blood serum is the supernatant liquid formed when blood clots; it can be used as a source of antibodies.*)

Combining form   Ser/o

📖 Word Exercise 6

Without using your Exercise Guide, build a word that means:

(a) the scientific study of sera

Serum investigations can lead to a patient being seronegative or seropositive for the presence of a particular antibody. For example, a person assessed as HIV-positive has antibodies in their blood to the human immunodeficiency virus. This means that the virus has entered their body and stimulated their immune system to make antibodies. If the virus is not destroyed by the immune system or inhibited by drug therapy, it will continue to replicate and lead to the development of AIDS.

Seronegative
showing a lack of antibody

Seropositive
showing the presence of a high level of antibody

Root

Py

(*From a Greek word* **pyon**, *meaning pus.*)

Combining form   Py/o

Pus is a yellow, protein-rich liquid, composed of tissue fluids containing bacteria and leucocytes. When a wound is forming or discharging pus, it is said to be **suppurating**. Pus is formed in response to certain types of infection.

 Word Exercise 7

Using your Exercise Guide, find the meaning of:

(a) **py**/aemia
    (Am. **py**/emia)

(b) **py/o**/genic

(c) **py/o**/rrhoea
    (Am. **py/o**/rrhea)

(d) **py/o**/poiesis

The immune response of the lymphatic system not only resists invasion by infective organisms but also functions to identify and destroy everything described as 'non-self', ie, foreign antigens that have entered the body, such as transplanted organs or body cells that have become malignant.

Patients infected with microorganisms, for example those who present with tonsillitis, experience swollen lymph nodes, and their blood counts indicate an increase in circulating white blood cells. The nodes swell because they contain plasma cells and T-cells forming clones of cells to fight the infection. Once the foreign cells have been destroyed, the nodes return to their normal size. The response of the body to the initial sensitization with the antigen is called the *primary response*.

An important feature of the immune response is that some activated B-cells develop into **memory B-cells** rather than plasma cells. These remain in the nodes and other lymphoid tissue ready to respond should the same antigen enter the body again. If the same antigen is contacted, the memory B-cells divide rapidly to produce plasma cells. These release large amounts of antibody, destroying the antigen before symptoms appear.

In a similar way, some **memory T-cells** remain in the lymphoid tissue and can be rapidly activated in response to another contact with the same antigen. The accelerated and increased response of the memory cells is called the *secondary response,* and it endows us with immunity.

Medical equipment and clinical procedures

Review the names of all instruments and clinical procedures mentioned in this unit, and then try Exercise 8. Make sure you know the meaning of the suffixes **-gram** and **-graphy**.

Word Exercise 8

Match each description in Column C with a term in Column A by placing the appropriate number in Column B.

Column A	Column B	Column C
(a) tonsillotome		1. X-ray picture of the splenic and portal veins
(b) lymphangiography		2. X-ray picture of the lymphatic system
(c) lymphadenography		3. an instrument used for cutting tonsils
(d) lymphogram		4. technique of making an X-ray of lymph vessels
(e) splenoportogram		5. technique of making an X-ray of the lymphatic system
(f) lymphography		6. technique of making an X-ray of lymph nodes

Other procedures used to investigate and treat disorders of the lymphatic system beside those mentioned in the word exercises include the following:

Bone marrow transplantation This follows the same procedure as HSCT mentioned previously except bone marrow cells are harvested and transplanted rather than stem cells. In allogenic transplants, the donor must have a tissue (HLA) type that matches the recipient. Patients are also treated with immunosuppressive drugs to suppress immunocompetent cells in the donor's tissue that may cause graft-versus-host disease (GVHD).

CD4+ cell count This is the measurement of the number of CD4+ cells in the blood of patients infected with HIV. A type of T-cell called a helper T-cell carries a CD4 glycoprotein (antigen) on its surface. Human immunodeficiency virus binds to the CD4 antigen and kills the T-cell bearing the protein. AIDS patients have inadequate numbers of CD4+ cells. If CD4+ falls below 250 cells/mm^3, the patient is treated with antiviral drugs (normal count is 500–1500 cells/mm^3).

Computed tomography (CT) A procedure that produces a series of X-rays showing multiple cross-sectional views of lymphoid organs.

ELISA (enzyme-linked immunosorbent assay) A screening test to detect anti-HIV antibodies in the bloodstream of patients who may have been exposed to the virus that causes AIDS. Antibodies to HIV appear in blood serum within two weeks of infection; if the test is positive, that is antibodies to HIV are detected, a more specific Western blot test is performed for confirmation of the result.

Haemopoietic stem cell transplantation (HSCT) In this procedure, diseased bone marrow cells are replaced with healthy bone marrow stem cells from a donor. Patients with leukaemia, lymphoma or multiple myeloma are suitable candidates for this treatment (Am. hemopoietic, leukemia).

The donor is given drug treatment to stimulate the growth of stem cells, which are then removed from their blood by leucapheresis (Am. leukapheresis). Meanwhile, the recipient's malignant cells are destroyed using a combination of chemotherapy and/or radiotherapy. The normal stem cells from the donor are then transplanted into the recipient where they divide to produce clones of normal blood cells and reinitiate the immune system. Allogenic HSCT involves two people: the donor and the patient. The donor must have a tissue (HLA) that matches the recipient to avoid rejection.

In the procedure known as autologous HSCT, the patient's own stem cells are collected, cleared of any diseased cells, stored and reinfused once chemotherapy is complete.

Histocompatibility testing The success of an organ or tissue transplant depends on histocompatibility; this means the tissue from the donor must be very similar to the tissue of the recipient so that it is not rejected. Tissue typing (or histocompatibility testing) is performed before any organ transplant takes place. A national register of donors with particular tissue types helps select appropriate donors.

HLA matching Human leucocyte antigens are chemicals (glycoproteins) found on the surface of almost all cells and were first discovered on leucocytes (Am. leukocytes). The proteins act as antigens and are of practical importance when donors and recipients are tissue-typed and matched for organ transplantation. Rejection occurs when donor and recipient HLAs do not match. These proteins are controlled by a group of genes referred to as the major histocompatibility complex (MHC).

Immunoelectrophoresis A test that detects the presence of abnormal levels of immunoglobulins in blood.

Viral load test A test that measures the amount of HIV in the bloodstream.

Western blot test A specific test for the presence of HIV antibodies.

ANATOMY EXERCISE

Now complete the Anatomy Exercise on page 78.

CASE HISTORY 6

The object of this exercise is to understand words associated with a patient's medical history.

To complete the exercise, do the following:

* Read through the passage on non-Hodgkin lymphoma; unfamiliar words are underlined, and you can find their meaning using the Word Help.

* Write the meaning of the medical terms shown in bold print on the lines that follow the Word Help.

Non-Hodgkin lymphoma

Mr F, a 48-year-old male, presented to his GP with a painless swelling in the right axilla. The lump had been present for at least two months before his consultation, and he had not been unduly concerned until he noticed a similar lump in his left axilla that appeared to be increasing in size. The patient indicated he had a good appetite and denied weight loss. There had been no change to his bowel and bladder habits, and apart from a recent cold and **tonsillitis**, he had not suffered any infection. He had smoked for 32 years and admitted moderate drinking. The only problem he mentioned was difficulty in sleeping; sometimes he would wake sweating copiously.

Examination revealed prominent lymph node enlargement in the right and left axillae and inguinal areas. The largest node was located in the right axilla, approximately 20 mm across. Examination of the head and neck also revealed enlarged cervical nodes, the largest approximately 15 mm across. The nodes were firm, tender and rubbery on palpation.

Cardiovascular and pulmonary examination was normal. He had **splenomegaly** that was palpable 30 mm below the left costal margin. His tonsils appeared swollen. It was evident from initial examination that Mr F was suffering from a generalized **lymphadenopathy** that did not appear to be associated with infection.

Mr F underwent axillary **nodal** biopsy, and his specimen was sent to **histopathology**. Examination of the tissue revealed a follicular, small, cleaved cell non-Hodgkin **lymphoma** (NHL). This was followed by a bilateral bone marrow trephine biopsy that demonstrated cells suspicious for lymphoma similar to those found in the nodes. The **lymphocytes** forming the tumour (Am. tumor) were classified as being of **B-cell** origin. Computed tomography (CT) was used to assess nodal enlargement, and he was referred to the Oncology Department for staging.

Mr F underwent four cycles of chemotherapy (R-CHOPS) and, since then, no disease is evident in his bone marrow, and his lymphadenopathy has regressed.

Word Help

axilla the armpit (plural axillae)

bilateral pertaining to two sides

biopsy removal and examination of living tissue

cervical pertaining to the neck

chemotherapy treatment with chemicals, ie, cytotoxic drugs that kill cancer cells

cleaved cut/separated (here refers to indentations in the nucleus of a lymph cell)

costal pertaining to the ribs

follicular pertaining to a follicle (here a well-defined collection of multiplying lymph cells)

GP general practitioner (family doctor)

inguinal pertaining to the groin

non-Hodgkin not Hodgkin lymphoma, a type of lymphoma named after Thomas Hodgkin (1798–1866, London, physician)

oncology study of tumours (Am. tumors)/cancers

palpation act of feeling with the fingers using light pressure

R-CHOPS type of chemotherapy regimen (using **R**ituximab, **C**yclophosphamide, **H**ydroxydaunorubicin, **O**ncovin and **P**rednisolone)

regressed reverted (towards former condition)

staging a system of classifying malignant disease that will influence its treatment

tomography technique of using X-rays to image a section through the body

trephine an instrument with a circular cutting edge that removes a disc of tissue

Now write the meaning of the following words from the Case History without using your dictionary lists:

(a) tonsillitis

(b) splenomegaly

(c) lymphadenopathy

(d) nodal

(e) histopathology

(f) lymphoma

(g) lymphocyte

(h) B-cell

(Answers to the Case History exercise are given in the Answers to Word Exercises on page 340.)

Quick Reference

Combining forms relating to the lymphatic system and immunology:

Aden/o	gland
Adenoid-	adenoid (a nasopharyngeal tonsil)
Cyt/o, -cyte	cell
-globulin	protein
Hist/i/o	tissue
Immun/o	immune
Lymph/o	lymph
Lymphaden/o	lymph node
Lymphangi/o	lymph vessel
Phag/o	eating/consuming
Plasma-	plasma cell
Py/o	pus
Ser/o	serum
Splen/o	spleen
Thym/o	thymus gland
Thymic/o	thymus gland
Tonsill/o	tonsil

Abbreviations

Some common abbreviations related to the lymphatic system are listed next. Note that some are not standard, and their meaning may vary from one healthcare setting to another. There is a more extensive list for reference on page 369.

AIDS	acquired immune deficiency syndrome
BM (T)	bone marrow (trephine)
HAART	highly active antiretroviral therapy (HIV treatment)
HL	Hodgkin lymphoma
HLA	human leucocyte antigen (Am. leukocyte)
Ig	immunoglobulin
LAS	lymphadenopathy syndrome
MAB, mAb, -mab	monoclonal antibody
NHL	non-Hodgkin lymphoma
NKT	natural killer T-cell
T & A	tonsillectomy and adenoidectomy

Pathology notes

Acquired immune deficiency syndrome

Acquired immune deficiency syndrome (AIDS) was first recognized in 1981. The condition is caused by the human immunodeficiency virus (HIV). HIV is a retrovirus containing RNA that once transcribed into DNA in the host cell directs it to produce new viruses. HIV infects vital cells in the immune system such as helper T-cells (specifically CD4+ cells that express the CD4 glyco-proteins on their surface), macrophages and dendritic cells. Once infected, the cells are destroyed and immunity is seriously impaired. When each T helper cell dies, it releases new retro-viruses that can spread the infection. As the HIV infection progresses, more and more CD4 lymphocytes are lost; this change is one of the principal clinical methods for monitoring AIDS. When helper T-cell function is impaired, infectious organisms and cancer cells can grow and spread much more easily than normal. Infections and tumours that rarely occur in healthy people such as *Pneumocystis carinii* pneumonia (a protozoal infection) and Kaposi sarcoma (a type of skin cancer) are frequently seen in AIDS patients. As their immune system is deficient, untreated AIDS patients usually die from one of these infections or cancers.

HIV is spread by direct contact of body fluids usually through sexual contact, blood transfusions, intravenous use of contaminated needles and breast-feeding by infectious mothers.

Allergy

The term allergy is used to describe hypersensitivity of the immune system to relatively harmless environmental antigens. Antigens that trigger an allergic response are called allergens. Almost any substance can be an allergen for some individuals. Before such a sensitization reaction occurs, a susceptible person must be exposed repeatedly to an allergen, triggering the production of antibodies. Exposure to the allergen causes antigen–antibody reactions that trigger the release of histamine, kinins and other inflammatory substances. In some cases, these substances may cause constriction of the airways, relaxation of blood vessels and irregular heart rhythms that can progress to a life-threatening condition called ana-phylactic shock. However, more typical allergy symptoms include a runny nose, conjunctivitis and urticaria (hives). Drugs called antihistamines are often used to relieve the symptoms of this type of allergy.

Anaphylaxis

This is a life-threatening condition resulting from an extreme hypersensitivity reaction to a previously encountered allergen such as a wasp sting.

Atopy

This is a familial (inherited) condition in which individuals have an increased tendency to develop an allergy such as eczema, asthma or rhinitis.

Autoimmunity

Autoimmunity is an inappropriate and excessive response to self-antigens. Disorders that result from autoimmune responses are called autoimmune diseases. Self-antigens are molecules that are native to a person's body and that are used by the immune system to identify the components of self. In auto-immunity the immune system inappropriately attacks these antigens. A common autoimmune disease is rheumatoid arthritis in which inflammatory changes affect joints, the heart, blood vessels and skin.

Isoimmunity

Isoimmunity is a normal but often undesirable reaction of the immune system to antigens from a different individual of the same species. Isoimmunity is important in two situations: pregnancy and tissue transplants. During pregnancy, antigens from a fetus may enter the mother's blood and sensitize her immune system. Antibodies that are formed as a result of this sensitization may then enter the fetal circulation and cause an inappropriate reaction. An example is erythroblastosis fetalis in which a Rhesus –ve mother makes antibodies to her Rhesus +ve fetus causing haemolysis (Am. hemolysis) and phagocytosis of her baby's red blood cells.

Isoimmunity is also of great importance in tissue or organ transplants. The immune system reacts against foreign antigens in grafted tissue causing a rejection syndrome.

Lymphoedema (Am. lymphedema)

Lymphoedema is an abnormal condition in which swelling of the tissues in the extremities occurs because of an obstruction of the lymphatics and accumulation of lymph. The most common causes are tumours and surgery.

Congenital lymphoedema (Milroy disease) due to deficient development of lymph vessels is more often seen in women between the ages of 15 and 25 years of age. The obstruction can be in the lymphatic vessels or in the lymph nodes themselves.

Lymphoma

Lymphoma is a term that refers to a tumour (Am. tumor) of the cells of lymphoid tissue. Lymphomas are often malignant but in rare cases can be benign. They usually originate in isolated lymph nodes but can involve lymphoid tissue in the liver, spleen and gastrointestinal tract. Widespread involvement is common because the disease spreads from node to node through the lymphatic vessels. The exact cause of these neoplasms is unknown. The two principal categories of lymphoma are Hodgkin lymphoma and non-Hodgkin lymphoma.

Hodgkin lymphoma a malignancy with an uncertain cause; some pathologists believe it originates as a viral-induced tumour of T-cells. Exposure to the Epstein-Barr virus that causes glandular fever is a known risk factor. The condition usually begins as painless, non-tender enlarged lymph nodes in the neck or axilla. Soon, lymph nodes in other regions enlarge in the same manner. If those near the trachea or oesophagus (Am. esophagus) swell, the increased pressure results in difficulty in breathing or swallowing. Lymphoedema (Am. lymphedema), anaemia (Am. anemia), leucocytosis (Am. leukocytosis), fever and weight loss occur as the condition progresses. Hodgkin lymphoma is potentially curable with radiation therapy provided it has not spread beyond the lymphatic system. Chemotherapy is used in addition to radiation therapy in more advanced cases.

Non-Hodgkin lymphoma the name given to a malignancy of lymphoid tissue other than Hodgkin lymphoma; examples include mantle cell lymphoma and Burkitt lymphoma. The cause is uncertain but has been hypothesized to be viral infection. Manifestations are similar to Hodgkin lymphoma, but there is usually a more generalized involvement of lymph nodes, and the central nervous system is often involved. Radiation and chemotherapy are treatments of choice.

Multiple myeloma

This is a malignant tumour of plasma cells (B-cell lymphocytes) that produce antibodies. Collections of abnormal plasma cells accumulate in the bone marrow where they interfere with the production of normal blood cells. The tumour cells usually produce one type of abnormal antibody that can impair the passage of blood through capillaries. Myeloma affects multiple places in the body where bone marrow is normally active, ie, spine, pelvis, ribs, shoulder and long bones of the arms and legs. Chemotherapy, steroids and biological therapies are the main treatments for myeloma; radiotherapy is also used to help control pain.

Associated words

Acquired immunity a type of immunity that results from exposure to an infectious disease or through vaccination

Active immunity a type of immunity that results from the development of antibodies in response to an antigen, as from exposure to an infectious disease or through vaccination

Allergen any substance that stimulates an allergic state (hypersensitivity reaction), eg, pollen

Antiserum a blood serum containing antibodies against specific antigens, injected to treat or protect against a specific disease, eg, for snakebite

Antitoxin an antibody formed in response to and capable of neutralizing a specific toxin of biological origin; an animal or human serum containing antibodies

Autoimmune disease condition in which the body develops antibodies and a cell-mediated response to its own tissues

Cluster of differentiation (CD) a system used for the identification and investigation of cell surface molecules; for example, a CD4 glycoprotein is a marker that identifies a helper T-cell

Histocompatibility compatibility between the tissues of different individuals, so that one accepts a graft from the other without giving an immune reaction

Human leucocyte antigen (HLA) a cell surface chemical first found on leucocytes that plays an important role in the regulation of the immune response

Hypersensitivity an abnormal, increased sensitivity to a particular antigen that results in an allergy such as asthma or anaphylaxis

Immunization the act of creating immunity by artificial means

Immunoassay the measurement of the concentration of substances by using antibodies

Immunosuppression the artificial prevention of the immune response by use of radiation or chemical agents

Immunotherapy the treatment of disease by inducing, enhancing, or suppressing an immune response

Inoculation the introduction of antigenic material into the body to stimulate the immune response

Natural immunity a person's own genetic ability to fight off disease

Passive immunity the short-term immunity that results from the introduction of antibodies from another person or animal, eg, the transfer of maternal antibodies through the placenta to a fetus and to the newborn in the first milk (colostrum)

Sensitization administration of an antigen to induce a primary immune response; exposure to an allergen that promotes the development of hypersensitivity

Stem cell an undifferentiated cell that is capable of giving rise to more cells of the same type and from which other kinds of cell arise by differentiation

Vaccination the introduction of a vaccine to produce immunity to a specific disease

Vaccine a suspension of attenuated (weakened) or killed microorganisms administered to stimulate immunity to a disease

Western blot a method of testing for HIV infection that causes AIDS

Tolerance the state marked by unresponsiveness of the immune system to a previously encountered antigen that can be harmful to the body

NOW TRY THE WORD CHECK

WORD CHECK

This self-check exercise lists all the word components used in this unit. First, write down the meaning of as many word components as you can. Then, check your answers using the Exercise Guide and Quick Reference box or the Glossary of Word Components (pp. 383–410).

Prefixes

anti-

auto-

macro-

Combining forms of word roots

aden/o

angi/o

cyt/o

-globulin

helc/o

hepat/o

hist/i/o

immun/o

lymph/o

lymphaden/o

lymphangi/o

phag/o

pharyng/o

plasm/a

port/o

py/o

reticul/o

ser/o

splen/o

thym/o

tonsill/o

Suffixes

-aemia
(Am. -emia)

-al

-cele

-eal

-ectasis

-ectomy

-genesis

-genic

-gram

-graphy

-ia

-ic

-itis

-ity

-logy

-lysis

-malacia

-megaly

-oma

-osis

-pathy

-pexy

-poiesis

-rrhagia

-rrhoea
(Am. -rrhea)

-tic

-tome

NOW TRY THE SELF-ASSESSMENT

SELF-ASSESSMENT

Test 6A

Next are some medical terms that refer to the anatomy of the lymphatic system. Indicate which part of the system they refer to by putting a number from the diagram (Fig. 38) next to each word.

(a) lymphaden/o

(b) splen/o

(c) thym/o

(d) tonsill/o

(e) lymphangi/o

Score [   ]

[5]

Test 6B

Prefixes, suffixes and combining forms of word roots

Match each meaning in Column C with a word component in Column A by inserting the appropriate number in Column B.

Column A	Column B	Column C
(a) aden/o		1. protein/ball
(b) angi/o		2. swelling/hernia/ protrusion
(c) anti-		3. immune
(d) auto-		4. self
(e) -cele		5. vessel
(f) -globin		6. pus
(g) -gram		7. cutting instrument
(h) helc/o		8. against
(i) immun/o		9. spleen
(j) lymphaden/o		10. ulcer
(k) -lysis		11. serum
(l) -malacia		12. tonsil
(m) port/o		13. lymph node
(n) py/o		14. gland
(o) -rrhoea (Am. -rrhea)		15. excessive flow
(p) ser/o		16. picture/tracing/ recording
(q) splen/o		17. condition of softening
(r) thym/o		18. disintegration/ breakdown
(s) -tome		19. portal vein
(t) tonsill/o		20. thymus gland

Score [   ]

[20]

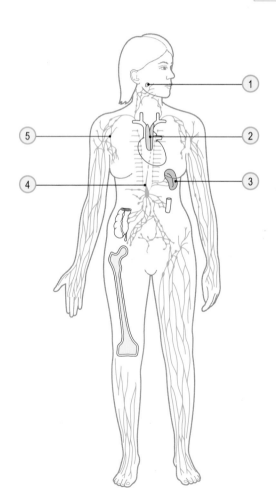

Figure 38   The lymphatic system.

Test 6C

Write the meaning of:

(a) lymphorrhoea
    (Am. lymphorrhea)

(b) splenic

(c) lymphadenectasis

(d) thymolysis

(e) serologist

Score

5

Test 6D

Build words that mean:

(a) tumour (Am. tumor) of
    lymph (tissue)

(b) X-ray examination of the
    lymph system

(c) removal of the spleen

(d) condition of bleeding /
    bursting forth of the spleen

(e) tumour (Am. tumor) of a
    lymph vessel

Score

5

Check answers to Self-Assessment Tests on page 361.

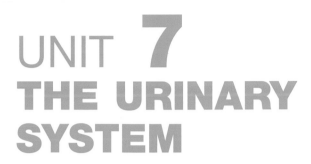

UNIT 7
THE URINARY SYSTEM

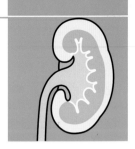

OBJECTIVES

Once you have completed Unit 7, you should be able to do the following:

- understand the meaning of medical words relating to the urinary system
- build medical words relating to the urinary system
- associate medical terms with their anatomical position
- understand common medical abbreviations relating to the urinary system

EXERCISE GUIDE

Use this list of word components and their meanings to complete the word exercises in this unit.

Prefixes

dys-	difficult/painful
hyper-	above normal/excessive
intra-	within/inside
oligo-	deficiency/few/little
poly-	many/much

Roots / Combining forms

albumin/o	albumin/albumen
azot/o	urea
calc/i	calcium
col/o	colon
enter/o	intestine
gastr/o	stomach
haemat/o	blood (Am. hemat/o)
hemat/o (Am.)	blood
hydr/o	water
lith/o	stone
metr/o	a measure
proct/o	anus/rectum
py/o	pus
sigmoid/o	sigmoid colon
trigon/o	trigone of the bladder

Suffixes

-al	pertaining to
-algia	condition of pain
-cele	swelling/protrusion/hernia
-clysis	infusion/injection/irrigation
-dynia	condition of pain
-ectasis	dilatation/stretching
-ectomy	removal of
-ferous	pertaining to carrying/bearing
-genesis	capable of causing/pertaining to formation
-gram	X-ray/tracing/recording
-graphy	technique of recording/making an X-ray
-ia	condition of
-iasis	abnormal condition
-ic	pertaining to
-itis	inflammation of
-lapaxy	empty / wash out / evacuate
-lithiasis	abnormal condition of stones
-logist	specialist who studies
-lysis	breakdown/disintegration
-meter	measuring instrument
-metry	process of measuring

-osis	abnormal condition / disease of	**-scope**	an instrument used to view/examine
-ous	pertaining to / of the nature of	**-scopy**	technique of viewing/examining
-pathy	disease of	**-stenosis**	condition of narrowing
-pexy	surgical fixation/fix in place	**-stomy**	to form a new opening or outlet
-phyma	tumour (Am. tumor) / boil	**-tome**	cutting instrument
-plasty	surgical repair/reconstruction	**-tomy**	incision into
-ptosis	falling/displacement/prolapse	**-tripsy**	act of crushing
-rrhagia	condition of bursting forth of blood / bleeding	**-triptor**	instrument to crush/fragment (using shock waves)
-rrhaphy	suturing/stitching	**-trite**	instrument to crush/fragment
-sclerosis	condition of hardening	**-uresis**	excrete in urine / urinate

 ANATOMY EXERCISE

When you have finished Word Exercises 1 to 12, look at the word components listed next. Complete Figure 39 by writing the appropriate combining form on each line, more than one component may relate to the same position. (You can check their meanings in the Quick Reference box on p. 101.)

Cyst/o	Ren/o	Urin/o
Glomerul/o	Ureter/o	Vesic/o
Nephr/o	Urethr/o	
Pyel/o		

The urinary system

The main components of the urinary system are the kidneys that remove metabolic wastes from the blood by forming them into urine. This yellow liquid is passed from the kidneys through the ureters to the urinary bladder where it is stored. Periodically, urine is passed out of the body through the urethra in the process of urination.

Besides removing waste substances that could be toxic to tissue cells, the kidneys maintain the volume of water in the blood and regulate its salt concentration and pH. The kidneys are therefore involved in homeostasis, ie, maintaining constant conditions within the tissue fluids of the body. The continuous activity of the kidneys is required to maintain life.

Use the Exercise Guide at the beginning of this unit to complete Word Exercises 1 to 12, unless you are asked to work without it.

Root

Ren

(*A Latin word* **ren***, meaning kidney.*)

Combining form   Ren/o

Word Exercise 1

Using your Exercise Guide, find the meaning of:

(a) **ren/o**[2]/**gastr**[3]/**ic**[1]

(b) **ren/o**/gram

(c) **ren/o**/graphy

Renography may show a renal calculus (from Latin *calcis,* small stone), ie, a kidney stone. The presence of a stone in a ureter leads to severe pain and is referred to as **renal colic**. Renal colic can also be caused by disorder and disease within a kidney.

Radioisotope renograms are useful in assessing kidney function. They are made following injection of radioisotopes into the bloodstream. The technique of making this type of recording is discussed in more detail in Unit 18.

Root

Nephr

(*From a Greek word* **nephros***, meaning kidney.*)

Combining form   Nephr/o

Word Exercise 2

Using your Exercise Guide, find the meaning of:

(a) **nephr/o**/ptosis

(b) hydr/o/**nephr**/osis

(c) **nephr/o**/cele

(d) **nephr**/algia

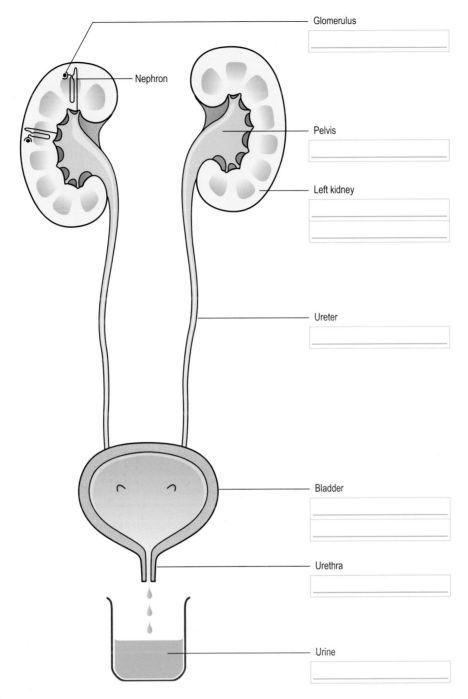

Glomerulus

Nephron

Pelvis

Left kidney

Ureter

Bladder

Urethra

Urine

Figure 39   The urinary system.

Using your Exercise Guide find the meaning of -ectomy, -lithia-sis, -pexy, -plasty and -tomy; then build words that mean:

(e) surgical fixation of a kidney
     (eg, floating kidney)

(f) surgical repair of a kidney

(g) incision into a kidney

(h) condition of stones in the
     kidney

(i)   removal of a kidney

Within each kidney, there are approximately one million kidney tubules or nephrons that do the work of the kidney (Fig. 39). At the beginning of each nephron is a **glomerulus**, a ball of capillaries surrounded by porous membranes that filter metabolic wastes from the blood. When glomeruli undergo pathological change, the filtering mechanism of the kidneys is seriously affected, reducing their ability to maintain homeostasis.

Using your Exercise Guide, find the meaning of:

(j) **glomerul**/itis
(suppurative)

(k) **glomerul/o**/pathy

(l) **glomerul/o**/sclerosis

Infections, diabetes, high blood pressure and disorders of the kidneys sometimes lead to chronic kidney disease (CKD). As it progresses, this results in the waste products of metabolism increasing in concentration within the blood and a failure to regulate water, mineral metabolism and pH. CKD can lead to end-stage renal failure or established renal failure (ERF), and at this stage the kidneys can no longer support the body's needs (ie, maintain homeostasis). The patient with ERF can be kept alive by administering one of the following procedures.

Haemodialysis (Am. hemodialysis)

This procedure involves diverting the patient's blood through a dialyser (Am. dialyzer), commonly called an artificial kidney (Fig. 40). To connect the patient to the machine an arteriovenous fistula (a communication between an artery and vein) is commonly created in the arm by surgery. This bypasses the capillaries and blood flows rapidly through the fistula. Blood is pumped from a vessel in the fistula into the dialyser where its waste products are removed, and it is returned to the body via another vessel. The patient must be connected to the dialyser for many hours per week and so cannot lead a normal life. (Dialysis means separating, ie, separating wastes from the blood.)

CAPD (continuous ambulatory peritoneal dialysis)

The patient is fitted with a peritoneal catheter (tube) (Fig. 41). Every 6 hours approximately 2 L of dialysing fluid is passed into the peritoneum. Toxic wastes diffuse into the dialysing fluid and are removed from the body when the fluid is changed. This procedure is repeated four times a day, 7 days a week. CAPD has been used on a long-term basis, but there is danger from peritonitis caused by infection.

Kidney transplant

A kidney can be transplanted between two individuals of the same species, ie, between two humans who are not closely related. This type of transplant or graft is known as a homotransplant or homograft (*homo* meaning the same, synonymous with allograft or allogeneic graft). The donor could be living and survive with one remaining kidney, or a victim of a fatal accident. The tissues of the donor and recipient have to undergo histocompatibility laboratory tests to ensure the recipient does not reject a donated kidney. A transplant may keep a patient alive for many years and avoids the inconvenience and dangers associated with CAPD and dialysis.

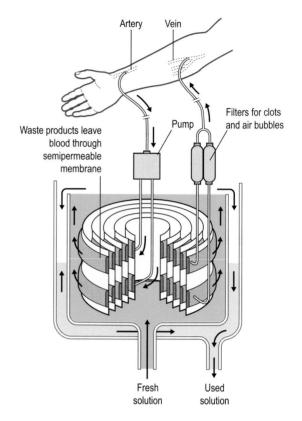

Figure 40   Haemodialysis (Am. hemodialysis).

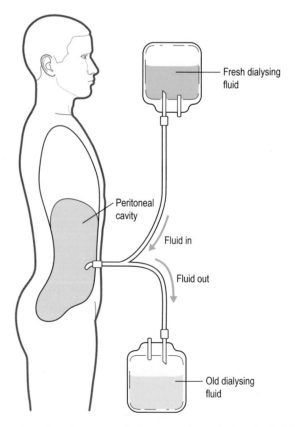

Figure 41   Continuous ambulatory peritoneal dialysis (CAPD).

Transplants between genetically identical twins are more successful. These are known as isografts (*iso* means same/equal) or syngrafts.

Root

Pyel

(*From a Greek word* **pyelos**, *meaning trough or basin. Here pyel/o means the renal pelvis, the space inside a kidney in which urine collects after its formation.*)

Combining form   Pyel/o

(Do not confuse this with py/o, meaning pus.)

Word Exercise 3

Without using your Exercise Guide, write the meaning of:

(a) **pyel/o**/nephr/itis

(This is due to a bacterial infection ascending from the urinary tract or entering the kidney from the blood.)

(b) **pyel/o**/lith/o/tomy

(c) **pyel/o**/nephr/osis

Without using your Exercise Guide, build words that mean:

(d) surgical repair of the renal pelvis

(e) X-ray picture of the renal pelvis

The technique of making an X-ray of the renal pelvis is known as **pyelo**graphy. It involves filling the pelvis with a radiopaque dye. There are several ways of doing this:

Intravenous pyelography (synonym intravenous urography) Here, the dye is injected into the bloodstream, and it eventually passes through the kidney pelvis (**intra**, meaning inside, **ven/o**, meaning vein).

Antegrade pyelography Here, the dye is injected into the renal pelvis (**ante**, meaning before/in front; **grad**, meaning take steps / to go (Latin)). It refers to the fact that the dye goes into the pelvis before it leaves the kidney. The dye is injected through a percutaneous catheter, ie, through the skin.

Retrograde (or ascending) pyelography (synonym retrograde or ascending urography) Here, the dye is injected into the kidney via the ureter, so it is being forced backwards up the ureter into the pelvis (**retro**, meaning backwards).

Root

Ureter

(*From a Greek word* **oureter**, *meaning ureter, the narrow tube that connects each kidney to the bladder. Urine flows through the ureters assisted by the action of smooth muscle.*)

Combining form   Ureter/o

Word Exercise 4

Without using your Exercise Guide, write the meaning of:

(a) **ureter/o**/cele

(b) **ureter/o**/cel/ectomy

(c) hydro**ureter**

Using your Exercise Guide, find the meaning of:

(d) **ureter/o**/rrhagia

(e) **ureter/o**/rrhaphy

(f) **ureter**/ectasis

(g) **ureter/o**/ren/o/ scopy

(h) **ureter/o**/stomy

Using your Exercise Guide, look up col/o, enter/o and -stomy; then, beginning with the underlined root, build words that mean:

(i) formation of an opening between a <u>ureter</u> and the intestine

(j) formation of an opening between a <u>ureter</u> and the colon

Root

Cyst

(*From Greek* **kystis**, *meaning bladder.*)

Combining form   Cyst/o

Note. We have already used cyst/o in Unit 2 with cholecyst/o, meaning the gallbladder (bile bladder). Here, we are using **cyst/o** alone to mean the urinary bladder, the organ that stores urine until it is expelled from the body.

Word Exercise 5

Without using your Exercise Guide, write the meaning of:

(a) **cyst**/itis

There are many causes of this acute or chronic condition including injury and infection. As the bladder is accessible from outside via the urethra, it is relatively easy for microorganisms to enter. Sometimes infections such as *Neisseria gonorrhoeae* and *Chlamydia* are transmitted into the urinary tract by sexual contact. Cystitis occurs more frequently in women because the female urethra is short and close to the anus (a source of bacteria). Symptoms include pelvic pain, an urge to urinate frequently and haematuria (Am. hematuria).

(b) **cyst/o**/lith/ectomy

(c) **cyst/o**/pyel/itis

(d) **cyst/o**/ptosis

Using your Exercise Guide, find the meaning of:

(e) **cyst/o**/scope

(f) **cyst/o**/proct/o/ stomy

Note. Meter (from Greek *metron*) means a measuring instrument, and **metr/o** a measure; **metry** (from Greek *metrein*) means the process of measuring. Without using your Exercise Guide and beginning with the underlined root, build words that mean:

(g) an instrument used to measure the bladder

(h) the technique of measuring the bladder

(i) a trace, or recording of bladder measurements (use metr/o)

A technique that applies an electric current to tissues, causing them to heat up, is known as **diathermy** (dia- meaning through and -*thermy* meaning heat). These can be combined here to make:

Cystodiathermy The process of applying heat through the bladder. The heat is produced by an electric current and is used to destroy tumours (Am. tumors) in the bladder wall.

Root

Vesic

(*From Latin* **vesica**, *meaning bladder.*)

Combining form   Vesic/o

Word Exercise 6

Without using your Exercise Guide, build words that mean:

(a) formation of an opening into the bladder

(b) incision into the bladder

Using your Exercise Guide, find the meaning of:

(c) **vesic/o**/clysis

(d) **vesic**/al

(e) **vesic/o**/sigmoid/o/ stomy

Without using your Exercise Guide, write the meaning of:

(f) **vesic/o**/ureter/al

Note. Vesico-ureteric reflux (VUR) is characterized by the abnormal flow of urine from the bladder to the upper urinary tract. It is more common in children and can lead to chronic infection and kidney damage.

Catheterization of the bladder is required following some surgical operations and when there is difficulty in emptying the bladder owing to a neuromuscular disorder or physical damage to the spinal cord. The procedure involves inserting a catheter through the urethra into the bladder (Fig. 42). A urinary **catheter** consists of a fine tube that allows urine to drain from the bladder into an external container. Some self-retaining catheters are held in position by means of an inflated balloon.

Root

Urethr

(*From Greek* **ourethro**, *meaning urethra, the tube through which urine leaves the body from the bladder.*)

Combining form   Urethr/o

Word Exercise 7

Without using your Exercise Guide, write the meaning of:

(a) **urethr/o**/metry

(b) **urethr/o**/trigon/itis

(Trigone refers to a triangular area at the base of the bladder, bounded by the openings of the ureters at the back and the urethral opening at the front.)

(c) **urethr/o**/pexy

Without using your Exercise Guide, build words that mean:

(d) condition of pain in the urethra

(e) condition of flow of blood from the urethra

(f) visual examination of the urethra

Using your Exercise Guide, find the meaning of:

(g) **urethr/o**/phyma

(h) **urethr/o**/tome

(i) **urethr/o**/stenosis

(j) **urethr/o**/dynia

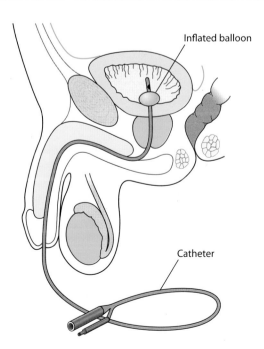

Figure 42   Catheterization.

Root

Urin

(*From a Latin word* **urina**, *meaning urine, the excretory product of the kidneys.*)

Combining forms   Urin/a/i/o

Word Exercise 8

Using your Exercise Guide, find the meaning of:

(a) **urin/i**/ferous

(b) **urin/a**/lysis

This word refers to the technique of analyzing urine. Detailed urinalysis is a valuable aid to the diagnosis of disease; for example, detecting the presence of high concentrations of glucose in the urine may indicate diabetes. Other components commonly analyzed are pH, specific gravity, ketone bodies, phenylketones, protein, bilirubin and solid casts of varying composition.

Without using your Exercise Guide, write the meaning of:

(c) urin/o/meter (used to estimate specific gravity of urine)

Root

Ur

(*From a Greek word* **ouron**, *meaning urine.*)

Combining form   Ur/o

(This combining form is also used to refer to the urinary tract and urination. Urodynamics is the study of the force and movement of urine in the urinary tract (bladder filling, emptying and voiding)).

Word Exercise 9

Without using your Exercise Guide, write the meaning of:

(a) **ur/o**/graphy

(This procedure is also performed by injecting dye directly into the urinary tract rather than into a vein.)

Using your Exercise Guide, find the meaning of:

(b) **ur/o**/logist

(c) **ur/o**/genesis

Inflated balloon

Catheter

(d) olig/**ur**/ia

(e) albumin/**ur**/ia

(f) azot/**ur**/ia

(g) poly/**ur**/ia

(h) dys/**ur**/ia

(i) haemat/**ur**/ia (Am. hemat/ur/ia)

(j) py/**ur**/ia

(k) hyper/calci/**ur**/ia

Note. The act of passing urine is known as micturition (from Latin *micturire*, meaning to pass water).

 ## Root

Lith

(*From a Greek word* **lithos***, meaning stone.*)

Combining form   Lith/o

Here **lith/o** refers to a kidney stone, which is a hard mass composed mainly of mineral matter present in the urinary system. Remember, a stone is sometimes called a **calculus** (plural **calculi**). Stones can prevent the passage of urine, causing pain and kidney damage. They need to be passed or removed because they can seriously affect the functioning of the kidneys.

Word Exercise 10

Without using your Exercise Guide, write the meaning of:

(a) **lith/o**/nephr/itis

(b) ur/o/**lith**/iasis

(c) **lith/o**/genesis

(d) nephr/o/**lith/o**/tomy

Using your Exercise Guide, find the meaning of:

(e) **lith/o**/trite

(f) **lith/o**/lapaxy

(g) **lith/o**/triptor

This instrument focuses high-energy shock waves generated by a high-voltage spark on to a kidney stone. No surgery is required, as the stone disintegrates within the body and is passed in the urine. The procedure for using this instrument is called extracorporeal shock wave lithotripsy (ECSL), *extra* meaning outside, *corporeal* meaning body.

(h) **lith**/o/tripsy

(i) **lith**/uresis

Figure 43A shows a stone blocking the proximal part of the ureter, causing the kidney pelvis to swell with urine (hydronephrosis). Figure 43B shows a stone blocking the distal part of the ureter causing the ureter to swell (hydroureter) along its length. Both conditions impede the flow of urine and can cause severe pain.

Medical equipment and clinical procedures

Before completing Exercise 11, review the names of all instruments and clinical procedures mentioned in this unit. Make sure you know the meanings of -graphy, -lapaxy, -meter, -scope, -scopy, -thermy, -tome, -tripsy, -triptor and -trite.

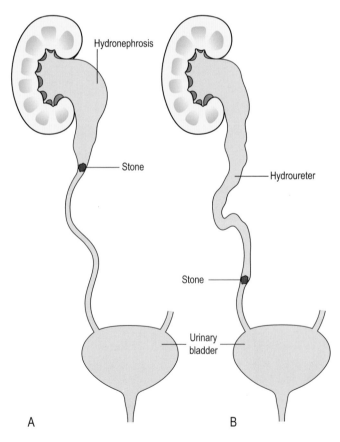

Figure 43   Ureterolithiasis. (A) Hydronephrosis caused by a stone blocking the proximal part of the ureter; (B) Hydroureter caused by a stone blocking the distal part of the ureter.

Word Exercise 11

Match each description in Column C with a term in Column A by placing the appropriate number in Column B.

Column A	Column B	Column C
(a) diathermy		1. an instrument used for crushing stones
(b) cystoscope		2. a device that separates wastes from the blood
(c) lithotriptor		3. an instrument used for cutting the urethra
(d) urinometer		4. visual examination of the ureter
(e) haemodialyser (Am. hemodialyzer)		5. an instrument that measures the pressure and capacity of the bladder
(f) ureteroscopy		6. an instrument used to view the urethra
(g) urethrotome		7. a device that destroys stones using shock waves
(h) cystometer		8. technique of heating a tissue by applying an electric current
(i) urethroscope		9. an instrument used for measuring the specific gravity of urine
(j) lithotrite		10. an instrument used to view the bladder

Column A	Column B	Column C
(c) lithotripsy		3. technique of making an X-ray picture of the urinary tract
(d) catheterization		4. a procedure that removes fluid and wastes from the blood
(e) urography		5. technique of viewing the ureter and kidney with an endoscope
(f) urodynamics		6. process of visualizing the renal pelvis on an X-ray
(g) litholapaxy		7. process of inserting a tube into a body cavity to allow passage of fluid
(h) ureterorenoscopy		8. process of breaking stones using shock waves (ultrasound)

Word Exercise 12

Match each description in Column C with a term in Column A by placing the appropriate number in Column B.

Column A	Column B	Column C
(a) retrograde pyelography		1. study of the force and movement of urine
(b) haemodialysis (Am. hemodialysis)		2. process of washing out the bladder following stone fragmentation

Other procedures widely used to investigate the urinary system besides those mentioned in the word exercises include:

Blood urea nitrogen (BUN) A laboratory test that measures the amount of nitrogenous waste (urea) in the blood, performed to check kidney function.

Computed tomography urography The technique of recording multiple cross-sectional X-ray images of the urinary tract; it is used to detect kidney stones and evaluate patients with haematuria (Am. hematuria).

Cystoscopy The technique of viewing the inside of the urinary bladder using an endoscope or cystoscope. A flexible fibreoptic cystoscope is used for examining the bladder and diagnosis; a rigid metal cystoscope is used to pass surgical instruments into the bladder to remove a tissue sample or carry out treatment.

Flow cystometry A clinical diagnostic procedure used to evaluate bladder function; specifically, it measures its contractile force when voiding urine. The resulting chart for analysis is called a cystometrogram.

KUB ultrasonography The technique of making an image of the kidneys, ureters (if distended) and bladder using high-frequency sound (ultrasound).

Micturition or voiding cystourethrography The radiographic and fluoroscopic study of the lower parts of the urinary tract. An image called a voiding cystourethrogram is made whilst the patient passes urine containing a contrast medium (visible on X-ray film). The test determines whether the flow of urine is normal when the bladder empties.

MRI urography The technique of using strong magnetic fields and radio waves (magnetic resonance imaging) to produce images of the kidney and surrounding structures in three planes.

Percutaneous renal biopsy The removal of renal tissue for microscopic examination by inserting a needle through the skin and muscles of the back into the kidney (a closed biopsy). Ultrasound or other imaging techniques are used to guide the needle into position. Biopsy samples can also be obtained directly when the kidney is exposed by surgical means (an open biopsy).

Renal angiography The technique of recording an image of the blood vessels within the kidney. A catheter is guided into the renal artery and a contrast medium is injected into the bloodstream whilst the X-rays are taken; the images can show obstructed or narrowed blood vessels.

ANATOMY EXERCISE

Now complete the Anatomy Exercise on page 92.

 CASE HISTORY 7

The object of this exercise is to understand words associated with a patient's medical history.

To complete the exercise:

* Read through the passage on urolithiasis; unfamiliar words are underlined, and you can find their meaning using the Word Help.

* Write the meaning of the medical terms shown in bold print on the lines that follow the Word Help.

Urolithiasis

Mr G, an engineer recently returned from working in the Middle East, was admitted to Accident and Emergency in pain and clutching his right side. He had been awoken during the night by an excruciating pain in his right flank radiating to the iliac fossa and right testicle. In the past two days, he had developed severe **urethral** pain and **dysuria** associated with **haematuria (Am. hematuria)**. Fluid intake

made the pain worse, and he had been vomiting. Mr G had recently been treated with antibiotics by his GP for bacteriuria and diagnosed as suffering from obstructive **uropathy**. His condition had become acute whilst waiting for his referral appointment. On admission, he required immediate analgesia for severe pain and was administered 10 mg morphine i.m. He was kept overnight for observation and transferred to the Urology Unit the following morning.

The next day a dull pain was still present, and examination revealed loin tenderness and an enlarged palpable hydronephrotic right kidney. A plain abdominal radiograph identified a single calculus in the line of the right ureter. Excretion urography (intravenous **pyelography**, IVP) confirmed the calculus to be obstructing the peliureteric junction. The kidney outline appeared enlarged but smooth with no anatomical abnormalities of the calyces.

Mr G underwent extracorporeal shockwave **lithotripsy** (ESWL), and the calculus was successfully fragmented and excreted. His urinary catheter was left in place for one day, and he was discharged on 50 mg diclofenac t.d.s. His recovery was unremarkable, and a follow-up KUB was arranged for two weeks through the Lithotripsy reception.

Mr G was advised that he should increase his fluid intake, particularly when he returned to the Middle East. It was recommended that a urine output of 2 to 2.5 L per day would be appropriate. Urine analysis indicated a slight **hypercalciuria**, and it was recommended that he restricted his intake of calcium and vitamin D. He was referred to the dietician for advice on food intake.

Word Help

analgesia condition of pain relief

calculus a stone or abnormal concretion (plural calculi)

calyces cup-shaped divisions of the renal pelvis (singular calyx)

catheter a tube for introducing or withdrawing fluid from the body

GP general practitioner (family doctor)

hydronephrotic pertaining to hydronephrosis (a kidney swollen with water)

iliac fossa pertaining to the concave, upper and anterior part of the sacropelvic surface of the iliac bone. A fossa is a depression/recess below the general surface of a part

i.m. intramuscular (here meaning an injection into muscle)

KUB kidneys, ureters and bladder (X-ray/examination)

pelviureteric pertaining to a renal pelvis and ureter

radiograph an X-ray picture

t.d.s. three times a day (ter die sumendum)

urography technique of recording/making an X-ray of the urinary tract

urology study of the urinary system (here it refers to a hospital department)

Now, write the meaning of the following words from the Case History without using your dictionary lists:

(a) urolithiasis

(b) urethral

(c) dysuria

(d) haematuria
    (Am. hematuria)

(e) uropathy

(f) pyelography

(g) lithotripsy

(h) hypercalciuria

(Answers to the Case History exercise are given in the Answers to Word Exercises on page 341.)

Quick Reference

Combining forms relating to the urinary system:

Albumin/o	albumin
Azot/o	urea/nitrogen
Cyst/o	bladder
Glomerul/o	glomerulus
Lith/o	stone
Nephr/o	kidney
Pyel/o	pelvis of kidney
Ren/o	kidney
Trigon/o	trigone
Ureter/o	ureter
Urethr/o	urethra
Urin/o	urine
Ur/o	urine/urinary tract
Vesic/o	bladder

Abbreviations

Some common abbreviations related to the urinary system are listed next. Note that some are not standard, and their meaning may vary from one healthcare setting to another. There is a more extensive list for reference on page 369.

ARF	acute renal failure
BUN	blood urea nitrogen
CKD	chronic kidney disease
CRF	chronic renal failure
CSU	catheter specimen of urine
Cysto	cystoscopy
ERF	established renal failure
GFR	glomerular filtration rate
HD	haemodialysis (Am. hemo-dialysis)
IVP	intravenous pyelogram
KUB	kidney, ureter, bladder (X-ray)
MSU	midstream urine
PCNL	percutaneous nephroli-thotomy
RP, RPG	retrograde pyelogram
UA	urinalysis
U & E	urea and electrolytes
UTI	urinary tract infection
VCU, VCUG	voiding cystourethrogram

Pathology notes

Autosomal dominant polycystic kidney disease (ADPKD)

This is the most common inherited kidney disease characterized by the development of multiple fluid-filled cysts in the kidneys. The cysts do not usually cause a problem until they grow large enough to interfere with kidney function; this usually happens in adulthood, but children can also be affected. Haemodialysis and transplantation are treatments for those with kidney failure (Am. hemodialysis).

Diabetic kidney disease

Renal failure is the cause of death in approximately 10% of all diabetics and up to 50% of cases of insulin-dependent diabetes mellitus (Type 1). In this condition, there is damage to large and small blood vessels in many parts of the body. The effects on the kidney include progressive glomerulosclerosis and atrophy of the renal tubules, acute pyelonephritis and nephrotic syndrome.

Glomerulonephritis (GN)

Glomerular disorders, collectively called glomerulonephritis, result from damage to the glomerular-capsular membranes that filter blood in the kidneys. Immune mechanisms, heredity, and other factors can cause this damage. Without successful treatment, glomerular disorders can progress to kidney failure.

Acute glomerulonephritis the most common form of kidney disease. It may be caused by a delayed immune response to streptococcal infection. If antibiotic treatment is not successful, it may progress to a chronic form of glomerulonephritis.

Chronic glomerulonephritis the general name for various noninfectious glomerular disorders that are characterized by progressive kidney damage leading to renal failure. Immune mechanisms are believed to be the major cause of this condition. Antigen–antibody complexes that form in the blood may lodge in the glomerular capsule membrane triggering a response. Less commonly, antibodies may form that directly attack the glomerular-capsular membranes.

Interstitial nephritis

This is characterized by inflammation of the connective tissue between the tubules within the kidney. It is caused by an autoimmune response or an allergic reaction to a drug, most commonly an antibiotic or antiinflammatory drug.

Kidney failure

Kidney failure, or renal failure, is simply the failure of the kidney to properly process blood and form urine. Renal failure can be classified as acute or chronic.

Acute renal failure (ARF) an abrupt reduction in kidney function that is characterized by oliguria and a sharp rise in nitrogenous compounds in the blood. Acute renal failure can be caused by various factors that alter blood pressure or affect glomerular filtration; examples include haemorrhage (Am. hemorrhage), severe burns, or obstruction of the lower urinary tract. If the underlying cause is attended to, recovery is usually rapid and complete.

Chronic renal failure (CRF) a slow progressive condition resulting from the gradual loss of nephrons. There are many diseases that result in a gradual loss of nephron function including infections, diabetes, glomerulonephritis, tumours, systemic autoimmune disorders and obstructive disorders.

Nephrotic syndrome

Nephrotic syndrome is not a disease in itself but a collection of signs and symptoms that accompany various glomerular disorders. When glomeruli are damaged, the permeability of the glomerular membrane is increased, and plasma proteins pass through into the filtrate. Proteinuria, hypoalbuminaemia (Am. hypoalbuminemia), hyperlipidaemia (Am. hyperlipidemia) and oedema (Am. edema) characterize this syndrome.

Renal calculi

Renal calculi, or kidney stones, are crystallized mineral deposits that develop in the renal pelvis or calyces. Many calculi form when minerals crystallize on the renal papillae and then break off into the urine. The solutes that form calculi include oxalates, phosphates, urates and uric acid, often deposited in layers.

If the stones are small enough, they simply pass through the ureters and urethra and are eventually voided with the urine.

Stag-horn calculi are large, branched stones that fill the pelvis and branched calyces. A large stone may obstruct the ureter, causing intense pain *(renal colic)* as rhythmical contractions in the wall of the ureter attempt to dislodge it. Hydronephrosis may occur if the stone does not move from its obstructing position.

Tumours (Am. tumors)

Tumours of the urinary system typically obstruct urine flow causing hydronephrosis in one or both kidneys. Most kidney tumours are malignant neoplasms called renal clear cell carcinomas; they usually occur in one kidney only. Bladder cancer occurs about as frequently as renal cancer. Bladder tumours are often multiple; their cause is unknown, but predisposing factors include cigarette smoking and exposure to chemicals used in the manufacture of aniline dyes and rubber.

Urinary incontinence

This is the involuntary voiding of urine due to defective voluntary control of the external urethral sphincter that controls the exit of urine from the body.

Retention and overflow incontinence may be due to disruption of the nerve input into the bladder. Such paralysis results in loss of normal control of micturition and is sometimes termed a neurogenic bladder. The condition is characterized by involuntary retention of urine, subsequent distention of the bladder and perhaps a burning sensation or fever. Once the bladder is full, the increased pressure opens the urethral sphincter and urine dribbles from the urethra.

Urge incontinence characterized by a sudden and intense urge to pass urine, the amounts voided are generally small and are sometimes accompanied by pain. The condition may be due to calculi, tumours and stress.

Wilms tumour (nephroblastoma)

A highly malignant tumour (Am. tumor) of the kidney arising from embryonic tissue that develops in early childhood.

Associated words

Anuria condition of cessation of excretion of urine, a condition of not excreting urine

Azotaemia condition of too much nitrogen in the blood (Am. azotemia)

Bed-wetting enuresis, involuntary passing of urine

Bougie a flexible cylindrical instrument used to dilate a passage

Diuresis condition of increased excretion of urine

Dysuria condition of painful urination (micturition)

Endourology a branch of urology that deals with minimally invasive surgical procedures (as opposed to open surgery) such as using small cameras and instruments inserted into the urinary tract

Enuresis incontinence of urine in the absence of disease

Glycosuria condition of glucose in the urine

Haematuria condition of blood in the urine (Am. hematuria)

Hesitancy difficulty in beginning the flow of urine

Homeostasis maintenance of a constant internal environment of the body, the process that keeps cells alive

Incontinence lack of voluntary control of urine or faeces (Am. feces)

Meatal stenosis condition of narrowing of the urinary opening of the urethra

Meatus an opening into a passage such as the urinary meatus at the opening of the urethra

Micturition the act of passing urine from the body

Neurourology a branch of urology concerned with nervous control of the genitourinary system, and of conditions causing abnormal urination

Nocturia condition of passing urine at night

Reflux flowing back, for example urine flowing back from the bladder to the kidney

Retention holding back, urinary retention is an inability to void urine

Rigor attack of intense shivering when heat regulation is disturbed, eg, by a kidney infection

Sediment abnormal particles present in the urine; they could be cells, casts, bacteria or crystals

Stent a hollow, flexible plastic tube, eg, ureteral stent inserted into the ureter between the kidney and bladder to relieve obstruction to the flow of urine

Stricture contraction or narrowing of a canal such as the urethra

Urgency an immediate need to void urine

Urination the act of discharging urine, micturition

Void to empty, for example passing urine from the bladder during micturition

NOW TRY THE WORD CHECK

WORD CHECK

This self-check exercise lists all the word components used in this unit. First, write down the meaning of as many word components as you can. Then, check your answers using the Exercise Guide and Quick Reference box or the Glossary of Word Components (pp. 383–410).

Prefixes

ante-	
dia-	
dys-	
hyper-	
intra-	
oligo-	
poly-	
retro-	

Combining forms of word roots

albumin/o	
azot/o	
calc/i	
col/o	
cyst/o	
enter/o	
gastr/o	
glomerul/o	
haem/o (Am. hem/o)	
hydr/o	
lith/o	
nephr/o	
proct/o	
pyel/o	
py/o	
ren/o	
sigmoid/o	
sten/o	
trigon/o	
ureter/o	
urethr/o	
urin/o	
ur/o	
ven/o	
vesic/o	

Suffixes

-al	
-algia	
-cele	
-clysis	
-dynia	
-ectasis	
-ectomy	
-ferous	
-genesis	

-gram	
-graphy	
-iasis	
-ic	
-itis	
-lapaxy	
-lithiasis	
-logist	
-lysis	
-meter	
-metry	
-osis	
-ous	
-pexy	
-phyma	

-plasty	
-ptosis	
-rrhage	
-rrhaphy	
-sclerosis	
-scope	
-scopy	
-stomy	
-thermy	
-tome	
-tomy	
-tripsy	
-triptor	
-trite	
-uresis	

NOW TRY THE SELF-ASSESSMENT

SELF-ASSESSMENT

Test 7A

Below are some combining forms that refer to the anatomy of the urinary system. Indicate which part of the system they refer to by putting a number from the diagram (Fig. 44) next to each word.

(a) ureter/o

(b) nephr/o

(c) glomerul/o

(d) pyel/o

(e) urethr/o

(f) lith/o

(g) cyst/o

(h) urin/o

Score [   ] 8

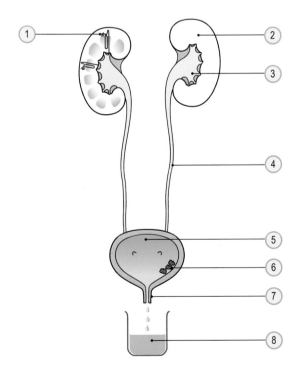

Figure 44   The urinary system.

Test 7B

Prefixes and suffixes

Match each meaning in Column C with a prefix or suffix in Column A by inserting the appropriate number in Column B.

Column A	Column B	Column C
(a) ante-		1. technique of breaking stones with shock waves
(b) -cele		2. measuring instrument
(c) -clysis		3. a crushing instrument
(d) dia-		4. abnormal condition of urine
(e) dys-		5. technique of measuring
(f) -ferous		6. backward
(g) -iasis		7. protrusion/swelling/hernia
(h) intra-		8. tumour (Am. tumor)/boil
(i) -lapaxy		9. before
(j) -meter		10. to fall/displace
(k) -metry		11. pertaining to carrying
(l) oligo-		12. abnormal condition of
(m) -phyma		13. too little/few
(n) poly-		14. difficult/painful
(o) -ptosis		15. infusion/injection into
(p) retro-		16. through
(q) -thermy		17. within/inside
(r) -tripsy		18. evacuation / wash out
(s) -trite		19. many
(t) -uresis		20. heat

Score [   ] 20

Test 7C

Combining forms of word roots

Match each meaning in Column C with a combining form of a word root in Column A by inserting the appropriate number in Column B.

Column A	Column B	Column C
(a) col/o		1. blood
(b) cyst/o		2. kidney (i)
(c) gastr/o		3. kidney (ii)
(d) glomerul/o		4. sigmoid colon
(e) haemat/o (Am. hemat/o)		5. pus
(f) lith/o		6. trigone / base of bladder
(g) nephr/o		7. urethra
(h) proct/o		8. bladder (i)
(i) pyel/o		9. bladder (ii)
(j) py/o		10. vein
(k) ren/o		11. stomach
(l) sigmoid/o		12. pelvis/trough
(m) sten/o		13. urine
(n) trigon/o		14. urine/urinary tract
(o) ureter/o		15. glomeruli (of kidney)
(p) urethr/o		16. ureter
(q) urin/o		17. colon
(r) ur/o		18. anus/rectum
(s) ven/o		19. stone
(t) vesic/o		20. narrowing

Score [20]

Test 7D

Write the meaning of:

(a) nephropyelolithotomy [　　　　　]

(b) ureterostenosis [　　　　　]

(c) cystourethrography [　　　　　]

(d) vesicocele [　　　　　]

(e) pyelectasis [　　　　　]

Score [5]

Test 7E

Build words that mean:

(a) dilatation of a ureter [　　　　　]

(b) formation of an opening between the sigmoid colon and ureter [　　　　　]

(c) technique of making an X-ray of the bladder (use cyst/o) [　　　　　]

(d) X-ray picture of the urinary tract [　　　　　]

(e) abnormal condition of hardening of the kidney [　　　　　]

Score [5]

Check answers to Self-Assessment Tests on page 361.

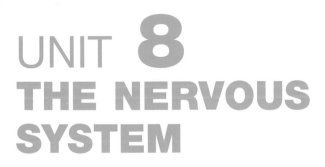

UNIT 8
THE NERVOUS SYSTEM

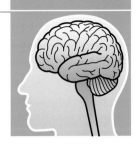

OBJECTIVES

Once you have completed Unit 8, you should be able to do the following:

- understand the meaning of medical words relating to the nervous system
- build medical words relating to the nervous system
- associate medical terms with their anatomical position
- understand common medical abbreviations relating to the nervous system

EXERCISE GUIDE

Use this list of word components and their meanings to complete the word exercises in this unit.

Prefixes

a-	without/not
acro-	extremities/point
agora-	open place
an-	without/not
di-	two/double
dys-	difficult/disordered
epi-	above/upon/on
hemi-	half
hyper-	above
hypo-	below
intra-	within/inside
macro-	large
meso-	middle
micro-	small
para-	beside/near
poly-	many
post-	after/behind
pre-	before / in front of
quadri-	four
sub-	under
tetra-	four

Roots / Combining forms

aqua-	water
cancer/o	cancer
ech/o	echo / reflected sound
electr/o	electrical
fibr/o	fibre (Am. fiber)
haemat/o	blood
hemat/o (Am.)	blood
hydro-	water
necr/o	death (dead tissue)
polio-	grey matter (of central nervous system)
py/o	pus
somat/o	body
syring/o	pipe/tube/cavity

Suffixes

-al	pertaining to
-algia	condition of pain
-cele	swelling/protrusion/hernia
-centesis	surgical puncture to remove fluid
-cyte	cell
-ectomy	removal of
-form	having the form of
-genic	pertaining to formation / originating in
-gram	X-ray picture/tracing/recording
-graph	usually an instrument that record
-graphy	technique of recording/making an X-ray
-gyric	pertaining to circular motion
-ia	condition of
-iatr(y)	specialized medical treatment or study
-ic	pertaining to / in pharmacology a drug
-itis	inflammation of

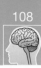

-ize	to cause to be / to become	-schisis	cleaving/splitting/parting
-logist	specialist who studies…	-sclerosis	condition of hardening
-logy	study of	-scopy	technique of viewing/examining
-malacia	condition of softening	-stomy	to form a new opening or outlet
-meter	measuring instrument	-therapy	treatment
-metry	process of measuring	-tic	pertaining to
-oma	tumour/swelling (Am. tumor)	-tomy	incision into
-osis	abnormal condition/disease of	-trauma	injury/wound
-ous	pertaining to	-trophy	nourishment/development
-pathy	disease of	-tropic	pertaining to affinity for / stimulating / changing in response to a stimulus
-phthisis	wasting away		
-plasia	condition of growth/formation (of cells)	-us	thing/structure
-rrhagia	condition of bursting forth of blood/bleeding		

 ANATOMY EXERCISE

When you have finished Word Exercises 1 to 21, look at the word components listed next. Complete Figs 45 and 46 by writing the appropriate combining form on each line. (You can check their meanings in the Quick Reference box on p. 120.)

Cephal/o	Gangli/o	Psych/o
Cerebr/o	Mening/i/o	Rachi/o
Crani/o	Myel/o	Radicul/o
Encephal/o	Neur/o	Ventricul/o

The nervous system

Humans have a complex nervous system with a brain that is large in proportion to their body size. The brain and spinal cord are estimated to contain at least 10^{10} cells with vast numbers of connections between them. The nervous system performs three basic functions:

- It receives, stores and analyzes information from sense organs such as the eyes and ears, making us aware of our environment. This awareness enables us to think and make responses that will aid our survival in changing conditions.

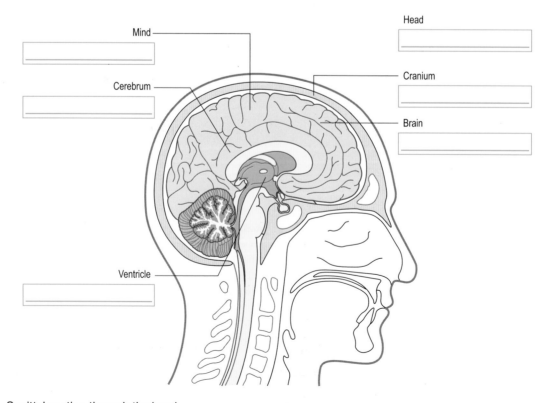

Figure 45 Sagittal section through the head.

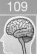

- It controls the physiological activities of the body systems and maintains constant conditions (homeostasis) within the body.
- It controls our muscles, enabling us to move and speak.

Because of its complexity, the nervous system has been difficult to study, and progress in understanding its common disorders has been slow. However, recently developed imaging techniques are improving the diagnosis and treatment of nervous disorders.

The structure of the nervous system

For convenience of study, physiologists have divided the system into the following:

Central nervous system (CNS)
The CNS consists of the brain and spinal cord.

Peripheral nervous system (PNS)
The PNS is composed of 12 pairs of cranial nerves and 31 pairs of spinal nerves that connect the CNS with sense organs, muscles and glands.

Autonomic nervous system (ANS)
The ANS describes certain peripheral nerves that send impulses to internal organs and glands.

We begin our study of medical terms by examining the cells that form the system.

Root

Neur

(*From a Greek word* **neuron**, *meaning nerve.*)

Combining form   Neur/o

Neurons are the basic structural units of the nervous system. They are specialized cells, elongated for the transmission of nerve impulses. Each neuron consists of a cell 'body' plus long extensions known as dendrons or dendrites and axons (Fig. 47). Axons conduct impulses away from the cell body, whilst dendrites conduct impulses towards the cell body. A **nerve fibre** (Am. fiber) is a general term for any process such as a dendrite or axon projecting from a cell body.

A **nerve** is a group of nerve fibres enclosed in a connective tissue sheath; it may contain both sensory and motor fibres.

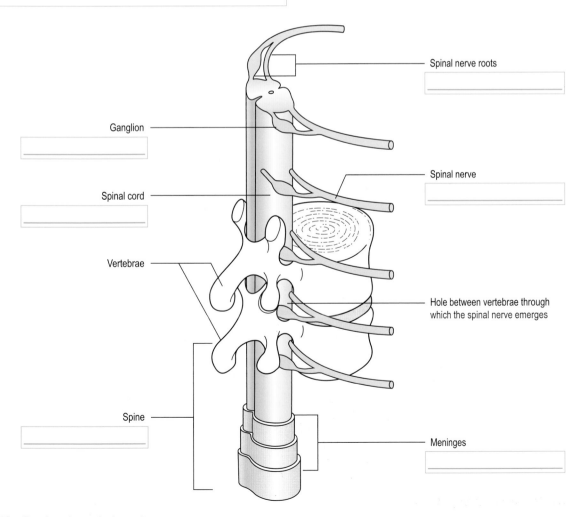

Ganglion

Spinal cord

Vertebrae

Spine

Spinal nerve roots

Spinal nerve

Hole between vertebrae through which the spinal nerve emerges

Meninges

Figure 46   Section through the spine.

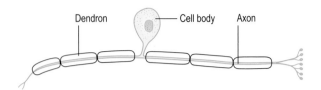

Figure 47   A sensory neuron.

There are three basic types of neuron:

The sensory neuron

The sensory neuron transmits nerve impulses from sense organs to the CNS (*sensory*, meaning pertaining to sensation).

The motor neuron

The motor neuron transmits nerve impulses away from the central nervous system to muscle cells or glands (*motor*, meaning pertaining to action).

The interneuron

The interneuron (also called an association neuron or connecting neuron) transmits nerve impulses from sensory neurons to motor neurons in the brain and spinal cord.

Note. As sensory neurons are transferring nerve impulses towards the CNS, they are sometimes referred to as **afferent** neurons (from Latin *affere*, to bring). Motor neurons are sometimes referred to as **efferent** neurons because they carry nerve impulses away from the CNS (from Latin *effere*, to carry away).

Use the Exercise Guide at the beginning of this unit to complete Word Exercises 1–21, unless you are asked to work without it.

 Word Exercise 1

Using your Exercise Guide, find the meaning of:

(a) **neur/o**/logy

(b) **neur/o**/pathy

(c) **neur**/algia

(d) **neur/o**^{2}/**fibr**^{3}/**oma**^{1}

(e) poly/**neur**/itis

(f) **neur/o**/genic

Using your Exercise Guide find the meaning of -logist, -malacia and -sclerosis; then build words that mean:

(g) hardening of a nerve

(h) condition of softening of a nerve

(i) a person who specializes in the study of nerves and their disorders

Using your Exercise Guide, find the meaning of:

(j) **neur/o**/phthisis

(k) **neur/o**/tropic

(l) **neur/o**/trauma

The neurons of the central nervous system are supported by another type of cell that sticks to them. These are known as **neuroglia** (glia is from a Greek word *glia*, meaning glue). **Neurogli/o** refers to a neurogliocyte, also spelt neuroglia-cyte. There are several types of glial cell, including astro-cytes, microglia, oligodendrocytes and ependymocytes.

Without using your Exercise Guide, write the meaning of:

(m) **neurogli/o**/cyte

(n) **neurogli**/oma

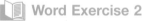 Root

Plex

(*From a Latin word* **plexus**, *meaning plait. Here plex/o means a nerve plexus, a network of nerves*.)

Combining form   Plex/o

 Word Exercise 2

Without using your Exercise Guide, write the meaning of:

(a) **plex/o**/pathy

(b) **plex/o**/genic

Root

Cephal

(*From a Greek word* **kephale**, *meaning head.*)

Combining form   Cephal/o

 Word Exercise 3

Using your Exercise Guide, find the meaning of:

(a) **cephal/o**/cele

(b) a/**cephal**/ous

(This refers to a condition seen in a nonviable embryo or fetus.)

(c) **cephal**/haemat/oma
(Am. **cephal**/hemat/oma)

(d) hydro/**cephal**/us

(Fig. 48 shows hydrocephalus; the condition is characterized by an excess of cerebrospinal fluid in the brain, resulting in an enlarged head, compression of the brain and, if not corrected, mental retardation.)

Using your Exercise Guide find the meaning of -gram, -ic, micro-, and -metry; then build words that mean:

(e) pertaining to a very small head

(f) X-ray picture of the head

(g) measurement of the head

Using your Exercise Guide, find the meaning of:

(h) macro/**cephal**/ic

(i) **cephal/o**/gyric

Root

Encephal

(*From a Greek word* **encephalos**, *meaning brain.*)

Combining form   Encephal/o

> Note. -**encephalon** means the brain and is used with prefixes to denote parts of the brain, eg, the met**encephalon**, the embryonic, anterior part of the hindbrain.

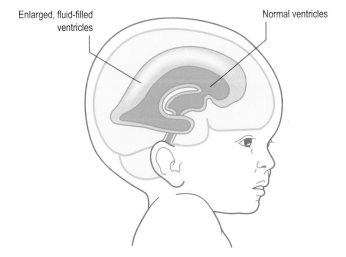

Enlarged, fluid-filled ventricles

Normal ventricles

Figure 48   Hydrocephalus.

📖 Word Exercise 4

Without using your Exercise Guide, write the meaning of:

(a) **encephal**/oma

Using your Exercise Guide, find the meaning of:

(b) **encephal/o**/py/osis

(c) an/**encephal**/ic

(d) electr/o/**encephal/o**/graph

(See Fig. 49)

This instrument records the electrical activity of the brain through electrodes placed on the surface of the scalp. The electroencephalogram is recorded on a computer and appears as a series of waves. Analysis of the waves can be used to localize intracranial lesions, diagnose epilepsy and brain tumours (Am. tumors), and confirm brain death.

Using your Exercise Guide, find the meaning of electr/o and -graphy; then beginning with the underlined root, build words that mean:

(e) technique of X-raying/recording the <u>brain</u>

(f) technique of making a trace/recording of the <u>electrical activity</u> of the brain

Without using your Exercise Guide, build words that mean:

(g) disease of the brain

(h) protrusion or hernia of brain

Using your Exercise Guide, find the meaning of:

(i) ech/o/**encephal/o**/gram (ultrasonic soundwaves are used)

(j) mes/encephalon

(k) polio/**encephal**/itis

Root

Cerebr

(*From a Latin word* **cerebrum**, *meaning brain. Here cerebr/o means the cerebrum of the brain or cerebral hemispheres.*)

Combining form   Cerebr/o

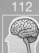

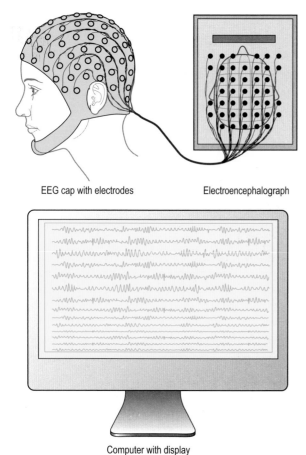

EEG cap with electrodes   Electroencephalograph

Computer with display

Figure 49 The electroencephalograph.

Note. The outer layer of the cerebrum is known as the cerebral cortex (*cortex* is from Latin, meaning rind/bark). It is extensively folded into fissures, giving it a large surface area. This part of the brain contains motor and sensory areas and is the site of consciousness and intelligence.

Word Exercise 5

Without using your Exercise Guide, build words that mean:

(a) hardening of the cerebrum

(b) condition of softening of the cerebrum

(c) pertaining to the cerebrum

Note. Cerebrovascular accident (CVA) or stroke occurs when vascular disease suddenly interrupts the flow of blood to the brain (*vascul/o* meaning vessel and *-ar* meaning pertaining to). An obsolete term, apoplexy, has also been used to mean stroke or CVA (see the Pathology Notes on stroke on page 122 and Fig. 50).

Root

Ventricul

(*From a Latin word* **ventriculum***, meaning ventricle or chamber. Here ventricul/o means ventricle, one of the cavities in the brain filled with cerebrospinal fluid.*)

Combining form   Ventricul/o

Word Exercise 6

Using your Exercise Guide find the meaning of -scopy and -tomy; then build words that mean:

(a) visual examination of the ventricles

(b) incision into the ventricles

Use the Latin root **cistern**, meaning a closed space serving as a reservoir for fluid, and your Exercise Guide to write the meaning of the following word. The closed space referred to here is the **subarachnoid space** outside the brain.

(c) **ventricul/o**/cistern/o/-stomy (this is an operation for hydrocephalus)

Root

Crani

(*From Greek* **kranion***, meaning skull. The bones of the skull protect the soft brain beneath.*)

Combining form   Crani/o

Word Exercise 7

Using your Exercise Guide find the meaning of intra-, -metry and -tomy; then build words that mean:

(a) incision into the skull

(b) the measurement of skulls

(c) pertaining to within the cranium (use -al)

Root

Gangli

(*From a Greek word* **ganglion***, meaning swelling. Here gangli/o means a ganglion, a knot of nerve cell bodies located outside the central nervous system.*)

Combining form   Gangli/o, note that the root -ganglion-is also used

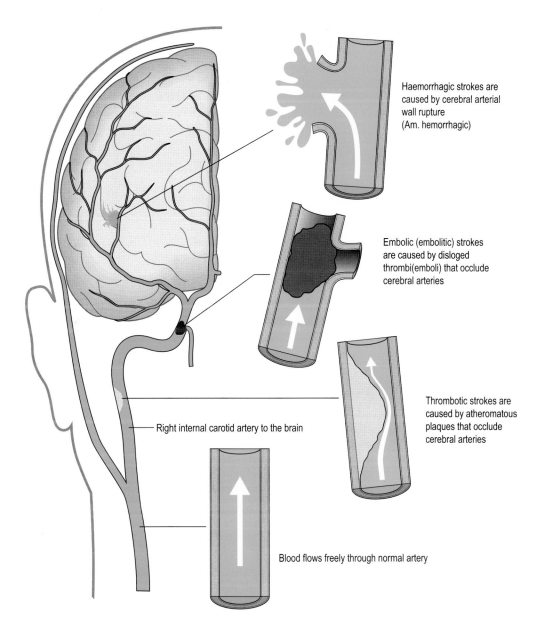

Figure 50 Three types of cerebrovascular accident (stroke). (Adapted from Ignatavicius DD, Workman ML, Medical-Surgical Nursing: Critical Thinking for Collaborative Care, 4th edition, 2002, Saunders.)

Haemorrhagic strokes are caused by cerebral arterial wall rupture (Am. hemorrhagic)

Embolic (embolitic) strokes are caused by disloged thrombi(emboli) that occlude cerebral arteries

Thrombotic strokes are caused by atheromatous plaques that occlude cerebral arteries

Right internal carotid artery to the brain

Blood flows freely through normal artery

Word Exercise 8

Using your Exercise Guide, find the meaning of:

(a) pre/**ganglion**/ic

(b) post/**ganglion**/ic

(c) **gangli/o**/form

Root

Mening

(*From a Greek word menigx, meaning membrane. Here mening/o means the meninges, the three membranes that surround the brain and spinal cord.*)

Combining forms   Mening/i/o

Word Exercise 9

Without using your Exercise Guide, build words using **mening/o** that mean:

(a) inflammation of the meninges

(b) hernia or protrusion of the meninges

Using your Exercise Guide, find the meaning of -rrhagia; then build a word that means:

(c) condition of bursting forth (of blood) from meninges

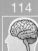

Without using your Exercise Guide, write the meaning of:

(d) **mening/o**/encephal/o/cele

(e) **mening/o**/encephal/itis

(f) **mening/o**/encephal/o/pathy

(g) **mening/i**/oma

The outer of the three membranes of the meninges is known as the **dura mater**. The injection of local anaesthetic into the spine above the dura, ie, into the epidural space, is known as an epidural block. It is often used for a forceps birth or caesarean (Am. cesarean) section delivery (epi- means above or upon).

Using your Exercise Guide, find the meaning of:

(h) epi/**dur**/al

(i) sub/**dur**/al haemat/oma
   (Am. hemat/oma) (see Fig. 51)

This is a common condition seen by neurologists following head injuries. It requires surgery via the cranium to seal leaking blood vessels and remove the blood clot. Surgery also relieves pressure on the brain tissue preventing further damage.

Note. Meningitis is a serious condition that can damage the nerves and brain. When meningitis is caused by the bacterial coccus *Neisseria meningitidis*, it is referred to as **meningococcal meningitis**. When the thick outer dura mater is inflamed, it is known as **pachymeningitis** (pachy- meaning thick); when the thinner meninges, the **pia mater** and the **arachnoid membrane** are inflamed, the condition is known as **leptomeningitis** (from a Greek word *leptos*, meaning thin/slender). Other organisms such as viruses, fungi and parasites can also cause meningitis.

Root

Radicul

(*From a Latin word* **radicula***, meaning root. Here radicul/o means the spinal nerve roots that emerge from the spinal cord.*)

Combining form   Radic/ul/o

Word Exercise 10

Without using your Exercise Guide, write the meaning of:

(a) **radicul/o**/ganglion/itis

(b) **radicul/o**/neur/itis

Another combining form **radic/o** is also derived from this root, eg,

(c) **radic/o**/tomy

Root

Myel

(*From a Greek word* **myelos***, meaning marrow. Here myel/o means the spinal cord, ie, the soft marrow within the spine. Note. Myel/o is also used to mean bone marrow and myelocyte.*)

Combining form   Myel/o

Word Exercise 11

Without using your Exercise Guide, write the meaning of:

(a) **myel/o**/mening/itis

(b) mening/o/**myel/o**/cele

(c) **myel/o**/radicul/itis

(d) **myel/o**/encephal/itis

(e) **myel/o**/phthisis

(f) polio/**myel**/itis

Without using your Exercise Guide, build words that mean:

(g) hardening of the spinal marrow

(h) condition of softening of the spinal marrow

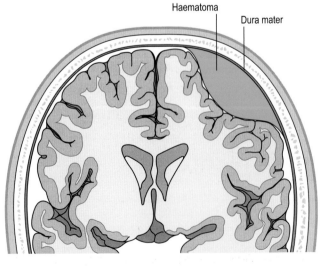

Figure 51   Subdural haematoma (Am. subdural hematoma).

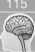

(i) technique of making an X-ray of the spinal cord

Using your Exercise Guide, find the meaning of:

(j) **myel/o**/dys/plasia

(k) **myel**/a/trophy

(l) syring/o/**myel**/ia

Note. Do not confuse myel/o meaning marrow or spinal cord with my/o meaning muscle.

Root

Rachi

(*From a Greek word* **rhachis**, *meaning spine.*)

Combining form   Rachi/o

Word Exercise 12

Using your Exercise Guide, find the meaning of:

(a) **rachi/o**/meter

(b) **rachi/o**/centesis

Rachiocentesis or rachicentesis (see Fig. 52) is performed to obtain a sample of cerebrospinal fluid (CSF) from the subarachnoid space in the lumbar region of the spinal cord. This procedure is commonly known as a **lumbar puncture** or **spinal tap**.

Using your Exercise Guide, find the meaning of:

(c) **rachi**/schisis

Synonymous with **spina bifida**, a congenital neural tube defect in which the vertebral arches (laminae) fail to unite in the midline. This leaves the meninges and part of the spinal cord exposed and protruding from the spine; it leads to physical and mental handicap. Spina bifida is associated with folic acid (vitamin B$_9$) deficiency in women of child bearing age. The condition can be detected by testing for alphafetoprotein in the amniotic fluid or by ultrasonography. Bifida means divided into two equal parts in the midline (from Latin *bi-* meaning two and *findere* meaning to cleave).

Root

Pleg

(*From Greek* **plege**, *meaning a blow. Here -pleg- means a paralysis. A stroke, also called a cerebrovascular accident, is often*

the cause of this condition when a blockage or haemorrhage (*Am.* hemorrhage) in the brain leads to destruction of cells that control motor activities.)

Combining form   -pleg-

Word Exercise 13

Using your Exercise Guide, find the meaning of:

(a) quadri/**pleg**/ia (paralysis of limbs)

(b) hemi/**pleg**/ia (paralysis of right or left side of the body)

(c) para/**pleg**/ia (paralysis of lower limbs)

(d) di/**pleg**/ia (paralysis of like parts on either side of body)

(e) tetra/**pleg**/ia

Note. The obsolete term **palsy** meaning paralysis is still used in **Bell palsy** (paralysis of the VIIth cranial nerve commonly called the facial nerve) and in **cerebral palsy**.

Root

Aesthesi

(*From Greek* **aisthesis**, *meaning perception or sensation. Here aesthes/i/o means sensation.*)

Combining forms   Aesthe/s/i/o, Esthe/s/i/o (*Am.*), aesthet-, esthet- (*Am.*)

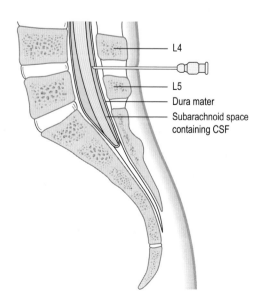

L4

L5

Dura mater

Subarachnoid space containing CSF

Figure 52   Lumbar puncture.

Note. An/**aesthes**/ia means a condition of being without sensation. In medicine, it is also used to mean a condition of loss of sensation due to the administration of a drug called an anaesthetic (Am. anesthetic). General and local anaesthetics are used to eliminate painful sensation during surgical procedures. General anaesthesia is the induction of a state of unconsciousness with the absence of pain over the entire body. Local anaesthesia is the loss of sensation and pain in the region to which the anaesthetic is injected or applied. The branch of medicine that studies anaesthesia, anaesthetics and perioperative medicine is called anaesthesiology (Am. anesthesiology).

 Word Exercise 14

Without using your Exercise Guide, write the meaning of:

(a) an/**aesthesi/o**/logist
(Am. an/**esthesi/o**/logist)

(b) an/**aesthet**/ist
(Am. an/**esthet**/ist)

(c) hemi/an/**aesthes**/ia (Am.
hemi/an/**esthes**/ia; refers
to one side of the body)

Using your Exercise Guide, find the meaning of:

(d) an/**aesthet**/ize
(Am. an/**esthet**/ize)

(e) hypo/**aesthes**/ia
(Am. hypo/**esthes**/ia)

(f) hyper/**aesthes**/ia
(Am. hyper/**esthes**/ia)

The term par**aesthes**ia (Am. par**esthes**ia) is used to mean any abnormal sensations, such as 'pins and needles' (from Greek word *para*, meaning near).

Without using your Exercise Guide, build words that mean:

(g) pertaining to following/
after anaesthesia
(Am. anesthesia)

(h) pertaining to before anaesthesia (Am. anesthesia)

Root

Narc

(*From a Greek word* **narke***, meaning stupor. Here narc/o means narcosis, an abnormally deep sleep induced by a drug (a narcotic). This is a different level of consciousness from anaesthesia (Am. anesthesia); patients are not oblivious to pain and can be woken up.*)

Combining form   Narc/o

 Word Exercise 15

Without using your Exercise Guide, write the meaning of:

(a) **narc**/osis

Using your Exercise Guide, find the meaning of:

(b) **narc/o**/therapy

Root

Alges

(*From a Greek word* **algesis***, meaning a sense of pain.*)

Combining forms   Alges/i/o

 Word Exercise 16

Without using your Exercise Guide, write the meaning of:

(a) **alges**/ia

(b) an/**alges**/ia

(c) hyper/**alges**/ia

(d) an/**alges**/ic
(a drug)

Psychiatry

Disorders that interfere with the normal functioning of the brain may affect behaviour and personality, ie, the mind. The study of the mind and treatment of its disorders is a specialist branch of medicine known as psychiatry. A psychiatrist is a person with medical qualifications who has specialized in the study and treatment of mental disease. Psychiatrists use the following terms.

Root

Psych

(*From Greek* **psyche***, meaning soul or mind. Here psych/o means the mind. The psyche is the human faculty for thought, judgement and emotion or, in other words, our mental life including both conscious and unconscious processes.*)

Combining form   Psych/o

 Word Exercise 17

Without using your Exercise Guide, write the meaning of:

(a) **psych/o**/logy

Note. A psychologist is not usually medically qualified and cannot treat disorders by means of drugs or surgery.

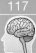

Psychologists study human behaviour: for example, an educational psychologist may study intelligence and behaviour of school children.

(b) **psych**/ic

(c) **psych/o**/pathy

Note. A psychopath is a person with a specific type of personality disorder in which he/she lacks empathy and in certain circumstances may display aggressive and antisocial behaviour. The term has a complex meaning in psychiatry.

(d) **psych**/osis

Note. A **psychosis** is a severe mental disorder in which thought and emotions are so impaired that contact is lost with external reality. **Psychoses** originate in the mind itself, in contrast to **neuroses** which are mental conditions believed to arise because of stresses and anxieties in the patient's environment. Neurotic comes from *neur/o* meaning nerves and *tic*, meaning pertaining to; in psychiatry it means pertaining to a neurosis.

(e) **psych/o**/tropic
(drug)

Using your Exercise Guide, find the meaning of:

(f) **psych/o**/somat/ic

(g) **psych**/iatry

▌Root

Phob

(*From a Greek word* **phobos**, *meaning fear. Here -phob- means an irrational fear or aversion to something.*)

Combining form   -phob-

📖 Word Exercise 18

Using your Exercise Guide, find the meaning of:

(a) acro/**phob**/ia

(b) agora/**phob**/ia

(c) aqua/**phob**/ia

(d) cancer/o/**phob**/ia

(e) necr/o/**phob**/ia

▌Root

Epilept

(*From Greek* **epileptikos**, *meaning a seizure. Here epilept/o means epilepsy, a state of disordered electrical activity in the brain that produces a 'fit' and unconsciousness.*)

Combining forms   Epilept/i/o

📖 Word Exercise 19

Without using your Exercise Guide, write the meaning of:

(a) **epilept/o**/genic

(b) post/**epilept**/ic

Using your Exercise Guide, find the meaning of:

(c) **epilept/i**/form

Modern treatments of mental disease involve drug treatments and occasionally surgery. One of the most useful physical methods of treatment that brings about improvement in depressive states, mania and stupor is **electro-convulsive therapy** (ECT). This involves the application of a high voltage to the head via electrodes placed on its surface to induce a seizure that has a beneficial anticonvulsive effect.

Medical equipment and clinical procedures

A patient showing signs and symptoms of disease of the nervous system will be referred to a neurologist. Much information about the state of health of the nervous system can be gained from relatively simple tests that assess the response of the body to various stimuli. One such test you are probably familiar with is the knee jerk reflex where the sensory nerve endings in the patella (knee cap) are tapped with a hammer (Fig. 53). In a healthy patient the response will be that muscles in the thigh will contract, causing the leg to jerk upwards. A normal reflex action will indicate that the nerve pathway from the knee through the spinal cord is working normally.

More detailed examinations of the nervous system require specialized equipment, described next. See Unit 18 for additional information on the imaging techniques listed here.

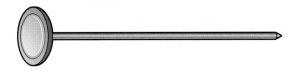

Figure 53   A tendon hammer.

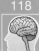
Computed tomography (CT)

This is a technique of making a recording using a **tomograph**, an X-ray machine that produces images of cross-sections through the body. The CT scan shows detailed images of brain structures and aids diagnosis of head injuries and diseases of the nervous system.

Magnetic resonance imaging (MRI)

This technique using nuclear magnetic resonance is particularly useful for imaging the soft tissue of the brain and spinal cord. The patient is placed in an intense magnetic field where hydrogen atoms in the nerve tissue are excited with radio waves, and signals from them are detected and computed into a picture. The procedure does not have the risks associated with X-rays.

Positron emission tomography (PET)

This is a technique of imaging the distribution of positron emitting radioisotopes administered to the body. Active brain cells take up some isotopes used in PET; this makes the technique particularly useful for studying brain metabolism.

Review the names of all instruments and clinical procedures mentioned in this unit, and then try Exercises 20 and 21.

 Word Exercise 20

Match each description in Column C with a term in Column A by placing the appropriate number in Column B.

Column A	Column B	Column C
(a) encepha-lography		1. an instrument used for testing reflexes
(b) positron emission tomography		2. an instrument that images serial sections of body using X-rays
(c) ventriculos-copy		3. measurement of the cranium
(d) tendon hammer		4. technique of imaging a section through the body using radioisotopes that emit positrons
(e) tomograph		5. technique of making an X-ray/ recording of the brain
(f) craniometry		6. technique of viewing ventricles

Word Exercise 21

Match each description in Column C with a term in Column A by placing the appropriate number in Column B.

Column A	Column B	Column C
(a) magnetic resonance imaging		1. technique of imaging serial sections of body using X-rays
(b) lumbar puncture		2. technique of making a recording of the electrical activity of the brain
(c) myelography		3. technique of imaging soft tissues of the brain and spinal cord without using X-rays
(d) computed tomography		4. technique of making a recording or image of the brain using ultrasound
(e) electroenceph-alography		5. technique of making an X-ray/ recording of the spinal cord
(f) echoencepha-lography		6. technique of removing cerebro-spinal fluid from spinal cord

Other procedures widely used to investigate the nervous system besides those mentioned in the word exercises include:

Cerebral angiography In this procedure a contrast medium visible on X-rays is injected into the bloodstream via the femoral artery in the groin. As the medium circulates through the brain, X-ray images are made that outline the blood vessels. Images that are taken before and after the dye is injected are electronically manipulated so that overlying tissues seen in the first image are removed from the final image giving a clear outline of the vessels; this is called intraarterial digital subtraction angiography.
Cerebrospinal fluid analysis Samples of cerebrospinal fluid removed during a lumbar puncture are tested for the presence of protein, blood cells, glucose, microorganisms, malignant cells and the presence of pigments in the laboratory; the CSF pressure is measured during the lumbar puncture procedure. These investigations are used to diagnose many conditions, including meningitis, Guillain–Barré syndrome, subarachnoid haemorrhages and multiple sclerosis.
Stereotaxic surgery This is a minimally invasive surgical procedure in which a stereotactic instrument is fixed to the

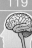

skull to guide probes that destroy or stimulate brain tissue. The instrument makes use of a three-dimensional coordinate system to locate precise targets in the brain and is used on patients with serious neurological or psychological problems.

ANATOMY EXERCISE

Now complete the Anatomy Exercise on page 108.

 CASE HISTORY 8

The object of this exercise is to understand words associated with a patient's medical history.

To complete the exercise:

- Read through the passage on cerebrovascular accident; unfamiliar words are underlined, and you can find their meaning using the Word Help.

- Write the meaning of the medical terms shown in bold print on the lines that follow the Word Help.

Cerebrovascular accident (stroke)

Mr H, a single, 56-year-old white male, became ill early in the day of admission whilst eating his breakfast. He had felt dizzy, developed a headache and complained of impaired vision in one eye. Signs of a right-sided **hemiplegia, hemiparaesthesia** and aphasia followed these symptoms. Three weeks prior to his illness, he had suffered a TIA in which he developed mild, right **hemisensory loss** in his arm and a sudden, transient hemianopia. His GP suspected a **cerebral** infarction or **intracranial** haemorrhage (Am. hemorrhage), and he was referred to the **Neurology** unit for assessment.

On admission in the evening, Mr H's right arm and leg were flaccid and **hyperreflexic**. A CT scan demonstrated a low-density area (an infarct) without a mass effect. There was a loud localized bruit in his neck, and digital subtraction angiography (DSA) detected a tight stenosis of the left internal carotid artery. Following diagnosis of a stroke caused by internal carotid artery occlusion, he was given anticoagulant therapy. Two weeks later, he underwent a successful internal carotid endarterectomy.

The long-term prognosis of Mr H's neurological deficit is uncertain. Three weeks following surgery, he showed signs of recovery and had sufficient language to be intelligible. He maintained a rigorous programme of physiotherapy (Am. physical therapy) and speech therapy following initial recovery. The occupational therapist visited his home and advised on the installation of aids that will assist his rehabilitation. Unfortunately, Mr H is severely depressed following his resignation as a structural engineer with a building company.

Word Help

aphasia condition of being without speech

bruit abnormal sound upon auscultation (listening to body sounds)

CT computerized tomography, a technique of imaging a 'slice' through the body using X-rays

DSA digital subtraction angiography. A technique of making two X-rays, one taken before an injection of dye into a blood vessel. A computerized image of the first X-ray is subtracted from the second, producing a clear image.

endarterectomy removal of the inside of a blood vessel to remove a blockage and open its lumen

flaccid relaxed, flabby and soft

GP general practitioner (family doctor)

haemorrhage (Am. hemorrhage) bursting forth of blood from a vessel

hemianopia loss of half the vision in each eye (loosely used to mean half the vision in one eye)

infarction process of forming an infarct, a piece of dead tissue formed by the failure of its blood supply

neurological pertaining to neurology; here it refers to the nervous system of the patient

occlusion state of being closed up

occupational therapist specialist in providing treatment/assistance aimed at helping people with physical and/or mental disability to become independent

physiotherapy (Am. physical therapy) employment of physical measures (massage, exercise, etc.) to restore function following injury or disease

rehabilitation reeducation that allows a sick or injured person to take his or her place in the world or gain some independence

stenosis abnormal condition of narrowing

TIA transient ischaemic (Am. ischemic) attack (ie, insufficient blood supply to the brain)

Now, write the meaning of the following words from the Case History without using your dictionary lists:

(a) cerebrovascular

(b) hemiplegia

(c) hemiparaesthesia (Am. hemiparesthesia)

(d) hemisensory loss

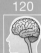
(e) cerebral

(f) intracranial

(g) neurology

(h) hyperreflexic

(Answers to the Case History exercise are given in the Answers to Word Exercises on page 343.)

Quick Reference

Combining forms relating to the nervous system:

Aesthesi/o	sensation (Am. esthesi/o)
Alges/i	sense of pain
Cephal/o	head
Cerebr/o	cerebrum/brain
Cistern/o	cistern / subarachnoid space
Crani/o	cranium
Dur/o	dura mater
Encephal/o	brain
Epilept/o	epilepsy
Esthesi/o (Am.)	sensation
Gangli/o	ganglion
Gli/a/o	glue-like/neuroglial cells
Mening/i/o	meninges
Motor-	action / moving / set in motion
Myel/o	marrow / spinal cord
Narc/o	stupor/numbness
Neur/o	nerve
Plex/o	network, eg, of nerves
Polio-	grey matter (of CNS) (Am. glay)
Psych/o	mind
Rachi/o	spine
Radicul/o	nerve root
Somat/o	body
Syring/o	tube/cavity
Ventricul/o	ventricle (of the brain)

Abbreviations

Some common abbreviations related to the nervous system and psychiatry are listed next. Note that some are not standard, and their meaning may vary from one healthcare setting to another. There is a more extensive list for reference on page 369.

ADHD	attention deficit hyperactivity disorder
CSF	cerebrospinal fluid
CVA	cerebrovascular accident
ECT	electroconvulsive therapy
EEG	electroencephalogram
ICP	intracranial pressure
KJ	knee jerk
LP	lumbar puncture
NCVs	nerve conduction velocities

OCD	obsessive compulsive disorder
PVS	persistent vegetative state
RTA	road traffic accident
SAH	subarachnoid haemorrhage (Am. hemorrhage)
SDH	subdural haematoma (Am. hematoma)
Sz	seizure
TBI	traumatic brain injury
TLE	temporal lobe epilepsy
TIA	transient ischaemic attack (Am. ischemic)

Pathology notes

Alzheimer disease (AD)

This is the most common form of dementia and was previously known as presenile dementia. It is characterized by progressive atrophy of the cerebral cortex accompanied by deteriorating mental functioning. The degeneration can progress to adversely affect memory, attention span, intellectual capacity, personality and motor control. Death usually occurs between two and five years after onset; Alzheimer disease is responsible for over 75% of all cases of dementia in people over 65 years of age.

Bipolar disorder

Bipolar disorder used to be called manic depression or manic depressive psychosis. As the names suggest, it is a type of mental illness in which the patient's mood alternates between phases of intense excitement and phases of depression. In between these phases, there can be periods of normality. The condition is also known as bipolar depression or bipolar affective disorder because of the alternation of the two states.

Brain tumour

Most primary brain tumours (Am. tumor) are gliomas or meningiomas developing from neuroglial cells or the meninges, respectively. Meningiomas are usually benign (noncancerous) and surrounded by a capsule but, as they grow, they compress the brain tissue. Malignant tumours such as glioblastoma mutiforme may spread into other parts of the brain. As tumours increase in size, they cause swelling (cerebral oedema, Am. edema) and hydrocephalus. Common early symptoms are headaches, fits (seizures), nausea, problems with vision and changes in mood and personality. Tumours called secondary brain tumours (or metastatic brain tumours) are cancers that have spread from somewhere else in the body such as the lung, breast or skin; they are more common than primary brain tumours.

Creutzfeldt–Jakob disease (CJD)

CJD is a poorly understood condition caused by an infectious heat-resistant particle known as a prion protein. Infection produces a rapidly progressive form of dementia that is always fatal. New variant CJD has been transmitted to humans from cattle meat infected with bovine spongiform encephalopathy (BSE).

Epilepsy

There are a number of seizure disorders known as epilepsies that result from disordered electrical activity of the brain. They are characterized by seizures or fits caused by a sudden abnormal electrical discharge by neurons.

Generalized seizures may be *tonic-clinic* (grand mal) or *absences* (petit mal). Tonic-clonic seizures are the most common type with loss of consciousness and convulsions. Absence seizures occur mainly in children and are characterized by a brief loss of consciousness without abnormal movements.
Partial seizures occur when the electrical disturbance is limited to a particular focus of the brain; they are manifested in a variety of ways. Consciousness is maintained, but there is an abnormal twitching movement, tingling sensations and hallucinations of vision, smell or taste. In *Jacksonian epilepsy*, the twitching movements may spread from one part of the body to another.

Guillain–Barré syndrome

Guillain–Barré syndrome is a rare, serious condition of the peripheral nervous system, it occurs when the body's immune system attacks the myelin sheath of the peripheral nerves. The cause is unknown, but most people develop the condition shortly after a viral or bacterial infection. Symptoms include tingling, numbness, muscle weakness and temporary progressive muscle paralysis. It may take a year to recover, and a small proportion of patients will be left with some disability.

Herpes zoster

Herpes zoster, also known as zoster and shingles, is caused by the reactivation of the varicella-zoster virus (VZV), the same virus that causes varicella or chickenpox, and it affects the peripheral nerves. Primary infection with VZV causes chicken pox; once the illness resolves, the virus remains dormant (latent) in the dorsal root ganglia near the spinal cord. VZV can reactivate later in a person's life and cause an infectious rash with painful blisters on one side of the body called herpes zoster. The reasons for reactivation of the virus are uncertain, but it is more likely to occur in people whose immune system is impaired due to ageing, immunosuppressive therapy or psychological stress.

Huntington chorea

Huntington chorea is an inherited disease characterized by involuntary, purposeless movements (chorea) that progresses to dementia and death. The initial symptoms of this disease first appear between the ages of 30 and 40 with death generally occurring by the age of 55.

Motor neuron disease

A group of disorders in which there is chronic progressive degeneration of the motor neurons. The most common type is amyotrophic lateral sclerosis (ALS), also called Lou Gehrig disease after a famous American baseball player who became a victim of the disease. The lesions develop in the cerebral cortex, brain stem and anterior horns of the spinal cord. It usually presents after the age of 50, and the cause is unknown; early signs are weakness and twitching of the small muscles of the hand, arm and shoulder girdle. The legs are affected later. As the disease progresses, the patient has difficulty eating and speaking and becomes immobile. Death is usually due to involvement of neurons in the respiratory centre of the medulla oblongata or from respiratory infection.

Multiple sclerosis

Multiple sclerosis is characterized by destruction of the myelin in the sheaths that surround neurons of the central nervous system and death of oligodendrocytes. Hard, plaque-like lesions replace the destroyed myelin, and inflammatory cells invade affected areas. As demyelination occurs, nerve conduction is impaired, and this leads to weakness, loss of coordination, visual impairment and speech disturbance. In most cases the disease is prolonged with remissions and relapses occurring over many years.

Parkinson disease

Parkinson disease is a progressive disease of the central nervous system with an unknown cause. Typically it affects victims around the age of 60 who show degeneration of dopamine-producing neurons in the substantia nigra region of the midbrain. Severe loss of dopamine results in symptoms of muscle tremor of the extremities, expressionless facial features, rigidity of voluntary muscles, a slow shuffling gait and stooping posture.

Schizophrenia

Schizophrenia is a general term for a group of psychotic disorders and is one of the major diagnostic categories of mental illness. Disintegration of personality, progressive loss of emotional stability, poor judgement and loss of contact with reality characterize the illness. A list of positive and negative symptoms called Schneider's first rank symptoms is used in the diagnosis and classification of schizophrenia. Positive symptoms for the disease include hallucinations and delusions or hearing voices and having strange thoughts. Negative symptoms include apathy, paucity of speech and social withdrawal. Types of schizophrenia include:

Catatonic schizophrenia characterized by prolonged rigid postures interspersed with outbursts of motor activity such as repeated movements.
Paranoid schizophrenia characterized by hallucinations and paranoid delusions; patients may suffer delusions of grandeur, persecution or jealousy.
Hebephrenic schizophrenia a form that occurs suddenly in young adults characterized by a general disintegration of the personality. There is thought disorder, meaningless behaviour, incoherence, giggling, peculiar mannerisms and delusions.

Sciatica

A type of neuritis characterized by severe pain along the path of the sciatic nerve and its pathways. A common cause is a prolapsed intervertebral disc.

Stroke (cerebrovascular accident)

A stroke or cerebrovascular accident (CVA) occurs when vascular (vessel) disease suddenly interrupts the flow of blood to the brain. There are two main causes: *cerebral infarction* and *spontaneous intracranial haemorrhage (Am. hemorrhage)*. Cerebral infarction is a result of atheroma complicated by thrombosis or blockage of an artery by an embolus. Spontaneous intracranial haemorrhage is commonly associated with a ruptured aneurysm or with high blood pressure (hypertension). Lack of oxygen to the brain tissue (hypoxia) often results in paralysis on one side of the body and disturbances of speech and vision. As cells in the cerebrum control voluntary movements of many parts of the body, paralysis of limbs and loss of speech are common symptoms of strokes. The severity of symptoms depends on the area of brain tissue damaged. Sometimes there is partial recovery, and the patient may be left with slight paralysis or weakness called a paresis, for example, a hemiparesis, slight paralysis on one side of the body.

Tourette syndrome

Tourette syndrome (named after Gilles de la Tourette, 1857–1904) is an inherited neuropsychiatric condition with early onset in childhood. It is characterized by repetitive, involuntary movements and vocalizations called tics. Usually multiple motor tics (eg, facial movements, grimacing, blinking, shrugging shoulders) and at least one phonic tic (eg, coughing, grunting, sniffing or shouting out words) are present. The cause is unknown, and although symptoms can be lifelong, most patients experience their worst tic symptoms in their late teens. Swearing (coprolalia), making rude gestures and repeating words of others (echolalia) often associated with Tourette syndrome affect only a small proportion of patients.

Associated words

Absence seizure a momentary absence of consciousness of thought or activity

Affect the observable expression of emotion or mood

Agitation restless, repeated activity arising from anxiety or frustration, eg, inability to sit still

Agnosia a condition of inability to recognize the significance of sensory stimuli (eg, recognize objects)

Aphasia condition of without speech (inability to speak)

Apraxia a condition of inability to perform purposeful movements

Aura a sensation that may precede an epileptic seizure or migraine, an aura can be auditory, visual or olfactory

Bradykinesia condition of slow voluntary movement

Causalgia condition of having an intense burning pain

Clonus a spasmodic rapid contraction and relaxation of muscle

Comatose in a state of unconsciousness from which the patient cannot be roused (in a coma)

Compos mentis Latin for of sound mind

Concussion a violent jarring or shaking from a blow usually applied to the brain that may alter consciousness

Confabulation the invention of events to fill in gaps in one's memory, a symptom of Korsakoff syndrome

Convulsion a fit or seizure with violent spasms of muscular contraction and relaxation

Delirium an abnormal mental state characterized by hallucinations

Delusion a false idea that cannot be corrected by reasoning

Dementia a condition of deterioration in mental functioning due to pathological changes in the brain

Demyelination process of losing the myelin sheath that lies around nerve fibres (Am. fibers)

Depression an affective disorder characterized by profound and persistent sadness and despair

Disorientation a state of confusion as to time, place or identity

Dopamine a neurotransmitter found in the central nervous system

Dyspraxia a condition of partial loss of ability to perform coordinated movements

Echolalia condition of involuntary repetition of phrases or words spoken by another person

Echopraxia condition of involuntary copying of the movements of others

Excitation the process of stimulating; the condition of being excited or responding to a stimulus

Gait manner of walking

Grand mal a form of epilepsy characterized by sudden loss of consciousness and tonic-clonic seizures

Hippus alternate contraction and dilation of the pupils seen in some nervous disorders

Hypochondria a condition of morbid preoccupation or anxiety about one's health

Ictal pertaining to, characterized by or caused by a stroke or epileptic seizure

Innervation the nerve supply to a part

Insight mental awareness, the recognition by patients that they are ill

Insomnia inability to sleep

Insult any trauma, irritation, poisoning or injury to the body, eg, a brain insult due to hypoxia

Intrathecal pertaining to within a sheath, refers to within the meninges in the subarachnoid space

Jerk a sudden muscular contraction, eg, a knee jerk used to test a nervous reflex action

Laceration a wound with torn and ragged edges, eg, tearing of the brain

Lassitude a feeling of extreme weakness and apathy

Lethargy condition of drowsiness or stupor that cannot be overcome by will

Mania a condition of extreme mental excitement, also used to denote an obsessive preoccupation with something

Melancholia a condition or state of extreme depression

Migraine a severe, unilateral, vascular headache often associate with nausea, vomiting and visual disturbance

Nutation involuntary nodding of the head

Obsession an idea that persists and recurs in an individual, a compulsive thought

Postictal pertaining to after a stroke or seizure

Tic a spasmodic twitching of muscles usually of the face, neck or shoulder

NOW TRY THE WORD CHECK

WORD CHECK

This self-check exercise lists all the word components used in this unit. First, write down the meaning of as many word components as you can. Then, check your answers using the Exercise Guide and Quick Reference box or the Glossary of Word Components (pp. 383–410).

Prefixes

a-

acro-

agora-

an-

di-

dys-

epi-

hemi-

hyper-

hypo-

lepto-

macro-

meso-

micro-

pachy-

para-

poly-

post-

pre-

quadri-

sub-

tetra-

Combining forms of word roots

aesthesi/o (Am. esthesi/o)

alges/i

cancer/o

cephal/o

cerebr/o

cistern/o

crani/o

cyt/o

dur/o

ech/o

electr/o

encephal/o

epilept/o

fibr/o

gangli/o

gli/a/o

haemat/o (Am. hemat/o)

hist/o

hydro-

iatr/o

mening/o

motor

myel/o

narc/o

necr/o

neur/o

plex/o

pneum/o

polio-

psych/o

py/o

rachi/o

radicul/o

somat/o

syring/o

ventricul/o

Suffixes

-al

-algia

-cele

-centesis

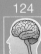

-cyte

-ectomy

-form

-genic

-gram

-graph

-graphy

-gyric

-ia

-ic

-ical

-itis

-ize

-logist

-logy

-malacia

-meter

-metry

-oma

-osis

-ous

-pathy

-phobia

-phthisis

-plasia

-plegia

-rrhagia

-schisis

-sclerosis

-scopy

-stomy

-therapy

-tomy

-tic

-trauma

-trophy

-tropic

-us

NOW TRY THE SELF-ASSESSMENT

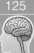

SELF-ASSESSMENT

Test 8A

Next are some combining forms that refer to the anatomy of the nervous system. Indicate which part of the system they refer to by putting a number from the diagrams (Figs 54 and 55) next to each word.

(a) crani/o

(b) encephal/o

(c) meningi/o

(d) neur/o

(e) rachi/o

(f) gangli/o

(g) ventricul/o

(h) radicul/o

(i) cephal/o

(j) myel/o

Score

10

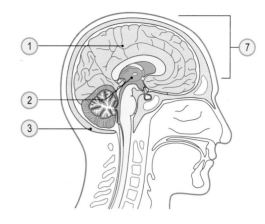

Figure 54   Sagittal section through the head.

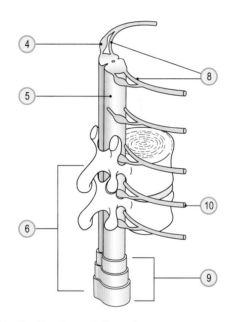

Figure 55   Section through the spine.

Test 8B

Prefixes

Match each meaning in Column C with a prefix in Column A by inserting the appropriate number in Column B.

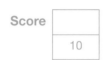

Column A	Column B	Column C
(a) a-		1. after/behind
(b) acro-		2. middle
(c) agora-		3. water (i)
(d) an-		4. water (ii)
(e) aqua-		5. thick
(f) di-		6. large
(g) epi-		7. without/not (i)
(h) hemi-		8. without/not (ii)
(i) hydro-		9. four (i)
(j) lepto-		10. four (ii)

Column A	Column B	Column C
(k) macro-		11. before / in front of
(l) meso-		12. many
(m) micro-		13. half
(n) pachy-		14. thin/slender
(o) para-		15. open space
(p) poly-		16. upon/above
(q) post-		17. small
(r) pre-		18. two/double

Column A	Column B	Column C
(s) quadri-		19. point/extremity
(t) tetra-		20. beside/near

Score

20

Column A	Column B	Column C
(s) somat/o		19. brain
(t) ventricul/o		20. sensation

Score

20

Test 8C

Combining forms of word roots

Match each meaning in Column C with a combining form of a word root in Column A by inserting the appropriate number in Column B.

Column A	Column B	Column C
(a) aesthesi/o (Am. esthesi/o)		1. spine
(b) cephal/o		2. mind
(c) cistern/o		3. grey matter (of CNS)
(d) crani/o		4. stupor / deep sleep
(e) dur/o		5. body
(f) encephal/o		6. membranes of CNS
(g) epilept/o		7. ganglion
(h) gangli/o		8. cranium/skull
(i) gli/a/o		9. ventricles of brain
(j) mening/o		10. head
(k) motor		11. dura mater
(l) myel/o		12. fit/seizure/ epilepsy
(m) narc/o		13. cistern / reservoir / subarachnoid space
(n) neur/o		14. root (of spinal nerve)
(o) polio-		15. nerve
(p) psych/o		16. marrow (of spine)
(q) rachi/o		17. pertaining to action
(r) radicul/o		18. flue (cell)

Test 8D

Suffixes

Match each meaning in Column C with a suffix in Column A by inserting the appropriate number in Column B.

Column A	Column B	Column C
(a) -centesis		1. condition of paralysis
(b) -form		2. abnormal condition / disease of
(c) -genic		3. technique of recording/making an X-ray
(d) -gram		4. pertaining to the body
(e) -graphy		5. pertaining to affinity for / stimulating
(f) -gyric		6. formation of an opening into
(g) -malacia		7. having characteristics or form of
(h) -osis		8. condition of increase in cell formation / number of cells
(i) -phobia		9. nourishment
(j) -phthisis		10. hardening
(k) -plasia		11. wasting away / decay
(l) -plegia		12. condition of softening
(m) -schisis		13. recording/tracing/ X-ray
(n) -sclerosis		14. puncture
(o) -somatic		15. treatment
(p) -stomy		16. splitting
(q) -therapy		17. condition of fear

Column A	Column B	Column C
(r) -trauma		18. pertaining to movement around a centre
(s) -trophy		19. formation / originating in
(t) -tropic		20. injury/shock

Score

20

Test 8E

Write the meaning of:

(a) neuromyelitis

(b) rachiotomy

(c) meningomalacia

(d) encephalomyelopathy

(e) ventriculoscope

Score

5

Test 8F

Build words that mean:

(a) disease of the meninges

(b) instrument for measuring the head

(c) inflammation of the spinal nerve roots and spinal cord

(d) condition of bursting forth (of blood) from the brain

(e) study of cells of the nervous system

Score

5

Check answers to Self-Assessment Tests on pages 361–362.

UNIT 9
THE EYE

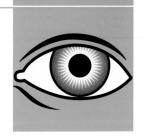

OBJECTIVES

Once you have completed Unit 9, you should be able to do the following:

- understand the meaning of medical words relating to the eye
- build medical words relating to the eye

- associate medical terms with their anatomical position
- understand common medical abbreviations relating to the eye

EXERCISE GUIDE

Use this list of word components and their meanings to complete the word exercises in this unit.

Prefixes

a-	without
ambly-	dull/dim
an-	without
an-iso-	not equal / unequal
bin-	two each / double
dia-	through
diplo-	double
dys-	difficult/painful
en-	in/within
ex-	out / out of / away from
hemi-	half
iso-	same/equal
mono-	one
pan-	all
presby-	old man / old age
uni-	one
xero-	dry

Roots / Combining forms

aden/o	gland
blast/o	immature germ cell / cell that forms…
blenn/o	mucus
chromat/o	colour
cyst/o	bladder or sac
electr/o	electrical
esthesi/o (Am.)	sensation
helc/o	ulcer
lith/o	stone

motor	action
my/o	muscle
myc/o	fungus
nas/o	nose
neur/o	nerve
py/o	pus
rhin/o	nose
ton/o	tone/tension

Suffixes

-al	pertaining to
-algia	condition of pain
-ar	pertaining to
-cele	swelling/protrusion/hernia
-centesis	puncture to remove fluid
-chalasis	slackening/loosening
-conus	cone-like protrusion
-dialysis	separating
-ectasis	dilatation/stretching
-ectomy	removal of
-edema (Am.)	swelling due to fluid
-erysis	drag/draw/suck out
-gram	X-ray/tracing/recording
-graph	usually an instrument that records
-graphy	technique of recording/making an X-ray
-gyric	pertaining to circular motion
-ia	condition of
-itis	inflammation of
-kinesis	movement
-logist	specialist who studies…

-malacia	condition of softening	-rrhaphy	suturing/stitching
-meter	measuring instrument	-rrhea (Am.)	excessive flow
-metrist	specialist who measures	-rrhoea	excessive flow (Am. rrhea)
-metry	process of measuring	-schisis	cleavage/splitting/parting
-mileusis	carving	-sclerosis	condition of hardening
-nyxis	perforation/pricking/puncture	-scope	an instrument used to view/examine
-oedema	swelling due to fluid (Am. edema)	-scopy	technique of viewing/examining
-oma	tumour/swelling (Am. tumor)	-spasm	involuntary muscle contraction
-osis	abnormal condition/disease/abnormal increase	-stenosis	condition of narrowing
		-stomy	formation of an opening into…
-pathy	disease of	-synechia	condition of adhering together
-pexy	fixation (by surgery)	-thermy	heat
-plasty	surgical repair / reconstruction	-tome	cutting instrument
-plegia	condition of paralysis	-tomy	incision into
-ptosis	falling/displacement/prolapse		

ANATOMY EXERCISE

When you have finished Word Exercises 1 to 21, look at the word components listed next. Complete Figs 56 and 57 by writing the appropriate combining form on each line. More than one component may relate to the same position. (You can check their meanings in the Quick Reference box on p. 139.)

Blephar/o	Irid/o	Papill/o
Choroid/o	Ir/o	Phac/o
Cor/e/o	Kerat/o	Phak/o
Corne/o	Lacrim/o	Pupill/o
Cycl/o	Ocul/o	Retin/o
Dacry/o	Ophthalm/o	Scler/o

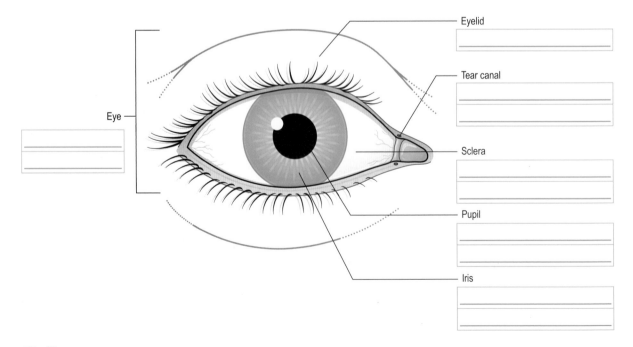

Figure 56   The eye.

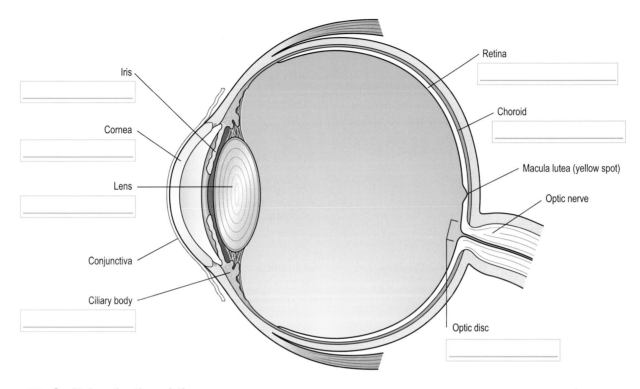

Figure 57   Sagittal section through the eye.

The eye

The eyes are our main sense organs. Light enters the eye through the pupil and transparent cornea; it passes through the lens and is focused onto the light-sensitive retina. In the retina, light stimulates receptors (rods and cones) that generate nerve impulses in sensory neurons; these impulses travel via neurons in the optic nerve to areas of the brain concerned with vision. In the visual cortex of the brain the impulses are interpreted as an image.

Use the Exercise Guide at the beginning of this unit to complete Word Exercises 1 to 21, unless you are asked to work without it.

 ## Root

Ophthalm

(*From a Greek word* **ophthalmos**, *meaning eye.*)

Combining form   Ophthalm/o

(Be careful with spelling ophth.)

Word Exercise 1

Using your Exercise Guide, find the meaning of -itis, -logist, myc/o, -osis, -plegia and -scope; then build words that mean:

(a) an instrument to view the eye

(b) a medically qualified person who specializes in the study of the eye and its disorders

(c) condition of paralysis of the eye

(d) inflammation of the eye (synonymous with ophthalmia)

(e) abnormal condition of fungal infection of the eye

Using your Exercise Guide, find the meaning of:

(f) **ophthalm**/algia

(g) **ophthalm/o**/gyric

(h) **ophthalm/o**[2]/**neur**[3]/**itis**[1]

(i)   pan/**ophthalm**/itis

(j)   **ophthalm/o**/ton/o/meter

(This instrument is used to detect raised pressure within the eye and is used in the diagnosis of glaucoma. Sometimes a **tonometer** is used alone, and **tonography** is used to mean the technique of using a tonometer.)

(k)   blenn/**ophthalm**/ia

(l)   xer/**ophthalm**/ia

(m)   en/**ophthalmos**

(n)   ex/**ophthalmos**

▌Root

Ocul

(*From Latin* **oculus**, *meaning of the eye.*)

Combining form   Ocul/o

📖 Word Exercise 2

Using your Exercise Guide, find the meaning of:

(a)   mon/**ocul**/ar

(b)   uni/**ocul**/ar

(c)   bin/**ocul**/ar

(d)   **ocul/o**/motor nerve

(e)   **ocul/o**/nas/al

(f)   electr/o-**ocul/o**/gram

(This is produced from an electrodiagnostic test; it also records eye position and movement.)

Without using your Exercise Guide, write the meaning of:

(g)   **ocul/o**/gyric

▌Root

Opt

(*From* **optikos**, *a Greek word meaning sight. The words optical and optician are derived from this root. Optical means pertaining to sight; optician refers to a person who makes and sells spectacles in accordance to an ophthalmic prescription.*)

Combining form   Opt/o

📖 Word Exercise 3

Without using your Exercise Guide, write the meaning of:

(a)   **opt/o**/meter

Using your Exercise Guide, find the meaning of:

(b)   **opt/o**/metry

(c)   **opt/o**/metrist

(d)   **opt/o**/my/o/meter

Orthoptics is the science of studying and treating muscle imbalances of the eye (squints). *Ortho* means straight or correct; therefore orthoptic means pertaining to straight or correct sight.

The combining form **optic/o** is also derived from the same root as **opt/o**. It also means pertaining to sight, but it is sometimes used to mean optic nerve, eg, optico-pupillary, pertaining to the pupil and optic nerve.

▌Root

Op

(*From Greek* **ops**, *also meaning eye. Here -op- is usually used in the suffix -opia to mean a condition of defective vision. Many focusing defects can be corrected by prescribing appropriate spectacles.*)

Combining form   -op- or -ops-, used in the suffixes
                        -opia and -opsia

📖 Word Exercise 4

Using your Exercise Guide, find the meaning of:

(a)   dipl/**op**/ia

(b)   presby/**op**/ia

(This refers to a condition in which the lens loses its elasticity in the elderly; it results in the gradual loss of the eye's ability to focus on nearby objects.)

(c)   ambly/**op**/ia

(d)   hemi/a/
       chromat/**ops**/ia

(e)   dys/**op**/ia

(f)   hemi/an/**op**/ia

Focusing a clear image on to the retina is essential for good vision. In the normal eye, light rays enter the eye and are focused into a clear upside down image on the retina. Our brain can easily invert the image in our conscious perception, but it cannot correct an image that is out of focus. There are several common words relating to errors of refraction using the suffix -opia that are difficult to understand from their word components, for example:

Hypermetropia or Hyperopia
A condition of long-sightedness in which light rays are focused beyond the retina (*hyper*, beyond/above/excess). The light rays when measured focus beyond the retina (*metr*, measure). This results in distant objects appearing in focus but near objects out of focus.

Myopia
A condition of short-sightedness. *My* comes from *myein*, meaning to close. Presumably, the eye tends to close when trying to view a distant object. Myopia is a condition in which the eyeball is elongated causing images of distant objects to focus in front of the retina rather than on it. Distant objects appear fuzzy, but near objects are seen in focus as the eye accommodates normally.

Emmetropia
A condition of normal/ideal vision Here, light falls directly on to the retina in its correct position, with no errors (*em* meaning in, *metr* meaning measure).

▌Root

Blephar
(*From a Greek word* **blepharon**, *meaning eyelid.*)

Combining form   Blephar/o

📖 Word Exercise 5

Without using your Exercise Guide, build a word that means:

(a) condition of paralysis of the eyelid

Using your Exercise Guide look up the meaning of -ptosis, -rrhaphy and -spasm, and then build words that mean:

(b) involuntary muscle contraction of the eyelid

(c) falling/displacement of the eyelid

(d) stitching/suturing of an eyelid

Using your Exercise Guide, find the meaning of:

(e) **blephar/o**/py/o/ rrhoea (Am. **blephar/o**/py/o/rrhea)

(f) **blephar/o**/aden/itis

(refers to meibomian glands lying in grooves on the inner surface of eyelids)

(g) **blephar/o**/synechia

(h) **blephar/o**/chalasis

▌Root

Scler
(*From Greek* **skleros**, *meaning hard. Here scler/o means the sclera, the tough, outer white part of the eye. The sclera is continuous with the transparent cornea at the front of the eye.*)

Combining forms   Scler/o

📖 Word Exercise 6

Using your Exercise Guide, find the meaning of:

(a) **scler/o**/tomy

(b) **scler**/ectasis

(c) **scler/o**/tome

▌Root

Kerat
(*From a Greek word* **keras**, *meaning horn. Here kerat/o means the cornea, the transparent, avascular membrane covering the front of the eye; it provides strength, refractive power and transmits light into the eye.*)

Combining form   Kerat/o

📖 Word Exercise 7

Without using your Exercise Guide, write the meaning of:

(a) scler/o/**kerat**/itis

(b) **kerat/o**/metry

(c) **kerat/o**/tome

Using your Exercise Guide, find the meaning of:

(d) **kerat/o**/plasty

(e) **kerat/o**/centesis

(f) **kerat/o**/helc/osis

(g) **kerat/o**/nyxis

(h) **kerat/o**/mileusis

(This is an operation that reshapes the cornea to correct a refractive error as in severe myopia or short-sightedness.)

(i) **kerat/o**/conus

(See Fig. 58.)

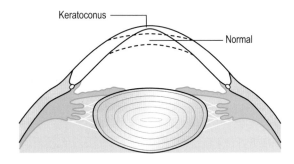

Keratoconus

Normal

Figure 58   Keratoconus.

The word cornea comes from the Latin word *corneus*, also meaning horny. Corneoplasty is synonymous with keratoplasty, an operation performed to replace a diseased or damaged cornea with a corneal graft.

Abnormal curvatures of the cornea cause light rays to focus on the retina unevenly. This is known as **astigmatism**.

The sclera and cornea are covered at the front of the eye with a delicate, transparent membrane that also lines the inner surface of the eyelids. This membrane is the **conjunctiva**; it is prone to irritation and infection, giving rise to **conjunctivitis**.

Root

Ir

(*From a Greek word* **iris**, *meaning rainbow. Here irid/o means the iris, a circular, coloured membrane surrounding the pupil of the eye. Contraction of its muscle fibres regulates the size of the aperture (pupil) within the iris, thereby regulating the amount of light entering the eye.*)

Combining forms   Ir/o, irid/o

Word Exercise 8

Without using your Exercise Guide and beginning with the underlined word, build words using irid/o that mean:

(a) falling / displacement of the <u>iris</u>

(b) inflammation of the cornea and <u>iris</u> (use kerat/o)

Using your Exercise Guide, find the meaning of:

(c) **irid/o**/kinesis

(d) **irid/o**/dialysis

(e) **irid/o**/cele

Without using your Exercise Guide, write the meaning of:

(f) scler/o/**ir**/itis

(g) **irid**/o/plegia

(h) kerat/o/**ir**/itis

Root

Cycl

(*From a Greek word* **kyklos**, *meaning circle. Here cycl/o means the ciliary body of the eye.*)

Combining form   Cycl/o

The ciliary body is a structure composed of smooth muscle fibres and secretory epithelial cells that lies behind the iris (see Fig. 57). It connects the circumference of the iris to the choroid (the middle layer of the eyeball), changes the shape of the lens and secretes a watery fluid, aqueous humor, into the anterior chamber. Study Fig. 59 that shows the anterior cavity in front of the lens and the posterior cavity behind the lens. The anterior cavity is subdivided into the anterior chamber in front of the lens and iris, and the posterior chamber between the iris and lens. The ciliary body continuously secretes aqueous humor into the anterior chamber. The fluid is drained into veins in the sclera at the same rate that it is produced. A raised intraocular pressure due to the accumulation of excess aqueous humor may result in **glaucoma**, a common disorder that causes pain and damage to the eye. The posterior cavity is filled with vitreous humor, a soft jelly-like material that maintains the spherical shape of the eyeball.

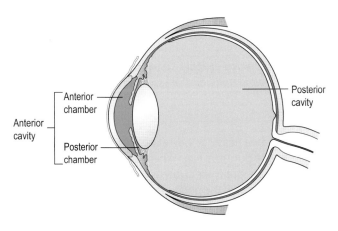

Figure 59   Sagittal section through the eye.

Root

Pupill

(*From a Latin word* **pupilla**, *meaning little girl-doll, so-called from the tiny image one sees of oneself reflected in the eye of another. Here pupill/o means the pupil, the small aperture that allows light to enter the eye.*)

Combining form   Pupill/o

 Word Exercise 11

Without using your Exercise Guide, write the meaning of:

(a) **pupill/o**/plegia

(b) **pupill/o**/metry

 Word Exercise 9

Without using your Exercise Guide, write the meaning of:

(a) irid/o/**cycl**/itis

(b) **cycl/o**/plegia

Using your Exercise Guide, find the meaning of:

(c) **cycl/o**/dia/thermy

Root

Goni

(*From a Greek word* **gonia**, *meaning angle. Here goni/o means the peripheral angle of the anterior chamber. This angle is observed when evaluating types of glaucoma.*)

Combining form   Goni/o

 Word Exercise 10

Without using your Exercise Guide, build words that mean:

(a) an instrument used to measure the angle of the anterior chamber

(b) an instrument used to view the angle of the anterior chamber

(c) an operation to make an incision into the angle of the anterior chamber (for glaucoma)

Root

Cor

(*From a Greek word* **kore**, *meaning the pupil of the eye.*)

Combining forms   Cor/e/o

 Word Exercise 12

Using your Exercise Guide, find the meaning of:

(a) iso/**cor**/ia

(b) an/iso/**cor**/ia

(c) **cor/e**/pexy

Without using your Exercise Guide, write the meaning of:

(d) **cor/e/o**/plasty

Root

Choroid

(*From a Greek word* **choroeides**, *meaning like a skin. Here choroid/o means the choroid, the middle pigmented vascular coat of the posterior five-sixths of the eyeball. The choroid absorbs light and stops reflections within the eye.*)

Combining form   Choroid/o

Word Exercise 13

Without using your Exercise Guide, write the meaning of:

(a) **choroid/o**/cycl/itis [   ]

(b) scler/o/**choroid**/itis [   ]

The word **uvea** from Latin *uva*, meaning grape, is used when referring to the pigmented parts of the eye. These parts include the iris, ciliary body and choroid. **Uve**itis refers to inflammation of all pigmented parts of the eye.

Root

Retin

(*From a Medieval/Latin word* **retina**, *probably derived from rete, meaning net. Here retin/o means the retina, the light-sensitive area of the eye. Light is focused on to the retina by the lens.*)

Combining form   Retin/o

Word Exercise 14

Using your Exercise Guide, find the meaning of:

(a) **retin/o**/blast/oma [   ]

(b) **retin/o**/malacia [   ]

(c) **retin/o**/schisis [   ]

(d) **retin/o**/pathy [   ]

(e) **retin/o**/scopy [   ]

Without using your Exercise Guide and beginning with the underlined root, build words that mean:

(f) picture/recording of the <u>electrical activity</u> of the retina [   ]

(g) inflammation of the <u>retina</u> and choroid [   ]

(h) inflammation of the <u>choroid</u> and retina [   ]

In the centre of the posterior portion of the retina along the visual axis is the **macula lutea** or yellow spot (see Fig. 57). The macula contains a central depression called the **fovea centralis** packed with photoreceptors called cones; this is the area of highest visual acuity producing our sharpest colour vision. If part of the macula or fovea is damaged, vision is reduced and central-vision blindness occurs. Age-related macular degeneration (AMD or ARMD) affects older adults and occurs in dry or wet forms; it is a major cause of blindness and visual impairment.

Root

Papill

(*From a Latin word* **papilla**, *meaning nipple-shaped. Here papill/o means the optic disc or optic papilla.*)

Combining form   Papill/o

Sensory neurons leaving the retina travel through the optic nerve at the back of the eye. Where the sensory neurons collect and form the optic nerve, there is a disc-shaped area in the retina (visible through the pupil). This area is known as the optic disc or optic papilla. **Papill/o** refers to the optic disc.

Word Exercise 15

Using your Exercise Guide, find the meaning of:

(a) **papill**/oedema (Am. **papill**/edema) [   ]

Without using your Exercise Guide and beginning with the underlined root, build a word that means:

(b) inflammation of the <u>retina</u> and optic disc [   ]

Root

Phak

(*From a Greek word* **phakos**, *meaning lentil. Here phac/o means the lens of the eye. The lens is a lentil-shaped crystalline structure surrounded by the lens capsule. The shape of the lens and its focus are changed by ligaments connected to muscles in the ciliary body. The ability to change focus of the lens is known as accommodation.*)

Combining forms   Phac/o or phak/o

Word Exercise 16

Without using your Exercise Guide, build words using phac/o that mean:

(a) condition of softening of a lens (ie, a soft cataract) [   ]

(b) instrument to view the lens (actually to view changes in its shape) [   ]

Using your Exercise Guide find the meaning of a-, -ia and -sclerosis; then build words that mean:

(c) hardening of a lens (ie, a hard cataract) [   ]

(d) condition of without a lens (use phak/o) [   ]

Using your Exercise Guide, find the meaning of:

(e) **phac/o**/cyst/ectomy

(f) **phac/o**/erysis

A common disorder of the lens is the development of a cataract, an opacity of the lens or lens capsule. There are many types of cataract; two common ones are hard cataracts that tend to form in the elderly and soft cataracts, that occur at any age. The lens can be removed by **phaco**emulsification. In this process, ultrasonic vibrations liquefy the lens, and it is then sucked out. The liquefied lens is replaced with an intraocular implant, ie, a plastic lens.

Root

Scot

(*From a Greek word* **skotos**, *meaning darkness. Here scot/o means a scotoma, a normal or abnormal blind spot in the visual field where vision is poor.*)

Combining forms   Scot/o, also used as scotoma-

Word Exercise 17

Without using your Exercise Guide, write the meaning of:

(a) **scot/o**/meter

(b) **scot/o**/metry

Using your Exercise Guide, find the meaning of:

(c) **scotoma**/graph

Root

Lacrim

(*From a Latin word* **lacrima**, *meaning tear. Here lacrim/o means tear or lacrimal apparatus.*)

Combining form   Lacrim/o

The eye is cleansed and lubricated by the lacrimal apparatus (Fig. 60) consisting of a gland, sac and ducts. The gland produces lacrimal fluid that washes over the eyeball and drains into the lacrimal sac through lacrimal ducts. The lacrimal sac, in turn, drains the fluid into the nose through the nasolacrimal duct.

Word Exercise 18

Without using your Exercise Guide and beginning with the underlined root, build words that mean:

(a) incision into the lacrimal apparatus

(b) pertaining to the nose and lacrimal apparatus (use nas/o)

Root

Dacry

(*From a Greek word* **dakryon**, *meaning tear. Here dacry/o means tear, lacrimal duct or lacrimal apparatus.*)

Combining form   Dacry/o

Word Exercise 19

Note. Dacryocyst/o means tear bladder, and it refers to the lacrimal sac.

Using your Exercise Guide, find the meaning of:

(a) **dacry**/o/cyst/o/graphy

(b) **dacry**/o/cyst/o/rhino/stomy

(c) **dacry**/o/lith

(d) **dacry**/o/stenosis

Without using your Exercise Guide, write the meaning of:

(e) **dacry**/o/cyst/o/blenn/o/rrhoea (Am. **dacry**/o/cyst/o/blenno/rrhea)

(f) **dacry**/o/cyst/o/py/osis

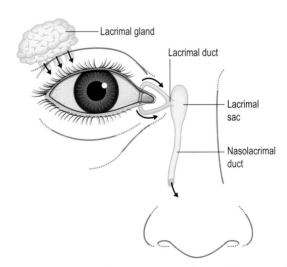

Figure 60   The lacrimal apparatus.

Medical equipment and clinical procedures

Review the names of all instruments and clinical procedures mentioned in this unit, and then try Exercises 20 and 21.

Word Exercise 20

Match each description in Column C with a term in Column A by placing the appropriate number in Column B.

Column A	Column B	Column C
(a) ophthalmo-scope		1. an X-ray picture of the lacrimal apparatus
(b) dacryocysto-gram		2. measurement of blind spots
(c) keratome		3. an instrument that measures tension within the eye
(d) pupillometry		4. an instrument used for visual examination of the eye
(e) optometry		5. an instrument used to cut the cornea
(f) scotometry		6. an instrument used for measuring the power of ocular muscles
(g) ophthalmoto-nometer		7. technique of measuring sight
(h) optomyometer		8. technique of measuring pupils (width)

 Word Exercise 21

Match each description in Column C with a term in Column A by placing the appropriate number in Column B.

Column A	Column B	Column C
(a) scler-otome		1. visual examination of the retina
(b) optometer		2. technique of recording raised pressure/tension in the eye
(c) keratometry		3. technique of making an X-ray of the lacrimal (tear) sac
(d) pupillometer		4. an instrument used to measure sight
(e) phacoscope		5. an instrument used to cut the sclera
(f) retinoscopy		6. measurement of the cornea (its curvature)
(g) tonography		7. an instrument used to view the lens
(h) dacryocyst-ography		8. an instrument that measures pupils (width)

Other procedures used to investigate and treat the eye besides those mentioned in the word exercises include:

Fluorescein angiography This is the technique of making a recording of blood circulation within the retina and choroid layers of the eye. In the procedure intravenous fluorescein angiography (IVFA), a fluorescent dye, is injected into a vein whilst a specialized camera takes images of the retina through dilated pupils. IVFA can detect diabetic and hypertensive retinopathy and confirm age-related macular degeneration as wet or dry.

Fundus photography The technique of making photographs of the inside of the eye using a fundus camera; the camera captures stereoscopic, colour images of the retina (Am. color).

LASIK Laser in situ keratomileusis is used to correct errors of refraction (myopia, astigmatism and hypermetropia) by re-shaping the cornea with an excimer laser that removes surface tissue. Surgeons cut across the cornea and raise a flap of tissue. The laser then reshapes the exposed surface, and the flap is replaced.

Ophthalmoscopy The technique of visual examination of the interior of the eye using an ophthalmoscope.

Scleral buckling In this procedure, fine bands of silicone rubber and sponge are sutured onto the outside of the eyeball to press the sclera towards the middle of the eye and push a detached, torn retina back into position.

Slit lamp microscopy In this procedure the anterior and posterior chambers of the eye are examined using a low-powered microscope (biomicroscope) and a high-intensity light source that can be focused into a thin beam. The eyelid and front of the eye can also be examined enabling the diagnosis of a variety of eye conditions.

Tonometry Technique of measuring tension in the eye; it is used to detect raised intraocular pressure, a sign of glaucoma.

Trabeculectomy a common type of surgery for glaucoma that lowers intraocular pressure. The procedure involves the removal of part of the trabecular meshwork that drains aqueous humor from the eye via the anterior chamber

ANATOMY EXERCISE

Now complete the Anatomy Exercise on page 130.

 CASE HISTORY 9

The object of this exercise is to understand words associated with a patient's medical history.

To complete the exercise:

- Read through the passage on optic neuritis; unfamiliar words are underlined, and you can find their meaning using the Word Help.

- Write the meaning of the medical terms shown in bold print on the lines that follow the Word Help.

Optic neuritis

Mr I, a 22-year-old physics researcher, consulted his **optometrist** complaining of **diplopia** whilst driving and reading. He had also experienced dizziness and **ophthalmalgia** when moving his eyes. He thought his inappropriate, old spectacles caused his symptoms. The optometrist observed **optic neuritis** involving the head of the optic disc (**papillitis**) and <u>perimetry</u> detected a central **scotoma**. She contacted Mr I's <u>GP</u>, and he was sent to the neurologist.

Examination revealed that the pupils were equal, round and reactive to light, but that there was a mild <u>paradoxic dilation</u> of the left pupil to the <u>swinging flashlight test</u>. <u>Vertical gaze</u> was normal. There was an abnormal **ocular** movement on <u>lateral gaze</u>; when he attempted to look left, his right eye failed to <u>adduct</u>, and although the left eye <u>abducted</u>, it showed a coarse horizontal <u>nystagmus</u>. When he looked to the right, there was no abnormality in the movement of the left eye, but the right eye failed to abduct. His abdominal reflexes were absent, and his <u>gait</u> was unsteady and wide.

Clinical examination indicated Mr I had lesions in the right medial longitudinal fasciculus (<u>MLF</u>) of the midbrain, producing an <u>internuclear</u> **ophthalmoplegia** and sixth nerve <u>palsy</u>. This was confirmed with an <u>MRI</u> scan that revealed small <u>periventricular foci</u> within the <u>pons</u> in the region of the MLF.

Mr I was informed that he had <u>multiple sclerosis</u> (MS) and received appropriate counselling for his condition.

Word Help

abducted to move away from the median line (an imaginary line running down the centre of the body)

adduct to move towards the median line or midline of the body

foci centre of disease process (visible on the MRI scan)

gait manner of walking

GP general practitioner (family doctor)

internuclear between nuclei (here nucleus refers to a collection of nerve cells that control eye movement)

lateral gaze looking to the side

MLF medial longitudinal fasciculus, a region of the midbrain that controls eye movement

MRI magnetic resonance imaging

multiple sclerosis nervous system disease characterized by loss of the myelin sheaths of nerve fibres and their

replacement with scar tissue; the sclerotic (hard) patches being found at numerous sites in the brain, spinal cord and optic nerves (synonymous with disseminated sclerosis)

nystagmus involuntary rapid jerky eye movement

palsy paralysis

paradoxic dilation contradictory occurrence (here the left pupil dilates in response to light)

perimetry measuring acuity (clearness of vision) throughout the visual field

periventricular pertaining to around a ventricle (a fluid-filled cavity in the brain)

pons part of the hind brain above the medulla

swinging flashlight test a test in which a flashlight is used to detect a pupillary defect

vertical gaze looking up and down

Now, write the meaning of the following words from the Case History without using your dictionary lists:

(a) optometrist

(b) diplopia

(c) ophthalmalgia

(d) optic neuritis

(e) papillitis

(f) scotoma

(g) ocular

(h) ophthalmoplegia

(Answers to the Case History exercise are given in the Answers to Word Exercises on page 345.)

Quick Reference

Combining forms relating to the eye:

Blephar/o	eyelid
Choroid/o	choroid
Chromat/o	colour
Conjunctiv/o	conjunctiva
Cor/e/o	pupil
Corne/o	cornea
Cycl/o	ciliary body
Dacry/o	tear / lacrimal apparatus / lacrimal ducts
Goni/o	angle (of anterior chamber)

Ir/o	iris
Irid/o	iris
Kerat/o	cornea
Lacrim/o	tear / lacrimal apparatus / lacrimal ducts
Ocul/o	eye
Ophthalm/o	eye
Optic/o	optic nerve
Opt/o	sight
Papill/o	optic disc
Phac/o	lens
Phak/o	lens
Pupill/o	pupil
Retin/o	retina
Scler/o	sclera
Scot/o	dark
Ton/o	tone/tension
Uve/o	uvea (pigmented part of eye)

Abbreviations

Some common abbreviations related to the eye are listed below. Note that some are not standard, and their meaning may vary from one healthcare setting to another. There is a more extensive list for reference on page 369.

Acc	accommodation of the eye
AMD	age-related macular degeneration
ENG	electronystagmogram/electronystagmography
EOM	extraocular muscles or extraocular movement
IOFB	intraocular foreign body
IOL	intraocular lens
IOP	intraocular pressure
OD	oculus dexter (right eye)
OS	oculus sinister (left eye)
OU	oculus uterque (both eyes together)
PERRLA	pupils equal, round, react to light and accommodation
POAG	primary open-angle glaucoma
PRK	photorefractive keratectomy
VA	visual acuity
VF	visual field

Pathology notes

Cataract

A cataract is a loss of transparency of the lens of the eye and is considered to be part of the aging process. Cataracts form because of changes to the protein fibres within the lens, making it appear white and opaque. With increasing loss of transparency, the detail and clarity of the image produced by the retina is lost, and focusing becomes difficult. Age-related cataracts develop because of long exposure to a variety of predisposing factors such as cigarette smoke, UV light, diabetes mellitus and systemic drug treatments with, for example, corticosteroids.

Chalazion

A cyst on the edge of the eyelid formed by retained secretion of the meibomian glands (tarsal glands).

Glaucoma

Glaucoma is an excessive intraocular pressure caused by an abnormal accumulation of aqueous humor within the eye. The condition is due to impaired drainage of fluid through the scleral venous sinus (canal of Schlemm) in the angle between the iris and cornea in the anterior chamber. As pressure against the retina and optic nerve increases, there is mechanical pressure against neurons in the optic nerve and compression of their blood vessels. Damage to the optic nerve impairs vision and can lead to permanent blindness. Glaucoma is treated with drugs, lasers and surgery.

Chronic open-angle glaucoma occurs mostly in people over 40 years of age and is usually bilateral. There is a gradual rise in intraocular pressure with progressive loss of vision; peripheral vision is lost first and may not be noticed until only central tunnel vision remains. As the optic disc atrophies due to damage to its neurons, vision is reduced. The condition eventually results in permanent blindness.

Primary angle-closure glaucoma occurs mostly in people over 40 years of age and usually affects one eye. A sudden obstruction in the outflow of aqueous humor from the eye and a consequent rise in pressure characterize the condition. Symptoms of an acute attack include sudden pain, photophobia, lacrimation and loss of vision. Miotic eye drops are used initially to constrict the pupil, thereby relieving the pressure on the scleral venous sinus. Recovery from repeated attacks may be incomplete, and vision is progressively impaired.

Congenital glaucoma may be due to abnormal development of the anterior chamber because of genetic abnormality or maternal infection, for example, with rubella virus (German measles).

Retinal detachment

Damage to the retina impairs vision because even a well-focused image cannot be perceived if some or all of the light receptors do not function properly. Retinal detachment is a painless condition that forms when a tear or hole in the retina allows fluid to accumulate between the layers of retinal cells or the retina and its supporting layers. Once a hole forms, more fluid collects and the detachment spreads. Patients experience floating spots and flashes of light when the eye moves due to random stimulation of light receptors. Causes include trauma to the head or eye, tumours (Am. tumors), haemorrhage (Am. hemorrhage) and cataract surgery. If left untreated, the retina may detach completely and cause total blindness in the affected eye. Retinal detachment is more common in patients with myopia.

Retinopathy

Diabetic retinopathy occurs in Type I and Type II diabetes mellitus and is characterized by small haemorrhages (Am. hemorrhages) and microaneurysms in retinal blood vessels that disrupt the supply of oxygen to the photoreceptors. The eye responds by building new abnormal blood vessels that can block vision and cause retinal detachment. Over a long period, diabetes mellitus may result in degeneration of the retina and permanent blindness.

Vascular retinopathy occurs when the central retinal artery or vein becomes blocked, causing sudden pain and unilateral loss of vision. Arterial occlusion is often due to an embolism. Venous occlusion is usually associated with arteriosclerosis or with venous thrombosis at another site. The retinal veins become distended, and retinal haemorrhage occurs.

Strabismus (squint)

A manifest (visible) condition in which the visual axes of the eyes are misaligned, and one eye deviates from the point of fixation when uncovered. This gives one the appearance of being cross-eyed because the eyes fail to move together. (The visual axis of the eye is an imaginary line passing from the object being looked at to the fovea centralis of the retina.)

Stye (hordeolum)

A stye is an acute bacterial infection of sebaceous or tarsal glands at the eyelid margin. The most common infectious organism is *Staphylococcus aureus*. Infection of the tarsal glands (meibomian glands) may block their ducts leading to the formation of a cyst called a chalazion that may damage the cornea.

Trachoma

A chronic inflammation of the eye caused by the coccoid bacterium *Chlamydia trachomatis*, also called granular conjunctivitis or Egyptian ophthalmia. In this condition, fibrous tissue forms in the conjunctiva and cornea leading to eyelid deformity and blindness. It is common in tropical regions where it is spread by flies and communal use of washing water, towels and clothing.

Associated words

Accommodation adjustment of the lens of the eye for viewing objects at different distances

Binocular vision blending the separate images from each eye into one composite image

Blind spot the area of the optic disc where the optic nerve fibres exit the eye and where there are no light-sensitive cells (Am. fibers)

Colour blindness the inability to see the difference between colours in the usual way, eg, red–green colour blindness (Am. color)

Cone a light-sensitive retinal receptor cell that provides sharp visual acuity and colour vision (Am. color)

Convergence turning of the eyes inwards so that they are both 'aimed' towards a near object being viewed

Dilation the act of temporarily enlarging the pupil with mydriatics to improve visualization of the interior of the eye

Drusen Yellow or white extracellular deposits that accumulate under the retina; they are composed of fat and protein, and the presence of numerous drusen is often a sign of age-related macular degeneration (singular druse)

Dry eye a condition that occurs when the eyes do not produce enough tears to keep the eye moist and comfortable

Ectropion the turning outward of the margin of the eyelid

Entropion the turning inward of the margin of the eyelid

Enucleation the removal of an eye

Epiphora persistent overflow of tears due to obstruction in the lacrimal passages

Esotropia a condition of eye misalignment in which one eye deviates towards the nose (inward) whilst the other fixates normally

Exotropia a condition of eye misalignment in which one eye deviates away from nose (outward) whilst the other fixates normally

Floaters Particles that float in the vitreous and cast shadows on the retina seen as moving spots or streaks

Fundus the furthest point at the back of the eye visible when viewed through the pupil with an ophthalmoscope

Hemianopsia condition of decreased vision or blindness in half the visual field of one or both eyes, usually on one side of the vertical midline

Hippus alternate contraction and dilation of the pupils seen in some nervous disorders

Hyphema haemorrhage within the anterior chamber of the eye (Am. hemorrhage)

Intraocular lens a plastic lens that is implanted into the lens capsule to replace the eye's natural lens

Intraocular pressure the fluid pressure inside the eye (tension) or the assessment of pressure inside the eye with a tonometer

Night blindness nyctalopia, a condition in which vision is weak or completely lost in dim light

Nystagmus involuntary, rapid movement of the eyeball

Patching covering an amblyopic patient's preferred eye, to improve vision in the other eye

Photophobia condition of abnormal intolerance of light

Pinguecula a small, yellow patch of connective tissue on the conjunctiva usually occurring in old age

Pterygium a wing-like membrane growing inwards from the conjunctiva over the cornea

Refraction a test to determine the refractive power of the eye; also, the bending of light as it passes from one medium into another

Rod a light-sensitive, specialized retinal receptor cell that works at low light levels (night vision)

Tunnel vision a condition in which visual fields are severely constricted and the patient lacks any peripheral vision

Visual acuity the clarity of vision, how well a person sees

Visual field the entire area that a person can see including peripheral vision

Now try the word check

WORD CHECK

This self-check exercise lists all the word components used in this unit. First, write down the meaning of as many word components as you can. Then, check your answers using the Exercise Guide and Quick Reference box or the Glossary of Word Components (pp. 383–410).

Prefixes

a-

ambly-

an-

bin-

dia-

diplo-

dys-

em-

en-

ex-

hemi-

hyper-

iso-

mono-

ortho-

pan-

presby-

uni-

xero-

Combining forms of word roots

aden/o

blast/o

blenn/o

blephar/o

choroid/o

chromat/o

conjunctiv/o

cor/e/o

cycl/o

cyst/o

dacry/o

electr/o

goni/o

helc/o

Ir/o

irid/o

kerat/o

lacrim/o

lith/o

-motor-

myc/o

my/o

my- (from myein)

nas/o

neur/o

ocul/o

ophthalm/o

optic/o

opt/o

papill/o

phak/o, phac/o

pupill/o

py/o

retin/o

rhin/o

scler/o

scot/o

sten/o

ton/o

uve/o

Suffixes

-al

-algia

-cele

-centesis

-chalasis

-conus

-desis

-dialysis

-ectasis

-ectomy

-erysis

-gram

-graph

-graphy

-gyric

-ia

-itis

-kinesis

-logist

-malacia

-meter

-metrist

-metry

-mileusis

-nyxis

-oedema
(Am. -edema)

-oma

-opia

-osis

-pathy

-pexy

-phobia

-plasty

-plegia

-ptosis

-rrhaphy

-rrhoea
(Am. -rrhea)

-schisis

-sclerosis

-scope

-scopy

-spasm

-synechia

-thermy

-tome

-tomy

NOW TRY THE SELF-ASSESSMENT

SELF-ASSESSMENT

Test 9A

Below are some combining forms that refer to the anatomy of the eye. Indicate which parts of the eye they refer to by putting a number from the diagrams (Figs 61 and 62) next to each word:

(a) irid/o

(b) scler/o

(c) pupill/o

(d) lacrim/o

(e) blephar/o

(f) phac/o

(g) papill/o

(h) retin/o

(i) kerat/o

(j) ophthalmoneur/o

Score

10

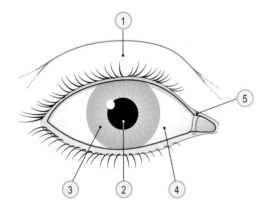

Figure 61   The eye.

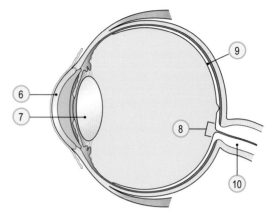

Figure 62   Sagittal section through the eye.

Test 9B

Prefixes and suffixes

Match each meaning in Column C with a prefix or suffix in Column A by inserting the appropriate number in Column B.

Column A	Column B	Column C
(a) ambly-		1. dragging / drawing / sucking out
(b) -chalasis		2. splitting
(c) -dialysis		3. swelling (due to fluid)
(d) diplo-		4. one (i)
(e) -erysis		5. one (ii)
(f) -graph		6. person who measures
(g) -gyric		7. old man, old age
(h) hemi-		8. all
(i) -kinesis		9. condition of sticking together
(j) -metrist		10. suturing/stitching
(k) -mileusis		11. condition of vision (defective)
(l) mono-		12. dulled /made dim
(m) -oedema (Am. -edema)		13. pertaining to a turning or circular movement

Column A	Column B	Column C
(n) -opia		14. instrument that records
(o) pan-		15. movement
(p) presby-		16. to carve
(q) -rrhaphy		17. slackening or loosening
(r) -schisis		18. separating
(s) -synechia		19. double
(t) uni-		20. half

Score

20

Test 9C

Combining forms of word roots

Match each meaning in Column C with a combining form of a word root in Column A by inserting the appropriate number in Column B.

Column A	Column B	Column C
(a) blephar/o		1. cone (shaped)
(b) choroid/o		2. cornea
(c) chromat/o		3. optic disc
(d) conjunctiv/o		4. iris (rainbow)
(e) -conus		5. pupil
(f) cycl/o		6. sight/vision
(g) dacry/o		7. pigmented area of eye (uvea)
(h) helc/o		8. retina
(i) irid/o		9. colour
(j) kerat/o		10. ulcer
(k) lacrim/o		11. lens
(l) ocul/o		12. ciliary body
(m) ophthalm/o		13. darkness/blind spot
(n) optic/o		14. choroid
(o) papill/o		15. eye (i)
(p) phak/o		16. eye (ii)
(q) pupill/o		17. eyelid
(r) retin/o		18. conjunctiva

Column A	Column B	Column C
(s) scotom/o		19. tear (i)
(t) uve/o		20. tear (ii)

Score

20

Test 9D

Write the meaning of:

(a) ophthalmoplasty

(b) retinopexy

(c) dacryopyorrhoea (Am. dacryopyorrhea)

(d) sclero-iritis

(e) oculomotor nerve

Score

5

Test 9E

Build words that mean:

(a) visual examination of the eye

(b) inflammation of the eyelid

(c) any disease of the cornea

(d) an instrument used to view the retina

(e) splitting of the iris

Score

5

Check answers to Self-Assessment Tests on page 362.

UNIT **10**
THE EAR

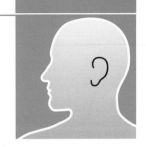

OBJECTIVES

Once you have completed Unit 10, you should be able to do the following:

- understand the meaning of medical words relating to the ear
- build medical words relating to the ear
- associate medical terms with their anatomical position
- understand common medical abbreviations relating to the ear

EXERCISE GUIDE

Use this list of word components and their meanings to complete the word exercises in this unit.

Prefixes

bin-	two of each / double
endo-	within/inside
macro-	large
micro-	small

Roots / Combining forms

electr/o	electrical
laryng/o	larynx
myc/o	fungus
pharyng/o	pharynx
py/o	pus
rhin/o	nose
ten/o	tendon

Suffixes

-al	pertaining to
-algia	condition of pain
-ar	pertaining to
-centesis	puncture to remove fluid
-eal	pertaining to
-ectomy	removal of
-emphraxis	blocking/stopping up
-genic	pertaining to formation / originating in
-gram	X-ray tracing/picture/recording
-graphy	technique of recording/making an X-ray
-ia	condition of
-itis	inflammation of
-logy	study of
-meter	measuring instrument
-metry	process of measuring
-osis	abnormal condition/disease / abnormal increase
-plasty	surgical repair/reconstruction
-rrhea (Am.)	excessive discharge/flow
-rrhoea	excessive discharge/flow (Am. -rrhea)
-sclerosis	condition of hardening
-scope	an instrument used to view/examine
-scopy	technique of viewing/examining
-stomy	formation of an opening / an opening
-tome	cutting instrument
-tomy	incision into

ANATOMY EXERCISE

When you have finished Word Exercises 1 to 14, look at the word components listed below. Complete Fig. 63 by writing the appropriate combining form on each line. (You can check their meanings in the Quick Reference box on p. 154.)

Auricul/o	Mastoid/o	Salping/o
Cochle/o	Myring/o	Tympan/o
Labyrinth/o	Ot/o	Vestibul/o

The ear

The ear is a major sense organ concerned with two important functions:

1. hearing
2. balance

The ear provides an auditory input into the brain. Sound waves in the air cause vibrations in the ear drum, and these are transmitted to the fluid-filled cochlea in the inner ear. The cochlea is the organ of hearing and contains special receptor cells that generate nerve impulses in response to sound. Nerve impulses from the cochlea are relayed via sensory neurons to auditory areas in the brain where they are interpreted as sounds. The possession of two ears enables us to sense the direction of sound.

The vestibular apparatus of the inner ear contains receptors that detect changes in velocity and position of the body. Sensory impulses from the vestibular apparatus are relayed via sensory neurons to centres in the cerebellum and other regions of the brain where they are used in the neural processes that allow us to maintain our balance and upright posture.

Use the Exercise Guide at the beginning of this unit to complete Word Exercises 1 to 14, unless you are asked to work without it.

Root

Ot

(*From Greek word* **ous**, *meaning ear*.)

Combining forms   Ot/o

Word Exercise 1

Using your Exercise Guide, find the meaning of -logy, -osis, py/o, -sclerosis and -scope; then build words that mean:

(a) the study of the ear

(b) instrument to view the ear (see Fig. 64)

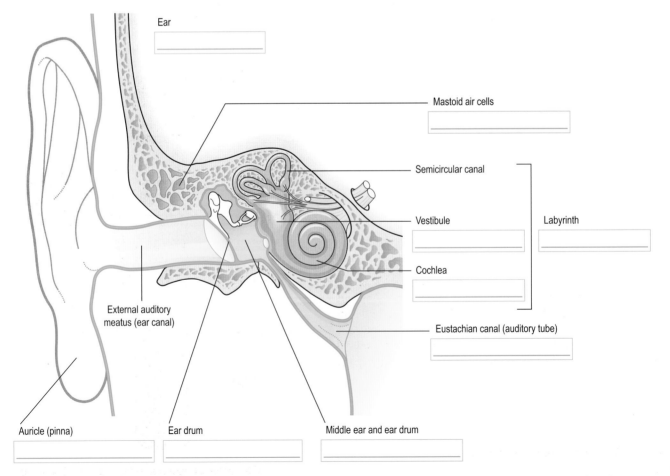

Figure 63   Section through the ear.

(c) condition of hardening of
the ear

(An inherited bone disorder that leads to progressive
hearing loss. Conductive deafness results from hard bone
formation around the footplate of the stapes, reducing its
ability to transmit vibrations across the middle ear to the
oval window.)

(d) condition of pus in the ear

Using your Exercise Guide, find the meaning of:

(e) **ot/o**/scopy

(f) **ot/o**/rhin/o/laryng/o/logy

(g) **ot/o**/myc/osis

(h) **ot/o**/py/o/rrhoea (Am.
ot/o/py/o/rrhea)

(i) micr/**ot**/ia

(j) macr/**ot**/ia

The ear can be divided into three areas, the external, middle
and inner ear. Infection and inflammation (**ot**itis) can occur in
any of these areas. The following terms are used to describe the
position of the inflammation:

Otitis externa
inflammation of the external ear
Otitis media
inflammation of the middle ear
Otitis interna
inflammation of the inner ear

Infection commonly begins in the middle ear because it is
connected to the **nasopharynx** by a short tube known as
the **eustachian tube** (**auditory tube** or **pharyngotympanic
tube**). This tube functions to equalize the pressure on either
side of the ear drum by allowing air into the middle ear but,
in doing so, it also provides an entrance for microorganisms
from the nose. See otitis in the Pathology Notes on page
155.

Root

Aur

(*From a Latin word* **auris**, *meaning ear.*)

Combining forms   Aur/i

Without using your Exercise Guide, build a word that means:

(a) an instrument used to
view the ear (see Fig. 64)

Viewing of the ear canal and tympanic membrane is
improved by using an **aural speculum** (Fig. 65), a device
that is inserted into the external ear before examining with
an **auriscope**.

The auriscope is used to examine the external ear canal
and the ear membrane. Occasionally, the ear canal can
become blocked by excessive amounts of wax produced
by the ceruminous glands in its lining. Earwax (cerumen)
can be removed by washing the ear with warm water using
an aural syringe (Fig. 66) or using wax solvents to bring
about ceruminolysis.

Using your Exercise Guide, find the meaning of:

(b) bin/**aur**/al

(c) end/**aur**/al

The Latin word *auricula* refers to the projecting part of the
external ear called the auricle or pinna (plural pinnae).

(d) bin/**auricul**/ar

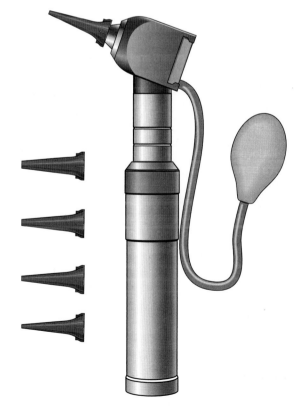

Figure 64   Otoscope/ auriscope. (Adapted from Dorland's
Illustrated Medical Dictionary, 32nd Edition, Saunders, 2011.)

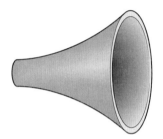

Figure 65   Aural speculum.

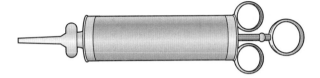

Figure 66   Aural syringe.

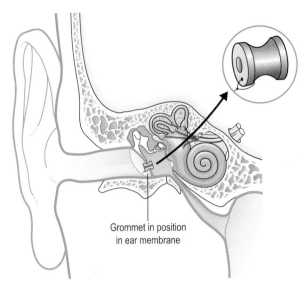

Grommet in position
in ear membrane

Figure 67   A grommet.

Root

Myring

(*A New Latin word* **myringa**, *meaning membrane. Here myring/o means the tympanic membrane or ear drum.*)

Combining forms   Myring/o

Word Exercise 3

Using your Exercise Guide find the meaning of -tome and -tomy; then build words that mean:

(a) incision into the ear
    membrane (this allows air
    to enter to aid drainage)

(b) instrument used to cut the
    ear membrane

Without using your Exercise Guide, build a word that means:

(c) abnormal condition of
    fungal infection of the ear
    membrane

Root

Tympan

(*From a Greek word* **tympanon**, *meaning drum. Here tympan/o means the tympanum, the name for the cavity of the middle ear and tympanic membrane combined.*)

Combining forms   Tympan/o

Word Exercise 4

Using your Exercise Guide, build words that mean:

(a) reconstructive surgery
    of the tympanum

(b) puncture of the tympa-
    num to remove fluid

(c) opening into the
    tympanum

Without using your Exercise Guide, write the meaning of:

(d) **tympan**/itis

(e) **tympan/o**/tomy

Sometimes the ear membrane is surgically punctured to assist the drainage of fluid from the middle ear (as in glue ear). Once an opening is made in the membrane, fluid drains through the eustachian tube (auditory tube) into the nasopharynx. A small plastic grommet (Fig. 67) can be fixed into the membrane to equalize the air pressure on either side of the membrane and allow drainage through the eustachian tube for an extended period. The grommet eventually falls out and the membrane heals.

Root

Salping

(*From Greek* **salpigx**, *meaning trumpet tube. Here salping/o means eustachian tube, the trumpet-shaped tube that connects the middle ear to the nasopharynx. The eustachian tube is also called the auditory tube or pharyngotympanic tube.*)

Combining forms   Salping/o

Word Exercise 5

Using your Exercise Guide, find the meaning of:

(a) **salping**/emphraxis [ ]

(b) **salping/o**/pharyng/eal [ ]

Within the middle ear, we find the smallest bones in the body, the ear ossicles (Fig. 68). These are named the **malleus**, **incus** and **stapes**. Their function is to transmit vibrations from the tympanic membrane to the oval window of the inner ear. Behind the oval window is a fluid-filled structure known as the **cochlea**, the organ of hearing. Within the cochlea are sensory hair cells (receptors) that respond to vibrations in the fluid by producing nerve impulses. The auditory area of the brain interprets nerve impulses from the cochlea as sound, enabling us to hear.

Root

Stapedi

(*From a Latin word* **stapes**, *meaning stirrup. Here stapedi/o means the stapes, the stirrup-shaped ear ossicle.*)

Combining forms   Staped/i/o

Word Exercise 6

Using your Exercise Guide, find the meaning of -ectomy, and then build a word that means:

(a) removal of the stapes [ ]

Using your Exercise Guide, find the meaning of:

(b) **stapedi/o**/ten/o/ tomy [ ]

Root

Malle

(*From a Latin word* **malleus**, *meaning hammer. Here malle/o means the malleus, the hammer-shaped ear ossicle.*)

Combining form   Malle/o

Word Exercise 7

Without using your Exercise Guide, write the meaning of:

(a) **malle/o**/tomy [ ]

Root

Incud

(*From a Latin word* **incus**, *meaning anvil. Here incud/o means the incus, the anvil-shaped ear ossicle.*)

Combining forms   Incud/o

Word Exercise 8

Without using your Exercise Guide, write the meaning of:

(a) **incud/o**/mall/eal [ ]

(b) **incud/o**/stapedi/al [ ]

(c) malle/o/**incud**/al [ ]

ANATOMY EXERCISE

Write the appropriate combining form for each ossicle on the lines of Fig. 68. Sometimes the small ear bones are referred to in a more general way, using **ossicul/o**, to mean ossicles, eg, **ossicul**ectomy for removal of one or more ossicles or **ossiculo**tomy for incision into the ear ossicles. The ossicles can be replaced by a plastic prosthesis that will transmit vibrations to the inner ear and restore hearing.

Root

Cochle

(*From a Latin word* **cochlea**, *meaning snail. Here cochle/o means the cochlea, the snail-shaped anterior bony labyrinth of the inner ear.*)

Combining form   Cochle/o

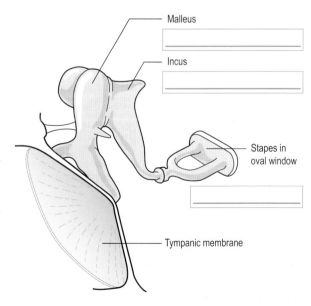

Malleus [ ]

Incus [ ]

Stapes in oval window

[ ]

Tympanic membrane

Figure 68   The ear ossicles.

Word Exercise 9

Using your Exercise Guide, find the meaning of electr/o, -graphy and -stomy; then build words that mean:

(a) an opening into the cochlea

(b) technique of recording the cochlea's electrical activity

Root

Labyrinth

(*From a Greek word* **labyrinthos**, *meaning maze or anything twisted or spiral-shaped. Here labyrinth/o means the labyrinth of the inner ear.*)

Combining form   Labyrinth/o

The inner ear consists of bony and membranous labyrinths. The bony labyrinth is a series of canals in the temporal bone filled with fluid. It consists of the cochlea (organ of hearing), vestibule and semicircular canals (organs of equilibrium).

The membranous labyrinth lies within the bony labyrinth and is also filled with fluid. Distension of the membranous labyrinth with excess fluid gives rise to **Meniere** disease, symptoms of which include vertigo (dizziness) and deafness (see the Pathology Notes on page 155).

The portions of the inner ear concerned with balance are collectively known as the **vestibular apparatus**.

Word Exercise 10

Without using your Exercise Guide, build words that mean:

(a) inflammation of a labyrinth

(b) removal of a labyrinth

Root

Vestibul

(*From the Latin word* **vestibulum**, *meaning entrance. Here vestibul/o means the vestibule, the oval cavity in the middle of the bony labyrinth.*)

Combining form   Vestibul/o

Word Exercise 11

Without using your Exercise Guide, write the meaning of:

(a) **vestibul/o**/tomy

Using your Exercise Guide, find the meaning of:

(b) **vestibul/o**/genic

Root

Mast

(*From a Greek word* **mastos**, *meaning breast. Here mastoid/o means the mastoid process or mastoid bone containing nipple-shaped air cells or air spaces. The mastoid process is a bone located behind the external ear.*)

Combining form   Mastoid/o

Word Exercise 12

Using your Exercise Guide, look up the meaning of -algia and build a word that means:

(a) condition of pain in the mastoid region

Without using your Exercise Guide and beginning with the underlined root, build words that mean:

(b) incision into the <u>mastoid</u> bone

(c) removal of tissue from the <u>mastoid</u> process

(d) inflammation of the <u>tympanum</u> and mastoid process

Root

Audi

(*From a Latin word* **audire**, *meaning to hear.*)

Combining forms   Audi/o

Word Exercise 13

Without using your Exercise Guide, build a word that means:

(a) the study of hearing

Using your Exercise Guide, find the meaning of:

(b) **audio**/meter

(c) **audio**/gram

(d) **audio**/metry

Note. An **audiometrist** is a technician specialized in the study of hearing. He or she tests and measures a patient's hearing ability (-*ist* meaning a specialist who...).

Medical equipment and clinical procedures

Review the names of all instruments and clinical procedures mentioned in this unit before completing Exercise 14.

Word Exercise 14

Match each description in Column C with a term in Column A by placing the appropriate number in Column B.

Column A	Column B	Column C
(a) audiometer		1. technique of measuring hearing
(b) audiometry		2. an instrument for viewing the ear
(c) aural speculum		3. technique of viewing the ear
(d) auriscope		4. a device for removing wax from the ear
(e) otoscopy		5. a device to aid drainage of fluid from the ear
(f) aural syringe		6. an instrument that measures hearing
(g) grommet		7. a device that holds the ear canal open

Other procedures used to investigate and treat the ear besides those mentioned in the word exercises include:

Audiometric testing An audiometer is a device that delivers 'pure tones' at different frequencies (Hertz) from low to high at different intensities (decibels) to determine a patient's hearing loss for each frequency. Air conduction testing uses earphones to send sounds through the auditory canal to the middle ear and inner ear. The patient indicates when they can hear sounds that are played to them during the test, and the data collected is presented as an audiogram indicating hearing ability at each frequency.

Cochlear implant surgery A cochlear implant is an electronic system that stimulates the auditory nerve in the cochlea. It can give a sensation of sound to a person who is profoundly deaf due to damaged sensory hair cells in the cochlea. An implant has two main components: an external component consisting of a microphone, speech processor and transmitter coil held behind the ear and an internal component consisting of a receiver/stimulator package surgically implanted into the mastoid bone. The electrical signals received from the external components are delivered to electrodes placed within the cochlea; the electrodes stimulate cells that innervate fibres (Am. fibers) of the auditory nerve, giving the sensation of hearing.

Tuning fork test Weber test–A vibrating tuning fork is placed in the middle of the forehead; the loudness of the sound in each ear is equal if hearing is normal. In patients with conductive deafness the sound is louder in the weaker ear; if the sound is louder in the better ear, it is likely to be sensorineural hearing loss.

Rinne test–A vibrating tuning fork is placed on the mastoid process behind the ear, and the patient indicates when they can no longer hear the sound. The still vibrating tuning fork is then moved to approximately 20 mm from the external auditory canal, and the patient is asked to indicate when they can no longer hear the sound. With normal hearing, air conduction should be greater than bone conduction, so the sound should be heard when they can no longer hear it against the mastoid; this is a positive Rinne test. A negative test is when the sound cannot be heard again, and bone conduction is therefore greater than air conduction; this indicates that something is inhibiting the passage of sound waves from the ear canal through the middle ear apparatus and into the cochlea (ie, conductive deafness is present).

ANATOMY EXERCISE

Now complete the Anatomy Exercise on page 148.

CASE HISTORY 10

The object of this exercise is to understand words associated with a patient's medical history.

To complete the exercise:

- Read through the passage on otitis media with effusion; unfamiliar words are underlined, and you can find their meaning using the Word Help.

- Write the meaning of the medical terms shown in bold print on the lines that follow the Word Help.

Otitis media with effusion (OME, glue ear)

Miss J, a 5-year-old child, presented to her GP with persistent **otalgia**. She had a previous history of acute otitis media with perforation in the left ear and had been treated with broad-spectrum antibiotics. Her parents were concerned that her hearing and speech were impaired. Miss J's nursery teacher reported that she was inattentive in class and seemed in a world of her own. Her mother had also noticed her snoring and had been worried about her breathing during a recent cold. Her tonsils were very large, she had a poor nasal airway, and she was breathing through her mouth; these are signs that are consistent with hypertrophy of the adenoid tissue.

Pneumatic **otoscopy** by her GP revealed <u>bilateral</u> otitis media with <u>effusion</u> (non<u>suppurative</u> OME), and she was referred to the **audiometrist** for a hearing assessment. She cooperated well and a pure-tone **audiogram** was obtained, indicating a mild loss of 20–30 dB in hearing threshold. Over the next 6 months, she received several courses of antibiotic therapy. Initially, there were signs of improvement, but her condition did not resolve, and she was referred to the <u>paediatric</u> **otology** clinic (Am. pediatric).

The consultant <u>otologist</u> confirmed the diagnosis. Her tympanic membranes were dull, retracted and lacked mobility. Fluid containing air bubbles was visible in the right ear, and she had a negative <u>Rinne test</u>.

Tympanometry revealed a flat <u>tympanogram</u> characteristic of glue ear with reduced <u>compliance</u> and a negative middle ear pressure. Her audiogram indicated <u>conductive deafness</u> across the entire frequency range of 35 to 40 dB.

Miss J underwent an <u>adenoidectomy</u> and <u>anterior</u>, bilateral **myringotomy** under general anaesthesia. A thick, <u>mucoid</u> secretion was <u>aspirated</u> from both ears and <u>grommets</u> (**tympanostomy** tubes) inserted into her tympanic membranes. Six months later the grommets were still in position, and her hearing and speech were much improved.

Word Help

acute symptoms/signs of short duration

adenoid resembling a gland (here it refers to the adenoids seen in the nasopharynx of children)

adenoidectomy removal of the adenoids (an enlarged pharyngeal tonsil)

anterior pertaining to towards the front

aspirated withdrawn by suction of fluid

bilateral pertaining to two sides

broad-spectrum affecting a wide range (of infective organisms)

compliance quality of yielding to pressure (here referring to the movement of the ear drum in relation to pressure)

conductive deafness deafness caused by impairment of conduction of sound waves through the normal route

decibel unit used for measurement of intensity of sound

effusion a fluid discharge into a part/escape of fluid into an enclosed space

GP general practitioner (family doctor)

grommet plastic tube inserted into the ear drum to ventilate the middle ear

hypertrophy increase in size of cells in a tissue (above normal growth/nourishment)

mucoid resembling mucus

otitis media condition of inflammation of the middle ear

otologist a specialist who studies the ear and its disorders

paediatric (Am. pediatric) pertaining to medical care and treatment of children

perforation a hole made through a membrane or similar tissue

pneumatic pertaining to air (pneumatic otoscopy refers to viewing the ear membrane whilst stimulating it with a puff of air to observe its movement)

Rinne test a test using a tuning fork for diagnosis of conductive deafness

suppurative having a tendency to produce pus

tympanogram a recording of the compliance and impedance of the tympanic membrane

Now write the meaning of the following words from the Case History without using your dictionary lists:

(a) otalgia

(b) otoscopy

(c) audiometrist

(d) audiogram

(e) otology

(f) tympanometry

(g) myringotomy

(h) tympanostomy

(Answers to the Case History exercise are given in the Answers to Word Exercises on page 346.)

Quick Reference

Combining forms relating to the ear:

Audi/o	hearing
Aur/i	ear
Auricul/o	pinna (the part of the ear outside the head) (plural pinnae)
Cochle/o	cochlea
Incud/o	incus (an ear ossicle)
Labyrinth/o	labyrinth (of inner ear)
Malle/o	malleus (an ear ossicle)
Mastoid/o	mastoid process / mastoid air cells

Myring/o	ear membrane (drum)
Ossicul/o	ossicle
Ot/o	ear
Salping/o	eustachian / auditory tube
Stapedi/o	stapes (an ear ossicle)
Tympan/o	ear drum / middle ear
Vestibul/o	vestibular apparatus (of inner ear)

Abbreviations

Some common abbreviations related to the ear are listed next. Note that some are not standard, and their meaning may vary from one healthcare setting to another. There is a more extensive list for reference on page 369.

AC	air conduction
AD	auris dextra (right ear)
AOM	acute otitis media
AS	auris sinistra (left ear)
ASOM	acute suppurative otitis media
CSOM	chronic suppurative otitis media
dB	decibel
EENT	eyes, ears, nose and throat
ENT	ear, nose and throat
ETD	eustachian tube dysfunction
ETF	eustachian tube function
OE	otitis externa
OM	otitis media
PE tube	pressure equalization tube
SOM	serous otitis media

Pathology notes

Cholesteatoma

Cholesteatoma is an uncommon but serious condition in which skin cells and purulent debris (including cholesterol) accumulate in the middle ear. The condition may be a result of chronic otitis media (middle ear infection) with perforation of the eardrum. During the healing process, skin from the ear canal grows into the middle ear and may damage the ossicles and surrounding bone. If left untreated, it can erode the roof of the middle ear and lead to inner ear infection and possibly meningitis. The cholesteatoma is removed by mastoidectomy or through the eardrum, but the procedure may result in conduction deafness.

Deafness

Hearing impairment can be classified into two main categories:

Conductive deafness due to impaired transmission of sound waves through the external and middle ear to the sensory receptors of the inner ear (the conduction pathway).

Sensorineural deafness also known as **nerve deafness** or **perceptive deafness** is the result of disease in the cochlea, vestibulocochlear nerve (cranial nerve VIII) or in the area of the brain concerned with hearing. Those affected usually perceive sound but cannot discriminate between different frequencies or understand what is being said. Sometimes patients have both conductive and sensorineural deafness in one ear; it is then known as **mixed deafness**.

Glue ear

Glue ear is an accumulation of thick, mucoid fluid behind the tympanic membrane in the middle that impairs hearing. Persistent glue ear is most common in children and is often accompanied by enlargement of the adenoids; it usually develops following an upper respiratory tract infection. Glue ear is also known as otitis media with effusion or as serous otitis media (see Otitis below).

Meniere disease

Meniere disease is a chronic inner ear disease characterized by recurrent tinnitus, deafness and vertigo; in 85% of cases, only one ear is affected. Nausea, vomiting and nystagmus (jerky eye movements) often accompany vertigo. The symptoms are caused by an increase in the amount of fluid in the membranous labyrinth of the inner ear. The accumulating fluid damages the part of the ear that controls balance (the labyrinth) and sometimes the organ of hearing (the cochlea) as well. The cause of the increased fluid accretion is unknown, but it tends to occur after 50 years of age.

Otitis

Otitis is an inflammation of the ear often caused by infection in one of its main regions:

Otitis externa or *external otitis* is usually due to an infection in the ear canal (external auditory meatus) often caused by the bacterium *Staphylococcus aureus*. More generalized inflammation may be due to fungi or allergic reactions to shampoos, hair dyes and dandruff.

Otitis media is an inflammation of the middle ear cavity between the eardrum and inner ear. *Acute otitis media* is usually caused by spread of microorganisms from an upper respiratory infection through the auditory tube or through a ruptured tympanic membrane. Infection leads to the accumulation of pus in the middle ear causing the eardrum to bulge and rupture; when the eardrum bursts, the purulent material is discharged. The condition is common in children and is accompanied by severe earache.

Serous otitis media, also known as *glue ear* or *secretory otitis media,* is a condition in which fluid collects in the cavity of the middle ear. It can be caused by blockage in the auditory tube by enlargement of the adenoids, swelling in the pharynx, tumours (Am. tumors), barotrauma and untreated otitis media. When the auditory tube becomes blocked, air in the middle ear is absorbed and a negative pressure develops causing the eardrum to bulge inwards. The reduced pressure causes a clear serous fluid to form in the cavity of the middle ear. In adults the condition causes discomfort and conductive hearing loss, but in young children speech development is also delayed and, as a result, behavioural problems may develop.

Otitis interna or *labyrinthitis* is the inflammation of the vestibular structures in the internal ear. The condition causes vertigo and is almost always caused by bacterial or viral infection. Other causes include head injury, development of cholesteatoma and inadequately treated otitis media.

Presbycusis

Presbycusis is a form of hearing impairment associated with the aging process. Degeneration of the sensory cells that detect sounds results in sensorineural deafness; this means the patient has difficulty perceiving certain frequencies. Perception of high frequencies is impaired first and later low frequencies. Patients have difficulty in following conversations as some frequencies are not perceived.

Tinnitus

Tinnitus is a ringing, buzzing or whistling noise heard in the ear in the absence of noise in the environment. In this condition the acoustic nerve transmits nerve impulses to the brain in the absence of vibrations from external sources. The condition is a symptom of many ear disorders including presbycusis, otosclerosis and exposure to continuous loud noise.

Vertigo

Vertigo is a sensation that one's self or one's surroundings are rotating or spinning in any plane. It results from a disturbance of the semicircular canals and/or their nerves in the inner ear. Labyrinthitis and Meniere disease can cause sudden vertigo that is often accompanied by vomiting and unsteadiness.

Vestibular schwannoma

Also called acoustic neuroma, this is a benign, primary, intracranial brain tumour (Am. tumor) that arises from the myelin forming cells on the vestibulocochlear nerve (cranial nerve VIII). Symptoms include tinnitus, hearing loss, difficulty with balance, facial pain and headache. The tumour is slow growing and does not spread to other parts of the body; treatment is most often with microsurgery or radiosurgery to remove or destroy part of the tumour.

Associated words

Acoustic relating to sound or hearing
Barotrauma trauma caused by environmental changes in air pressure, especially to the ear following an explosion
Decibel a unit used to express intensity of sound (loudness)
Dysequilibrium any disturbance of balance

Endolymph fluid of the membranous labyrinth of the inner ear
External auditory meatus an opening or passage into the ear (synonym external acoustic meatus, ear canal and auditory canal)
Hertz (Hz) a unit of frequency that is defined as one cycle per second. Human hearing is in the range of 20–20,000 Hz, though there is considerable variation between individuals
Hyperacusis condition of having an exceptionally acute sense of hearing
Hypoacusis condition of having a diminished sense of hearing
Otalgia condition of pain in the ear; earache
Otorrhoea (Am. Otorrhea) discharge or excessive flow from the ear, especially pus
Presbycusis bilateral hearing loss associated with aging
Suppurative the formation and discharge of pus
Threshold the decibel level of the softest sound one is able to hear

NOW TRY THE WORD CHECK

WORD CHECK

This self-check exercise lists all the word components used in this unit. First, write down the meaning of as many word components as you can. Then, check your answers using the Exercise Guide and Quick Reference box or the Glossary of Word Components (pp. 383–410).

Prefixes

bin-	
endo-	
macro-	
micro-	

Combining forms of word roots

audi/o	
aur/i	
auricul/o	
cochle/o	
electr/o	
incud/o	
labyrinth/o	
laryng/o	
malle/o	
mastoid/o	

myc/o	
myring/o	
ossicul/o	
ot/o	
pharyng/o	
py/o	
rhin/o	
salping/o	
stapedi/o	
ten/o	
tympan/o	
vestibul/o	

-sclerosis	
-scope	
-stomy	
-tome	
-tomy	

NOW TRY THE SELF-ASSESSMENT

Suffixes

-al	
-algia	
-ar	
-aural	
-centesis	
-eal	
-ectomy	
-emphraxis	
-externa	
-genic	
-gram	
-ia	
-interna	
-ist	
-itis	
-media	
-logy	
-meter	
-metry	
-osis	
-plasty	
-rrhoea (Am. -rrhea)	

SELF-ASSESSMENT

Test 10A

Next are some combining forms that refer to the anatomy of the ear. Indicate which part of the system they refer to by putting a number from the diagram (Fig. 69) next to each word.

(a) ot/o

(b) myring/o

(c) tympan/o

(d) nasopharyng/o

(e) ossicul/o

(f) labyrinth/o

(g) cochle/o

(h) mastoid/o

(i) salping/o

(j) vestibul/o

Score

10

Test 10B

Prefixes and suffixes

Match each meaning in Column C with a prefix or suffix in Column A by inserting the appropriate number in Column B.

Column A	Column B	Column C
(a) -al		1. incision into
(b) -ar		2. excessive flow / discharge
(c) -aural		3. external
(d) bin-		4. instrument that cuts
(e) -eal		5. condition of hardening
(f) -emphraxis		6. internal
(g) endo-		7. middle
(h) -externa		8. pertaining to (i)
(i) -gram		9. pertaining to (ii)
(j) -ia		10. pertaining to (iii)
(k) -interna		11. small
(l) macro-		12. in/within
(m) -media		13. abnormal condition / disease of
(n) -metry		14. pertaining to the ear
(o) micro-		15. picture/X-ray/ tracing
(p) -osis		16. two of each / double
(q) -rrhoea (Am. -rrhea)		17. condition of
(r) -sclerosis		18. large
(s) -tome		19. to block / stop up
(t) -tomy		20. measurement

Score

20

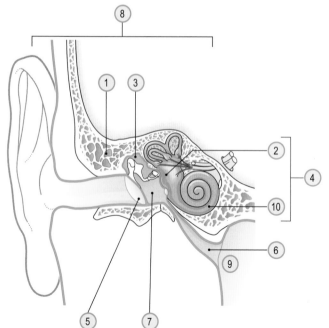

Figure 69   Section through the ear.

Test 10C

Combining forms of word roots

Match each meaning in Column C with a combining form of a word root in Column A by inserting the appropriate number in Column B.

Column A	Column B	Column C
(a) audi/o		1. stapes
(b) aur/i		2. larynx
(c) auricul/o		3. nose
(d) incud/o		4. eustachian tube
(e) labyrinth/o		5. ear (i)
(f) laryng/o		6. ear (ii)
(g) malle/o		7. pinna / part of the ear outside the head
(h) mastoid/o		8. ear drum / middle ear
(i) myc/o		9. vestibular apparatus
(j) myring/o		10. malleus
(k) ossicul/o		11. fungus
(l) ot/o		12. hearing
(m) pharyng/o		13. ear membrane
(n) py/o		14. tendon
(o) rhin/o		15. incus
(p) salping/o		16. pharynx
(q) stapedi/o		17. mastoid
(r) ten/o		18. ear bones / ossicles
(s) tympan/o		19. pus
(t) vestibul/o		20. labyrinth of inner ear

Score

20

Test 10D

Write the meaning of:

(a) otolaryngology

(b) tympanosclerosis

(c) stapediovestibular

(d) tympanomalleal

(e) mastoideocentesis

Score

5

Test 10E

Build words that mean:

(a) pertaining to the vestibule and cochlea

(b) removal of the ear membrane

(c) surgical repair of the ear

(d) condition of pain in the ear

(e) originating in the middle ear

Score

5

Check answers to Self-Assessment Tests on pages 362–363.

Test your recall of the meanings of word components in Units 6–10 by completing the appropriate self-assessment tests in Unit 22 on pages 326–328.

UNIT **11**
THE SKIN

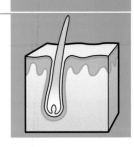

OBJECTIVES

Once you have completed Unit 11, you should be able to do the following:

* understand the meaning of medical words relating to the skin
* build medical words relating to the skin
* associate medical terms with their anatomical position
* understand common medical abbreviations relating to the skin

EXERCISE GUIDE

Use this list of word components and their meanings to complete the word exercises in this unit.

Prefixes

a-	without
an-	without/not
auto-	self
crypto-	hidden
dys-	difficult/painful
epi-	above/upon/on
hyper-	above/excessive
hypo-	below/deficient
intra-	within/inside
pachy-	thick
para-	beside/near
sub-	under/below
xantho-	yellow
xero-	dry

Roots / Combining forms

aden/o	gland
aesthe/s/i/o	sensation/sensitivity (Am. esthesi/o)
esthe/s/i/o (Am.)	sensation/sensitivity
lith/o	stone
motor	action
myc/o	fungus
phyt(e)	plant (fungus)
schiz/o	split/cleft

Suffixes

-al	pertaining to
-auxis	increase
-cyte	cell
-ia	condition of
-ic	pertaining to
-itis	inflammation of
-logist	specialist who studies
-lysis	breakdown/disintegration
-oma	tumour/swelling (Am. tumor)
-osis	abnormal condition / disease / abnormal increase
-phagia	condition of eating
-plasty	surgical repair/reconstruction
-poiesis	formation
-rrhexis	break/rupture
-rrhea (Am.)	excessive discharge/flow
-rrhoea	excessive discharge/flow (Am. -rrhea)
-schisis	splitting/parting/cleaving
-tic	pertaining to
-tome	cutting instrument
-trophy	nourishment/development
-tropic	pertaining to stimulating / affinity for

ANATOMY EXERCISE

When you have finished Word Exercises 1–9, look at the word components listed below. Complete Figure 70 by writing the appropriate combining form on each line; more than one component may relate to the same position. (You can check their meanings in the Quick Reference box on p. 168.)

Derm/o	Melan/o	Seb/o
Hidraden/o	Pil/o	Trich/o
Kerat/o		

The skin

The skin can be regarded as the largest organ in the body; it consists of two layers: the outer **epidermis** and the inner **dermis**. The skin protects us from the environment and plays a major role in thermoregulation. In its protective role, it prevents the body dehydrating, resists the invasion of microorganisms and provides protection from the harmful effects of ultraviolet light. Cells in the epidermis enable the surface of the skin to continuously regenerate, and the presence of elastic fibres and collagen fibres in the dermis make the skin tough and elastic.

Use the Exercise Guide at the beginning of this unit to complete Word Exercises 1–9, unless you are asked to work without it.

Root

Derm

(*From a Greek word* **derma**, *meaning skin.*)

Combining forms Derm/o, derm/a/t/o, *also used as the* suffix *-derma*

The medical specialty concerned with the diagnosis and treatment of skin disease is known as **dermatology**.

Word Exercise 1

Using your Exercise Guide, find the meaning of:

(a) **dermat**/osis _____

Actinic dermatoses are conditions in which the skin is abnormally sensitive to sunlight (from a Greek word *aktis*, meaning ray; they are also known as photodermatoses or solar keratoses).

(b) epi/**dermis** _____

The **epidermis** forms the outer layer of the body, and it functions to protect the underlying layer called the **dermis**. Note the dermis and epidermis form the skin; the underlying (subcutaneous) fatty tissue often studied with them is not regarded as part of the true skin.

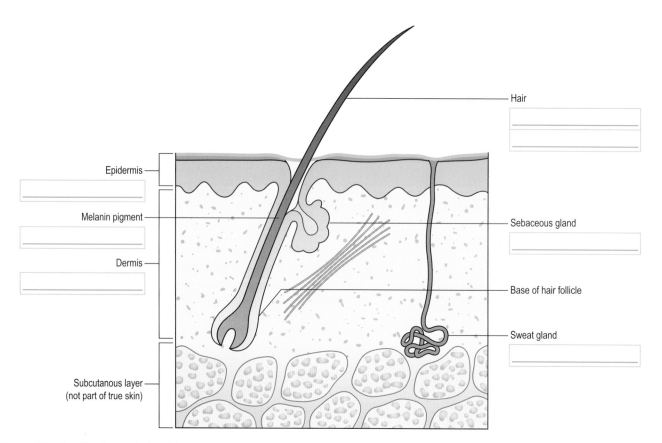

Figure 70 Section through the skin.

The epidermis can be subdivided into five distinct layers, the outermost forming a layer of tough dead cells (scales), known as the stratum corneum. At the surface, the cells of the epidermis fit together like the scales of a fish; for this reason, it is known as a stratified **squamous** epithelium (squamous from Latin *squama*, meaning scale of a fish or reptile). The word epithelium (combining form epitheli/o) refers to a type of tissue formed from one or more layers of cells that cover and line internal and external surfaces of the body. As the epidermis consists of many layers of cells, it is described as a stratified epithelium.

(c) **dermat/o**/phyte

(d) pachy/**derma**

(e) xanth/o/**derma**

(f) **dermat/o**/auto/plasty

(g) xer/o/**derm**/ia

(h) **dermat/o**/logist

Using your Exercise Guide look up -al, hypo-, -ic, intra-, myc/o, -osis, sub- and -tome; then build words that mean:

(i) abnormal condition of fungi in the skin (use dermat/o)

(j) an instrument to cut skin for grafts (use derm/a)

(k) pertaining to below the skin (use derm/a)

(l) pertaining to within the skin (use derm/a)

Note. There are a few words in use derived from *cutis*, the Latin for skin, for example cutaneous, pertaining to the skin (from cutane/o meaning skin and -ous meaning pertaining to). The word cuticle means a small skin (from cuti- meaning skin and -cle meaning small), but it is used to mean the narrow band of epidermis that extends from the nail wall onto the nail surface.

Root

Kerat

(*From a Greek word* **keras**, *meaning horn. Here kerat/o means the epidermis, the outer, horny layer of the skin. Note that kerat/o is also used to mean the cornea of the eye.*)

Combining form   Kerat/o

Word Exercise 2

Without using your Exercise Guide, write the meaning of:

(a) actinic **kerat**/osis (actinic means pertaining to the sun's rays)

Using your Exercise Guide, find the meaning of:

(b) hyper/**kerat/o**/tic

(c) **kerat**/oma

(d) **kerat/o**/lysis

Note. There is no way of telling whether a medical term containing the root *kerat* refers to the cornea or epidermis except by noting the context in which it is written.

The cells of the outer layer of the epidermis are said to be **keratinized** because they contain the waterproof protein **keratin** that gives the epidermis its ability to protect the underlying dermis. (The combining form **keratin/o** refers to the protein keratin.)

Other disorders of the epidermis include the following:

Ichthyosis

A condition in which there is abnormal keratinization, giving rise to a dry, scaly skin that has the appearance of fish skin (from Greek **ichthy/o**, meaning fish or fish-like).

Acanthosis

A condition of thickening of the prickle cell layer of the epidermis (**acanth/o** from Greek, meaning spike).

The skin appendages

The multiplication of cells in the basal layer of the epidermis gives rise to the appendages of the skin: hairs, sebaceous glands, sweat glands and nails. Here, we use terms associated with each appendage:

Root

Pil

(*From a Latin word* **pilus**, *meaning hair. Hairs grow from depressions in the epidermis and dermis known as hair follicles.*)

Combining form   Pil/o

Word Exercise 3

Using your Exercise Guide, find the meaning of:

(a) **pil/o**/motor nerve

(This nerve stimulates the arrector pili muscles to contract, causing erection of the hair in cold conditions.)

A technique known as electrolysis is used to destroy hairs permanently by heating the base of a hair to destroy its dividing cells. The heating is achieved by passing an electric current through the hair follicle. This technique is also used by beauty therapists for the removal of excess hair and is known as e**pil**ation (e- meaning out from, ie, the hair out of its follicle).

Hairs can also be removed by using a de**pil**atory paste that dissolves hair (de- meaning away). The hairs regrow following depilation as the base of the hair is not destroyed.

Alopecia or baldness may be hereditary, as in the case of male-pattern baldness, or due to disease or damage caused by drug treatment such as chemotherapy. (From a Greek word *alopex* meaning fox, the disease resembling the mange of foxes).

Root

Trich

(*From a Greek word* **trichos**, *meaning hair.*)

Combining form   Trich/o

Word Exercise 4

Without using your Exercise Guide, write the meaning of:

(a) **trich/o**/phyt/osis

(b) **trich**/osis

Using your Exercise Guide, find the meaning of:

(c) **trich/o**/aesthes/ia (Am. **trich/o**/esthes/ia)

(d) schiz/o/**trich**/ia

(e) **trich/o**/rrhexis

Root

Seb

(*From a Latin word* **sebum**, *meaning fat or grease. Here seb/o means sebum, the oily secretion of the sebaceous glands, or sebaceous gland.*)

Combining form   Seb/o

The sebaceous glands open directly on to the skin or more usually into the side of a hair follicle (a pilo**seb**aceous follicle). They produce an oily secretion known as sebum that lubricates and waterproofs the hair and skin. Sebum is mildly bacteriostatic and fungistatic, enabling the skin to resist infection.

Excessive production of sebum at puberty gives rise to **acne vulgaris**, a condition in which the skin becomes inflamed and develops pus-filled pimples.

Word Exercise 5

Using your Exercise Guide, find the meaning of:

(a) **seb/o**/rrhoea
    (Am. **seb/o**/rrhea)

(b) **seb/o**/lith

(c) **seb/o**/tropic

Root

Hidr

(*From a Greek word* **hidros**, *meaning sweat.*)

Combining form   Hidr/o

Word Exercise 6

Without using your Exercise Guide, write the meaning of:

(a) **hidr**/osis

(b) hyper/**hidr**/osis

Using your Exercise Guide, find the meaning of:

(c) **hidr/o**/poiesis

(d) an/**hidr**/osis

(e) **hidr**/aden/itis

Sweat glands are also known by their Latin name of sudoriferous glands (*sudor* meaning sweat, *ferous* meaning pertaining to carrying).

Root

Onych

(*From a Greek word* **onychos**, *meaning nail.*)

Combining form   Onych/o

Word Exercise 7

Using your Exercise Guide, find the meaning of:

(a) **onych/o**/crypt/osis

(b) **onych**/auxis

(c) **onych/o**/dys/trophy

(d) **onych**/a/trophy

(e) par/**onych**/ia

(f) **onych/o**/schisis

(g) **onych/o**/phagia

Without using your Exercise Guide, build words that mean:

(h) breaking down/
disintegration of nails

(In this condition, the nail comes away from the nail bed.)

(i) fungal condition of nails

(j) inflammation of nails (synonymous with **onych**ia)

Without using your Exercise Guide, write the meaning of:

(k) **onych/o**/rrhexis

(l) an/**onych**/ia

(m) pachy/**onych**/ia

Root

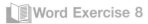

Melan

(*From a Greek word* **melas**, *meaning black. Here melan/o means melanin, a black pigment found in skin, hair and the choroid of the eye.*)

Combining form   *Melan/o*

Word Exercise 8

Without using your Exercise Guide, build words that mean:

(a) a pigment cell

(b) abnormal condition of
excessive black/pigment

Without using your Exercise Guide, write the meaning of:

(c) **melan**/oma

Malignant melanoma is on the increase, and this is believed to be mainly the effect of solar damage caused by excessive sun-bathing. Sometimes a melanoma develops from a pigmented naevus (mole). Melanomas are highly malignant, and once the tumour (Am. tumor) cells have spread, they become difficult to eradicate. Malignant melanoma can be fatal unless treated early in its development. A five-year survival rate is related to the depth of the tumour in the skin at first presentation.

Note. Naevus (plural naevi; Am. nevus, plural nevi) is the medical name for a mole or birthmark on the body. Naevi arise from melanocytes or developmental abnormalities of blood vessels.

Medical equipment and clinical procedures

Suspicious lesions of skin need to be examined microscopically for signs of malignancy. Small samples of skin are removed during an excision **biopsy** (*bio* meaning life, *opsis* meaning vision; therefore biopsy means observation of living tissue). These are then sectioned and stained in the histology laboratory. The biopsy tissue is examined by a histologist or pathologist to determine whether the cells are **benign** or **malignant** (benign means innocent or harmless; malignant means virulent and dangerous to life).

Benign lesions can be removed if they are causing a problem or are unsightly. Malignant lesions threaten life and are treated by surgical excision, radiotherapy and chemotherapy.

Other terms used for lesions that appear in skin disease are listed in the following table:

Bulla	a large watery blister (plural bullae)
Comedone/comedo	an accumulation of sebum in the outlet of a hair follicle; comedones may be closed, forming whiteheads, or open, forming blackheads
Cyst	a sac with a membranous wall enclosing fluid or semisolid matter
Erosion	wearing away of the epidermis
Fissure	a split, crack or crack-like sore in the skin
Keloid	an overgrowth of scar tissue that occurs after injury or surgery
Macule	a nonpalpable flat area of skin showing a change in colour (often red)
Nodule	a solid, round swelling or protuberance approx. 10 mm or more in diameter
Papule	a small circular, solid elevation of the skin (synonym pimple)

Polyp	a stalked (pedunculated) tumour (Am. tumor) arising from a mucous membrane
Pustule	a small swelling of the skin containing pus
Ulcer	an open sore in the skin often suppurating (forming pus)
Vesicle	a small blister containing clear fluid (serum)
Weal/wheal	a smooth superficial swelling (red or white) characteristic of urticaria or nettle stings
Wen	a sebaceous cyst filled with sebum due to a blocked opening of a sebaceous gland

Treatment of skin disorders using lasers

Developments in physics have led to the development of medical **lasers** that play a prominent role in the treatment of skin disorders. Here, we examine a selection of their applications to dermatology. First, we need to understand the meaning of the acronym laser.

LASER is built from the first letter of each of the following words: **L**ight **A**mplification by **S**timulated **E**mission of **R**adiation.

A laser is a device that produces an intense, coherent beam of monochromatic light in the visible region. All the light waves in the beam are in phase and do not diverge, so it can be targeted precisely (see Fig. 71).

The medical laser transfers energy in the form of an intense beam of light to the tissue undergoing treatment. When the laser beam strikes the tissue, it is heated and destroyed (**thermolysis**) in a fraction of a second. Some lasers can heat tissues to over 100°C, resulting in their complete vaporization.

The extent of destruction of a tissue depends on the presence of chemicals in cells that absorb the light. These are known as **chromatophores**. There are three main chromatophores found in tissues: water, melanin and haemoglobin. A skin lesion containing a large amount of melanin, such as a mole, can be specifically targeted and destroyed by a laser with little destruction of the surrounding tissue.

There are many types of medical laser, each one emitting a beam of specific wavelength. The wavelength of the radiation emitted depends on the medium used by the laser, which may be a gas, liquid or solid. In the laser, the atoms of the medium are excited electrically and are stimulated to emit energy in the form of light. Besides laser light, other forms of radiation are used to treat chronic skin disorders. Here are three examples of lasers used by dermatologists:

Type of laser	Medium	Wavelength	Chromatophore	Use
CO_2	Carbon dioxide gas	Infrared 10–600 nm	Water	Vaporizes and cuts tissue. Coagulates blood vessels. Bloodless surgery as it seals up cut vessels. Used to incise tissue and excise a variety of lesions
Argon	Ionized argon gas	Blue-green 488–514 nm	Melanin haemoglobin	Penetrates epidermis and coagulates underlying pigments. Used to remove vascular and pigmented navei (Am. nevi), and polyps
Pulsed dye	Various synthetic dyes	585–595 nm	Haemoglobin	Removing tattoo inks, vascular lesions, moles, port wine stains, etc.

Treatment of psoriasis

Psoriasis is a common chronic skin condition in which there is an increased rate of production of skin cells. The excess skin cells form plaques of silvery scales that continuously flake off, exposing erythematous (reddened) skin that shows pinpoint bleeding. A large proportion of a dermatologist's time may be concerned with this disorder as it affects approximately 2% of the population. There is no cure, and therapies are aimed at reducing the scaling and inflammation. A treatment originally developed for psoriasis is called:

PUVA (Psoralen Ultra Violet A light)

This is a form of **photochemotherapy** that uses a **psoralen** to sensitize the skin to light before it is irradiated with ultraviolet

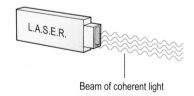

Beam of coherent light

Figure 71   Laser.

light (longwave A). After administration of the psoralen (taken orally), the patient is placed in a chamber illuminated with ultraviolet light. The treatment is convenient for patients; their skin shows dramatic improvement, and the effect lasts for several months. Unfortunately, there is a risk of developing skin cancer because of excessive exposure to UVA.

Review the names of all instruments and clinical procedures mentioned in this unit, and then try Exercise 9.

Word Exercise 9

Match each description in Column C with a term in Column A by placing the appropriate number in Column B.

Column A	Column B	Column C
(a) excision biopsy		1. removal of hair
(b) dermatome		2. an instrument that destroys tissue using a beam of coherent light
(c) medical laser		3. destruction of tissue by heating with an electric current
(d) PUVA		4. removal of living tissue from the body
(e) epilation		5. an instrument used for cutting a thin layer of skin (for grafts)
(f) electrolysis		6. technique of exposing photosensitized skin to light

Other procedures used to investigate and treat the skin besides those mentioned in the word exercises include:

Cryotherapy Also called cryosurgery, the procedure uses liquid nitrogen to freeze and destroy tissue; it is used to remove actinic keratoses, warts and nonmelanoma tumours (Am. tumor).
Curettage The use of a sharp, spoon-shaped device to scrape away a skin lesion.
Mohs micrographic surgery A procedure used to treat nonmelanoma skin cancers in areas where it is important to minimize the removal of healthy tissue. Each time a piece of tissue is removed, it is checked for the presence of malignant cells.
Photodynamic therapy In this procedure the patient takes a nontoxic, light-sensitive drug that targets malignant or other diseased cells. The cells are then selectively exposed to light from a laser or other source. On exposure the drug becomes

toxic and destroys the cells. PUVA is a form of photodynamic therapy but is often classified as a separate technique.
Skin test In this test an allergen is applied to the skin to observe the patient for signs of the rash of contact dermatitis. The allergen can be applied on a piece of gauze pressed against the skin (patch test), pricked into the skin with a needle (skin prick test or scratch test) or injected under the skin (intradermal test).

ANATOMY EXERCISE

Now complete the Anatomy Exercise on page 162.

CASE HISTORY 11

The object of this exercise is to understand words associated with a patient's medical history.

To complete the exercise:

- Read through the passage on psoriasis; unfamiliar words are underlined, and you can find their meaning using the Word Help.

- Write the meaning of the medical terms shown in bold print on the lines that follow the Word Help.

Psoriasis

Mrs K, a 48-year-old woman, presented at the **dermatology** clinic with chronic plaque psoriasis and accompanying arthropathy. She had developed guttate psoriasis at the age of 12 following severe tonsillitis. This was self-limiting, but shortly after psoriatic patches appeared on her legs and arms and then on the trunk. Since then the condition has persisted with exacerbations on her scalp, knees and arms, and over the last 5 years, she has developed arthritis in her distal interphalangeal finger joints.

Mrs K's condition was reviewed by the **dermatologist**. She had developed large **hyperkeratotic** plaques on her trunk and extremities. Her scalp was also affected with some degree of erythema extending beyond the hair margin. Mrs K indicated that the severity of her arthritis seemed to parallel the worsening of her **cutaneous** lesions.

Her nails were pitted with opaque yellow areas within the nail plates. Several nails were showing signs of **onycholysis** with **keratinous** debris under their free edges. Following assessment, Mrs K underwent a course of PUVA using 8-methoxypsoralen twice weekly for 6 weeks. She experienced drying of the skin and pruritus but showed considerable improvement. At the present, she is receiving a single maintenance treatment every 3 weeks, and her fair skin is being examined for presence of malignant **epitheliomas** (non**melanoma** skin cancer being the major, slight, long-term risk factor).

Word Help

arthritis inflammation of the joints

arthropathy diseased joints

chronic pertaining to long term, continued

distal further away from point of attachment

erythema relating to erythema (reddening of the skin)

exacerbations increased severity of symptoms

guttate marked or covered with drop-like spots

interphalangeal pertaining to between the bones of the fingers or toes

lesion a pathological change in a tissue

malignant dangerous, life-threatening

8-methoxypsoralen (8-mop) a psoralen (drug) that sensitizes the skin to light

plaque a flat area, a patch

pruritus itching

psoriasis a chronic inflammatory disease of the skin exhibiting red patches in the epidermis covered with silvery scales

psoriatic pertaining to psoriasis

PUVA administration of a **p**soralen (a drug that sensitizes the skin to light) followed by exposure to **u**ltra**v**iolet light **A**

Now write the meaning of the following words from the Case History without using your dictionary lists:

(a) dermatology

(b) dermatologist

(c) hyperkeratotic

(d) cutaneous

(e) onycholysis

(f) keratinous

(g) epithelioma

(h) melanoma

(Answers to the Case History exercise are given in the Answers to Word Exercises on page 347).

Quick Reference

Combining forms relating to the skin:

Acanth/o	spiny
Cutane/o	skin
Derm/at/o	skin/dermis
Epitheli/o	epithelium
Hidr/o	sweat
Hidraden/o	sweat gland
Ichthy/o	fish/fish-like
Kerat/o	epidermis
Keratin/o	keratin
Melan/o	melanin
Onych/o	nail
Pil/o	hair
Seb/o	sebum / sebaceous gland
Squam/o	scaly
Trich/o	hair

Abbreviations

Some common abbreviations related to the skin are listed below. Note that some are not standard, and their meaning may vary from one healthcare setting to another. There is a more extensive list for reference on page 369.

BCC	basal cell carcinoma
Bx	biopsy
DLE	discoid lupus erythematosus
Ez	eczema
KS	Karposi sarcoma
LMM	lentigo maligna melanoma
MM	malignant melanoma
NMSC	nonmelanoma skin cancer
SC, s.c.	subcutaneous
SCC	squamous cell carcinoma
SED	skin erythema dose
SLE	systemic lupus erythematosus
SSM	superficial spreading melanoma
ST	skin test
STD	skin test dose
STU	skin test unit
ung	ointment (unguentum)

Pathology notes

Acne vulgaris

A common condition in adolescents caused by increased levels of sex hormones after puberty. It develops when sebaceous glands in hair follicles become blocked and infected, leading to inflammation and the formation of pustules. In severe cases, permanent scarring may result. The most common sites are the face, chest and upper back.

Burn

A burn is an injury caused by thermal, chemical, electrical or radiation energy. A scald is a burn caused by contact with a hot liquid or steam. Burns are classified as the following: **epidermal burn**, **superficial partial thickness burn** (epidermis and papillary dermis), **deep partial thickness burn** (epidermis and entire papillary dermis), **full thickness burn** (involving the entire thickness of the skin and possibly subcutaneous tissue) and **full thickness burn +** (involving the entire skin and underlying structures such as muscle and bone).

Cellulitis

This is an acute infection of the connective tissue in the deeper layers of the skin and underlying tissue; it is characterized by redness of the affected area, pain and swelling. Cellulitis can have a wide range of causes, but the majority of cases are caused by streptococcal or staphylococcal bacteria and in rare cases by fungal infection. Without antibiotic treatment, abscesses may form, and the infection can spread to the blood and other parts of the body.

Decubitus ulcer

Decubitus ulcers are also known as *pressure sores* or *bedsores* and are caused by lying in one position for long periods. They occur in areas where the skin is compressed between a bony prominence and a hard surface such as a bed or chair. When this occurs, blood flow to a local area is reduced causing necrosis, ulcer formation and sloughing of the skin. If infection occurs, this can result in septicaemia (Am. septicemia). Frequent changes in body position and soft support cushions help prevent decubitus ulcers.

Dermatitis

Dermatitis is used synonymously with the term *eczema* and describes inflammation of the skin that can be acute or chronic. In acute dermatitis, there is redness, swelling and exudation of serous fluid usually accompanied by itching, crusting and scaling. If the condition becomes chronic, the skin thickens and may become leathery due to excessive scratching, and infection may complicate the condition.

Atopic dermatitis a predisposition that brings about hypersensitivity to allergens, often affecting children who also suffer from hay fever or asthma.
Contact dermatitis caused by direct contact of the skin with irritants such as cosmetics, detergents, synthetic rubber, nickel and other chemicals.

Eczema

Eczema is used synonymously with the term dermatitis and describes an inflammation of the skin that can be acute or chronic. See dermatitis above.

Furuncle

Furuncles are also known as boils; they are localized staphylococcal infections of hair follicles characterized by large, inflamed, pus-filled lesions. A group of untreated boils may fuse into an even larger lesion called a *carbuncle*.

Impetigo

This is a highly contagious bacterial condition that results from staphylococcal or streptococcal infection and occurs most often in young children. Impetigo starts as a reddish discolouration (Am. discoloration) called erythema, but it soon develops into vesicles (blisters) with yellowish crusts. Impetigo is most commonly caused by *Staphylococcus aureus.* Superficial pustules develop, usually around the nose and mouth; occasionally the infection becomes systemic and life-threatening.

Karposi sarcoma

A viral-induced malignant disease characterized by the growth of new blood vessels. The lesions appear as red, blue or brown nodules that are common on the ankle, trunk and nose. Originally common in tropical Africa, it is now seen in individuals who are immunologically compromised, such as those with AIDS.

Necrotising fasciitis

This is an uncommon infection involving deep soft tissue such as the dermis, subcutaneous tissue and fascia of connective tissue and muscle. Commonly called flesh-eating disease, it is difficult to diagnose in its initial stages as it mimics cellulitis. Early symptoms are pain, tenderness and symptoms of systemic illness out of proportion to the local signs. Later the skin becomes discoloured, and the tissues start to break down. Many types of bacteria can cause this condition, including *Streptococcus pyogenes*, *Staphylococcus aureus*, *Clostridium perfringens* and *Vibrio vulnificus.* Since 2001, MRSA methicillin-resistant *S. aureus* has been observed with increasing frequency; it is difficult to treat and life-threatening.

Tumours (Am. tumors)

Excessive exposure to the sun can result in skin cancer; there are three basic forms:

Basal cell carcinoma (BCC) also called *rodent ulcer* accounts for over 75 percent of all skin cancers. It occurs on exposed parts, especially those of the face, nose, eyelids and cheek. It begins as a small, firm, flat nodule and grows slowly, eventually forming a shallow ulcer with raised edges. The ulcer is locally destructive, destroying deeper tissue as it grows. Fortunately, basal cell carcinomas do not spread (metastasize) to other parts of the body.
Squamous cell carcinoma (SCC) also begins in the epidermis and is derived from keratinocytes. High proportions of squamous carcinomata arise on skin damaged by sunlight or chemicals. Initially, the skin thickens, and the lesion becomes hyperkeratotic and ulcerated. If the tumour is not promptly removed, there will be metastatic spread into local lymph nodes and beyond.
Malignant melanoma a malignant tumour of epidermal melanocytes; it is the leading cause of death from skin disease

because it can spread rapidly. Melanoma is most common in white females over the age of 30, and its development may be related to severe sun exposure, genetic factors and unknown chemical carcinogens.

Urticaria (hives)

Urticaria is also known as *nettle rash* because the itching and weals that develop on the skin resemble the effects of the stinging nettle *(Urtica dioica)*. It is often due to allergic reaction to certain foods, food additives or drugs such as antibiotics.

Verruca

A wart, for example, *verruca plana*, the common wart that infects the hands, knees and face, and *verruca plantaris*, a flat wart infecting the sole of the foot (see wart).

Vitiligo

This is a skin disease characterized by loss of pigment (depigmentation). There is an absence of melanocytes in affected areas, producing white patches. It is associated with autoimmune disease of the endocrine system, and in some cases, there is an inherited component.

Wart

Warts or verrucas are nipple-like neoplasms of the epidermis caused by infection with the human papilloma virus. Common sites of infection are the hands, face and soles of the feet. Transmission of warts generally occurs through direct contact with warts on the skin of an infected person. Freezing, drying, laser therapy or application of chemicals (keratolytics) can remove them (see verruca).

Associated words

Abrasion a superficial injury to the skin

Abscess a localized collection of pus in a cavity formed by disintegration of tissues

Actinic of light able to cause photochemical reactions (as in the skin)

Albinism an inherited condition characterized by a lack of melanin in the skin, hair and eyes

Boil a furuncle, a painful inflamed nodule formed in the skin, due to staphylococci entering the skin through a hair follicle

Callus a thickened patch of the horny layer of the epidermis formed on the palms or soles of the feet due to excess friction

Cicatrix the scar of a healed wound or ulcer

Corium the dermis, the layer under the epidermis

Crust a collection of dried sebum and cellular debris formed by drying of a bodily exudate

Cuticle a narrow band of epidermis extending onto the nail surface from the nail wall, also called the eponychium

Desquamation the peeling or shedding of the outer parts of the epithelium of the skin

Dysplastic pertaining to abnormal development of tissue, in size, shape or organization of cells

Ecchymoses condition of bluish-black patches (bruises) on the skin

Erosion breaking down of the surface of a tissue, usually by ulceration

Eruption process of breaking out or becoming visible, eg, a red rash on the skin

Erythema reddening of the skin

Excoriation process of abrading the skin

Exfoliation the splitting off from the surface of dead tissue in thin, flaky layers

Exudate a fluid containing protein and cell debris that oozes from blood vessels and is deposited in tissues

Fungating the process of producing a fungus-like growth

Gangrene death of a tissue associated with a loss of blood supply

Glabrous pertaining to smooth and bare (skin)

Lesion any injury or morbid change in a tissue such as the skin

Lichenification process of producing irregular areas of thickened skin

Morbid diseased, disordered or pathological

Pallor paleness of the skin

Petechiae condition of small pinpoint haemorrhages in the skin (Am. hemorrhages)

Purpura red or purple spots (petechiae) or patches (ecchymoses) due to bleeding into the skin

Rash a superficial, temporary eruption on the skin

Scabies a contagious parasitic infection of the skin caused by a mite *Sarcoptes scabei*

Scleroderma an autoimmune disease marked by hardening of connective tissue in the skin and other organs

Slough to shed or cast off, eg, necrotic tissue such as dead skin

Telangiectasis condition of having dilated blood vessels, eg, in the skin where they are known as spider veins

Tinea infection of the skin caused by fungi, also known as ringworm because of the ring-like patches that develop as the infection recedes

NOW TRY THE WORD CHECK

WORD CHECK

This self-check exercise lists all the word components used in this unit. First, write down the meaning of as many word components as you can. Then, check your answers using the Exercise Guide and Quick Reference box or the Glossary of Word Components (pp. 383–410).

Prefixes

a-

an-

auto-

crypto-

dys-

epi-

hyper-

hypo-

intra-

pachy-

para-

sub-

xantho-

xero-

Combining forms of word roots

acanth/o

aden/o

aesthesi/o

(Am. esthesi/o)

cutane/o

cyt/o

dermat/o

epitheli/o

hidr/o

ichthy/o

kerat/o

keratin/o

lith/o

melan/o

-motor-

myc/o

onych/o

phyt(e)

pil/o

schiz/o-

seb/o

squam/o

trich/o

Suffixes

-auxis

-ia

-ic

-itis

-logist

-logy

-lysis

-oma

-osis

-ous

-phagia

-plasty

-poiesis

-rrhexis

-rrhoea
(Am. -rrhea)

-schisis

-tic

-tome

-trophy

-tropic

NOW TRY THE SELF-ASSESSMENT

SELF-ASSESSMENT

Test 11A

Below are some combining forms that refer to the anatomy of the skin. Indicate which part of the system they refer to by putting a number from the diagram (Fig. 72) next to each word:

(a) hidraden/o

(b) seb/o

(c) trich/o

(d) melan/o

(e) kerat/o

(f) dermat/o

Score

6

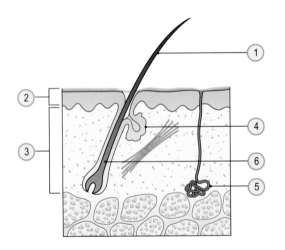

Figure 72   Section through the skin.

Test 11B

Prefixes and suffixes

Match each meaning in Column C with a prefix or suffix in Column A by inserting the appropriate number in Column B.

Column A	Column B	Column C
(a) a-		1. cutting instrument
(b) auto-		2. above / above normal
(c) -auxis		3. breakdown/ disintegration
(d) crypto-		4. within
(e) dys-		5. condition of eating/ swallowing
(f) hyper-		6. thick
(g) hypo-		7. nourishment
(h) intra-		8. hidden/concealed
(i) -lysis		9. dry
(j) -oma		10. formation/making
(k) pachy-		11. break/rupture
(l) -phagia		12. pertaining to affinity for / stimulating
(m) -poiesis		13. difficult/painful
(n) -rrhexis		14. tumour or swelling (Am. tumor)
(o) -schisis		15. yellow
(p) -tome		16. below / below normal
(q) -trophy		17. increase
(r) -tropic		18. without/not
(s) xantho-		19. self
(t) xero-		20. splitting

Score

20

Test 11C

Combining forms of word roots

Match each meaning in Column C with a combining form of a word root in Column A by inserting the appropriate number in Column B.

Column A	Column B	Column C
(a) aden/o		1. horny/epidermis
(b) dermat/o		2. pertaining to action
(c) hidr/o		3. fungus
(d) kerat/o		4. hair (i)
(e) lith/o		5. hair (ii)
(f) -motor-		6. nail
(g) myc/o		7. skin
(h) onych/o		8. plant
(i) phyt/o		9. sweat
(j) pil/o		10. sebum
(k) seb/o		11. gland
(l) trich/o		12. stone

Score [12]

Test 11D

Write the meaning of:

(a) dermatophytosis

(b) keratinocyte

(c) trichoanaesthesia (Am. trichoanesthesia)

(d) hidradenoma

(e) epidermomycosis

Score [5]

Test 11E

Build words that mean:

(a) inflammation of the skin

(b) abnormal condition of nails

(c) condition of nails blackened with melanin

(d) study of skin

(e) condition of thick nails

Score [5]

Check answers to Self-Assessment Tests on page 363.

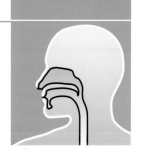

UNIT **12**
THE NOSE AND MOUTH

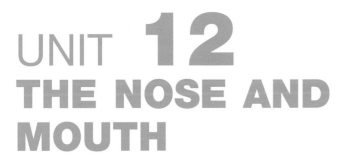

OBJECTIVES

Once you have completed Unit 12, you should be able to do the following:

- understand the meaning of medical words relating to the nose and mouth
- build medical words relating to the nose and mouth
- associate medical terms with their anatomical position
- understand common medical abbreviations relating to the nose and mouth

EXERCISE GUIDE

Use this list of word components and their meanings to complete the word exercises in this unit.

Prefixes

a-	without
dys-	difficult/painful
endo-	within/inside
intra-	inside
macro-	large
ortho-	straight/correct/normal
peri-	around
poly-	many
post-	after
prosth-	adding (replacement part)

Roots / Combining forms

aden/o	gland
aer/o	air/gas
angi/o	vessel
bronch/o	bronchi / bronchial tree
bucc/o	cheek
dynam/o	force
laryng/o	larynx
man/o	pressure
myc/o	fungus
nas/o	nose
ot/o	ear
pharyng/o	pharynx
trich/o	hair
tympan/o	middle ear / ear drum

Suffixes

-agogue	agent that induces/promotes
-al	pertaining to
-algia	condition of pain
-cele	swelling/protrusion/hernia
-dynia	condition of pain
-eal	pertaining to
-ectomy	removal of
-genic	pertaining to formation/originating in
-gram	X-ray tracing/picture/recording
-graphy	technique of recording/making an X-ray
-ia	condition of
-ic	pertaining to
-ics	art or science of / a specialty / a field of knowledge
-ist	specialist
-itis	inflammation of
-lith	stone
-logy	study of
-meter	measuring instrument
-metry	process of measuring
-osis	abnormal condition / disease of
-pathy	disease of
-phagia	condition of eating
-phonia	condition of having voice
-phyma	tumour/boil (Am. tumor)
-plasty	surgical repair/reconstruction
-plegia	condition of paralysis

-rrhagia	condition of bursting forth (of blood)	**-scope**	an instrument used to view/examine
-rrhaphy	stitching/suturing	**-scopy**	technique of viewing/examining
-rrhea (Am.)	excessive flow	**-stomy**	formation of an opening into…
-rrhoea	excessive flow (Am. -rrhea)	**-tomy**	incision into
-schisis	cleaving/splitting/parting	**-us**	thing / structure / anatomical part

ANATOMY EXERCISE

When you have finished Word Exercises 1 to 18, look at the word components listed below. Complete Figures 73 and 74 by writing the appropriate combining form on each line; more than one component may relate to the same position. (You can check their meanings in the Quick Reference box on p. 183.)

Antr/o	Labi/o	Sial/o
Cheil/o	Nas/o	Sin/o
Faci/o	Odont/o	Stomat/o
Gingiv/o	Palat/o	Uvul/o
Gloss/o	Ptyal/o	
Gnath/o	Rhin/o	

The nose and mouth

Receptors for the sense of smell are located in the olfactory epithelium, which is in the roof of the nasal cavity. For us to smell a substance, it must be volatile so it can be carried into the nose, and then it must dissolve in the mucus covering the receptors. Humans can distinguish between 2000 and 4000 different odours (Am. odors).

Receptors for taste are located on the taste buds of the tongue. When a substance is eaten, four types of receptor can be stimulated, producing sensations for sweet, bitter, salty and sour. The sense of taste is known as **gustation**.

In this unit we will look at terms associated with the mouth and nose.

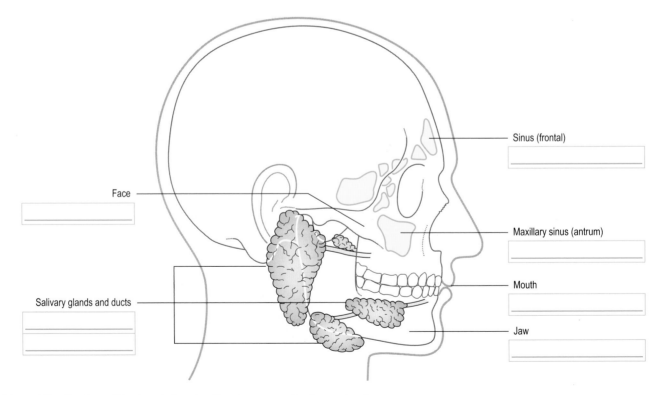

Figure 73   Section of the head showing the sinuses and salivary glands.

Use the Exercise Guide at the beginning of this unit to complete Word Exercises 1 to 18, unless you are asked to work without it.

Root

Stomat
(*From a Greek word* **stomatos**, *meaning mouth.*)

Combining form   Stomat/o

Word Exercise 1

Using your Exercise Guide, find the meaning of:

(a) **stomat/o**/logy

(b) **stomat/o**/rrhagia

(c) **stomat/o**/pathy

Using your Exercise Guide, find the meaning of -dynia, myc/o and -osis; then build words that mean:

(d) condition of pain in the mouth

(e) abnormal condition of fungi in the mouth

Root

Or
(*From a Latin word* **oris**, *meaning mouth.*)

Combining form   Or/o

Word Exercise 2

Using your Exercise Guide, find the meaning of:

(a) **or**/al

(b) intra/-**or**/al

(c) **or/o**[2]/pharyng[3]/eal[1]

(d) **or/o**/nas/al

Root

Gloss
(*From a Greek word* **glossa**, *meaning tongue.*)

Combining form   Gloss/o

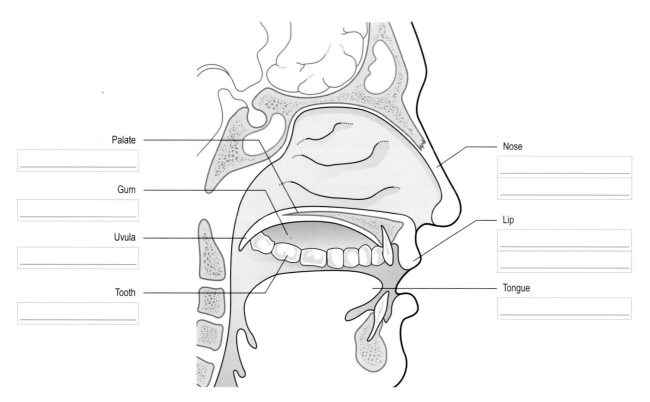

Palate

Gum

Uvula

Tooth

Nose

Lip

Tongue

Figure 74   Sagittal section of the nasal cavity and mouth.

Word Exercise 3

Without using your Exercise Guide and beginning with the underlined root, build words that mean:

(a) the study of the <u>tongue</u>

(b) condition of pain in the <u>tongue</u> (use -dynia or -algia)

(c) pertaining to the <u>tongue</u> and pharynx (use -eal)

Using your Exercise Guide, find the meaning of:

(d) **gloss/o**/plegia

(e) **gloss/o**/trich/ia

(f) **gloss/o**/cele

(g) macro/**gloss**/ia

(h) **gloss/o**/plasty

A Latin combining form lingu/o is also used to mean tongue, language or relationship to the tongue, eg, lingual, pertaining to the tongue, sublingual, under the tongue.

Disorders of the mouth, tongue, pharynx and palate give rise to problems with, eg, eating, swallowing and talking.

Dysphagia

A condition of difficulty in eating (from Greek *phagein* to eat).

Dyslalia

A condition of difficulty in talking (from Greek *lalein* to talk).

Root

Sial

*(From a Greek word **sialon**, meaning saliva. Here sial/o means saliva, salivary gland or salivary duct. Three pairs of salivary glands secrete saliva into the mouth. Saliva lubricates the food and contains amylase, an enzyme that begins the digestion of starch.)*

Combining form   Sial/o

 Word Exercise 4

Using your Exercise Guide, find the meaning of:

(a) **sial/o**/aden/ectomy

(b) **sial/o**/angi/o/graphy

(c) poly/**sial**/ia

(d) **sial/o**/gram

Using your Exercise Guide look up -lith; then build a word that means:

(e) a stone in the saliva (salivary duct or salivary gland)

Using your Exercise Guide, find the meaning of:

(f) **sial**/agogue (a drug)

(g) **sial/o**/aer/o/phagia

Root

Ptyal

*(From a Greek word **ptyalon**, meaning saliva.)*

Combining form   Ptyal/o

 Word Exercise 5

Using your Exercise Guide, find the meaning of:

(a) **ptyal**/o/genic

(b) **ptyal**/o/rrhoea (Am. **ptyal**/o/rrhea)

Root

Gnath

*(From a Greek word **gnathos**, meaning jaw.)*

Combining form   Gnath/o

 Word Exercise 6

Without using your Exercise Guide and beginning with the underlined root, build words that mean:

(a) condition of pain in the <u>jaw</u>

(b) plastic surgery of the <u>jaw</u>

(c) study of the jaw (and chewing apparatus)

(d) pertaining to the <u>mouth</u> and jaw (use -ic)

Using your Exercise Guide, find the meaning of:

(e) **gnath/o**/dynam/o/meter

(f) **gnath/o**/schisis (refers to
the upper jaw and palate,
a cleft palate)

(g) **gnath**/itis

Root

Cheil

(*From a Greek word* **cheilos***, meaning lip.*)

Combining form   Cheil/o

 ### Word Exercise 7

Without using your Exercise Guide, write the meaning of:

(a) **cheil/o**/stomat/o/plasty

(b) **cheil/o**/schisis

Using your Exercise Guide, find the meaning of:

(c) **cheil/o**/rrhaphy

Without using your Exercise Guide, build a word that means:

(d) inflammation of the lip

Root

Labi

(*From a Latin word* **labium***, meaning lip.*)

Combining form   Labi/o

Word Exercise 8

Using your Exercise Guide, find the meaning of:

(a) **labi/o**/gloss/o/laryng/eal

Without using your Exercise Guide and beginning with the underlined root, build a word that means:

(b) pertaining to the <u>lips</u>, tongue
and pharynx (use -eal)

Root

Gingiv

(*From a Latin word* **gingiva***, meaning gum.*)

Combining form   Gingiv/o

 ### Word Exercise 9

Without using your Exercise Guide, build words that mean:

(a) inflammation of the gums

(b) removal of gum (usually
performed for pyorrhoea
(Am. pyorrhea), the flow of
pus a result of periodontal
disease)

Without using your Exercise Guide, write the meaning of:

(c) labi/o/**gingiv**/al

Root

Palat

(*From Latin* **palatum***, meaning the palate.*)

Combining form   Palat/o

 ### Word Exercise 10

Without using your Exercise Guide and beginning with the underlined root, build words that mean:

(a) condition of paralysis of
the soft <u>palate</u>

(b) a split <u>palate</u> (cleft palate)

Using your Exercise Guide, find the meaning of:

(c) post/**palat**/al

Root

Uvul

(*From a Latin word* **uvula***, meaning grape. Here uvul/o means
the uvula, the central tag-like structure extending downwards
from the soft palate.*)

Combining form   Uvul/o

 ### Word Exercise 11

Without using your Exercise Guide and beginning with the underlined word, build words that mean:

(a) removal of the <u>uvula</u>

(b) surgical repair of the
<u>uvula</u>, palate and pharynx

Root

Phas

(*From a Greek word* **phasis**, *meaning speech.*)

Combining form   Phas/i/o

Word Exercise 12

Using your Exercise Guide, find the meaning of:

(a) a/**phas**/ia

(b) dys/**phas**/ia

There are many varieties and causes of aphasia. Two common types are:

Motor aphasia

A condition often due to a stroke that results in an inability to move the muscles involved in speech in the normal way. (The word **aphonia** is also used to refer to a loss of voice.)

Sensory aphasia

A condition caused by brain damage that results in an inability to recognize spoken (or written) words.

Root

Odont

(*From a Greek word* **odontos**, *meaning tooth.*)

Combining form   Odont/o

Word Exercise 13

Without using your Exercise Guide, build words that mean:

(a) the scientific study of teeth (dentistry)

(b) any disease of teeth

(c) condition of pain in a tooth (toothache)

Using your Exercise Guide, find the meaning of:

(d) peri/**odont**/ics (includes all tissues supporting teeth)

(e) end/**odont**/o/logy (includes the tooth pulp and roots)

(f) orth/**odont**/ics

(g) orth/**odont**/ist

(h) prosth/**odont**/ics

A prosthesis is an artificial replacement for a body part (plural -prostheses). Prosthodontics is the branch of dentistry that specializes in the replacement of lost teeth and associated structures.

Root

Rhin

(*From a Greek word* **rhinos**, *meaning nose.*)

Combining form   Rhin/o

We have already used rhin/o when studying the breathing system. Here, we use the same combining form with new suffixes.

Word Exercise 14

Using your Exercise Guide, find the meaning of:

(a) **rhin/o**/phonia

(b) **rhin/o**/man/o/meter

(c) **rhin/o**/phyma

(d) **rhin/o**/scopy

(e) ot/o/**rhin/o**/ laryng/o/logy

Without using your Exercise Guide, write the meaning of:

(f) **rhin/o**/rrhagia (also known as epistaxis)

Note. There is also a Latin word **nasus** meaning nose; its combining form nas/o is used in several exercises in this unit.

Root

Sinus

(*A Latin word meaning a hollow or a cavity. Here sin/o means a sinus, a cavity in a bone of the skull.*)

Combining forms   Sin/o, sinus

Word Exercise 15

Using your Exercise Guide, find the meaning of:

(a) **sin**/us

(b) **sin/o**/bronch/itis

Without using your Exercise Guide, write the meaning of:

(c) **sinus**/itis

This condition affects the membrane lining the paranasal sinuses (the air-filled cavities surrounding the nose). Micro-organisms spread from the nose or pharynx to infect the mucous membranes lining the sinuses of the maxillary, sphenoidal, ethmoidal and frontal bones of the skull. The primary viral infection is often followed by secondary bacterial infection with *Staphylococcus aureus, Streptococcus pyogenes* or *Streptococcus pneumoniae.* The congested linings may block the drainage channels from the sinuses, preventing the expulsion of the accumulating pus. When this occurs, there is a feeling of tension and pain in the affected area. Other symptoms include fever, stuffy nose and loss of the sense of smell. If there are repeated attacks or if recovery is not complete, the infection may become chronic.

(d) **sin/o**/gram

Note. A **mucocele** is a mucus-filled swelling that forms in a paranasal sinus, eg, in an ethmoid sinus or frontal sinus. A mucocele forms when the ostium (opening) of a sinus is obstructed, preventing normal sinus drainage. Obstruction may be due to infection, allergy, trauma or the growth of a cyst or tumour (Am. tumor).

Root

Antr

*(From a Greek word **antron**, meaning cave. Here antr/o means antrum, in particular the antrum of Highmore, also known as the superior maxillary sinus.)*

Combining form   Antr/o

Word Exercise 16

Using your Exercise Guide and beginning with the underlined root, build words that mean:

(a) an instrument used to view the <u>antrum</u>

(b) pertaining to the <u>antrum</u> and tympanum

Without using your Exercise Guide, write the meaning of:

(c) **antr/o**/tomy (usually performed to drain out infected fluid)

(d) **antr/o**/nas/al

(e) **antr/o**/cele

Using your Exercise Guide, find the meaning of:

(f) **antr/o**/bucc/al

(g) **antr/o**/stomy

Root

Faci

*(From a Latin word **facies**, meaning face.)*

Combining form   Faci/o

Word Exercise 17

Without using your Exercise Guide, write the meaning of:

(a) **faci**/al

(b) **faci/o**/plegia

(c) **faci/o**/plasty

Medical equipment and clinical procedures

Review the names of all instruments and clinical procedures mentioned in this unit before completing Exercise 18.

Word Exercise 18

Match each description in Column C with a term in Column A by placing the appropriate number in Column B.

Column A	Column B	Column C
(a) antro-scope		1. an instrument that measures the force of the jaws
(b) sialoangi-ography		2. technique of recording the tongue (movement in speech)
(c) gnathody-namometer		3. an instrument for viewing the maxillary sinus (antrum)

Column A	Column B	Column C
(d) rhinoma-nometer		4. an artificial part of the body, eg, a false tooth
(e) prosthesis		5. technique of making an X-ray/recording of salivary ducts
(f) glossogra-phy		6. an instrument that measures air pressure in the nose

Other procedures used to investigate and treat the nose and mouth besides those mentioned in the word exercises include:

Computed tomography (CT) This procedure uses X-rays to produce images in three planes and outlines the anatomy of the nasal cavity and paranasal sinuses.

Functional endoscopic sinus surgery (FESS) This is the main surgical treatment of sinusitis, nasal polyps and chronic sinus problems. FESS uses nasal endoscopes through the nostrils to avoid cutting the skin and is performed using general anaesthesia (Am. anesthesia).

Magnetic resonance imaging (MRI) MRI scans are the primary choice in looking at cancers of the nasal cavities and paranasal sinuses. They are better than CT scans in distinguishing fluid from tumour, and sometimes they can help tell the difference between a benign and malignant tumour. MRI improves the differentiation of soft tissue but cannot define bony anatomy as well as the CT scan (Am. tumor).

Rhinomanometry The technique of measuring nasal airflow and pressure; it is used to evaluate nasal obstruction.

ANATOMY EXERCISE

Now complete the Anatomy Exercise on page 176.

 CASE HISTORY 12

The object of this exercise is to understand words associated with a patient's medical history.

To complete the exercise:

* Read through the passage on acute sinusitis; unfamiliar words are underlined, and you can find their meaning using the Word Help.

* Write the meaning of the medical terms shown in bold print on the lines following the Word Help.

Acute sinusitis

Mrs L, a 28-year-old mother, was brought into Accident and Emergency late at night; her husband was concerned that she was seriously ill. She was recovering from a viral **rhinitis**

when, on the morning of admission, she was stricken with an excruciating frontal headache with pain in her cheek and upper teeth. She felt dizzy, and her right cheek was hot and tender to touch. There was no immediate history of any dental problems.

She was examined by the casualty registrar and found to have an elevated temperature and pulse. **Rhinoscopy** demonstrated reddened, oedematous mucous (Am. edematous) membranes and signs of a mucopurulent discharge from the middle meatus. Questioning of the patient revealed she had hyposmia and in the previous three days had become embarrassed by a cacosmia emanating from her nose.

A CT scan demonstrated fluid in her right maxillary sinus and excluded any orbital or intracranial involvement. A diagnosis of acute maxillary **sinusitis** was made by the registrar, and she was prescribed decongestants and started on a course of antibiotic therapy. A sample of the discharge from her nose was sent to the microbiology laboratory for culture and sensitivity testing. Before leaving A and E, she was given appropriate analgesia for her headache and referred to the department of **Otorhinolaryngology**.

Mrs L's follow up medical treatment with antibiotics and decongestants had limited success, and her condition became chronic with a purulent nasal and **postnasal** discharge. Pus from the maxillary sinus was removed by **antral** washout (antral lavage) following proof puncture through the nasal wall of the maxillary antrum. This was repeated on four occasions before the consultant advised surgery and the formation of an **intranasal antrostomy**. Functional endoscopic sinus surgery (FESS) was used to improve drainage of the maxillary sinus through its natural ostium.

Following her operation, Mrs L showed great improvement; mucosal activity and the self-cleaning mechanism of her sinuses was restored.

Word Help

acute symptoms/signs of short duration

analgesia condition of without pain/prescribing of drugs that reduce pain

cacosmia condition of stench or unpleasant odour (Am. odor)

chronic lasting/lingering for a long time

CT computed tomography

culture and sensitivity testing growing microorganisms in the laboratory and testing them for sensitivity to antibiotics

decongestant a drug used for the relief of congestion

endoscopic pertaining to (using) an endoscope, ie, an instrument used to visually examine the body cavities

intracranial pertaining to within the cranium

hyposmia condition of reduced sense of smell (below normal)

maxillary sinus the sinus/antrum (air space) in the facial bone known as the maxilla

meatus a passage or opening

mucopurulent containing pus and mucus

mucosal pertaining to the mucosa (here the mucous membrane lining the maxillary sinus)

mucous pertaining to or containing mucus (a viscous secretion)

oedematous pertaining to accumulation of fluid in a tissue (Am. edematous)

orbital pertaining to the orbit of the eye (bony eye socket)

ostium a natural mouth or opening

proof evidence (here proving the antrum is infected)

purulent containing pus

Gingiv/o	gum
Gloss/o	tongue
Gnath/o	jaw
Labi/o	lip
Laryng/o	larynx
Lingu/o	tongue
Nas/o	nose
Odont/o	tooth
Or/o	mouth
Palat/o	palate
Phag/o	eating/consuming
Pharyng/o	pharynx
Ptyal/o	saliva / salivary gland / salivary duct
Rhin/o	nose
Sial/o	saliva / salivary gland / salivary duct
Sin/o	sinus
Sinus-	sinus
Stomat/o	mouth
Uvul/o	uvula

Now, write the meaning of the following words from the Case History without using your dictionary lists:

(a) rhinitis

(b) rhinoscopy

(c) sinusitis

(d) otorhinolaryngology

(e) postnasal

(f) antral

(g) intranasal

(h) antrostomy

(Answers to the Case History exercise are given in the Answers to Word Exercises on page 348.)

Quick Reference

Combining forms relating to the nose and mouth:

Aden/o	gland
Antr/o	antrum / maxillary sinus
Bucc/o	cheek
Cheil/o	lip
Faci/o	face

Abbreviations

Some common abbreviations related to the nose and mouth are listed next. Note that some are not standard, and their meaning may vary from one healthcare setting to another. There is a more extensive list for reference on page 369.

BUC, Buc, bucc	buccal (pertaining to the cheek or mouth cavity)
CL/CP	cleft lip and cleft palate
Dmft	decayed missing filled teeth (deciduous)
DMFT	decayed missing filled teeth (permanent)
FESS	functional endoscopic sinus surgery
ging	gingiva (gums), gingivitis
Nas	nasal
NP	nasopharynx
NPO	non per os (nothing by mouth)
OH	oral hygiene
Os	mouth
po/PO	per os (by mouth)
RCT	root canal treatment
RPD	removable partial denture

Pathology notes

Allergic rhinitis (hay fever)

Allergic rhinitis is an allergy triggered by airborne substances that cause inflammation of the mucous membrane lining the nasal cavity. In this condition, atopic hypersensitivity develops to foreign proteins (antigens) that have been inhaled. Allergens commonly associated with allergic rhinitis include scales, hair and feathers from animals, pollen grains and mites in house dust. The immediate exaggerated immune response triggers the release of histamine and other chemicals that cause inflammation, rhinorrhoea (Am. rhinorrhea), reddening of the eyes and excessive secretion of tears.

Angular cheilitis

Angular cheilitis is an inflammation in the fold of tissue at the corner of the mouth that develops into a painful crack. The condition usually develops in the elderly or debilitated people if they do not wear their dentures and the folds remain moist. The moisture allows the growth of microorganism such as *Candida albicans* and *Staphylococcus aureus* that cause inflammation.

Aphthae

Aphthae are small ulcers that occur singly or in groups on the inside of the cheek or lip or underneath the tongue. The cause is uncertain, but they have been associated with streptococcal infection, minor injury, vitamin B deficiency and iron deficiency. Recurrent mouth ulceration with accompanying inflammation is known as aphthous stomatitis.

Cleft lip

Cleft lip is a vertical split, usually off centre (Am. center) in the upper lip; it may be a minor notch in the lip or a substantial split extending up to the nose. In some cases the upper gum may also be cleft and the nose crooked. The term harelip is used in the rare cases that the cleft is in the midline of the upper lip. Cleft lip is often associated with failure of the two halves of the palate to join; see cleft palate.

Cleft palate

During embryonic development, the roof of the mouth (hard palate) develops as two separate halves. Before birth, the right and left halves fuse along the midline of the body. If fusion is incomplete, a cleft palate occurs; the opening can be minor or substantial. A cleft palate creates a gap between the mouth and nasal cavity.

Dental caries (tooth decay)

Formation of dental caries is a result of gradual softening (demineralization) of the dentine and enamel of a tooth. If untreated, bacteria and other organisms will infect the tooth causing inflammation and death of its pulp. This may lead to the formation of an abscess in the bone surrounding the roots and the pain of toothache. Demineralization of teeth is caused by the action of acid formed by bacteria breaking down sugars in the mouth or by ingested fruit acid.

Erythroplakia

A slow-growing lesion that appears as a red and flat or eroded area in the lining of the mouth. The mucous membrane thins and appears red because the underlying capillaries are more visible. Erythroplakia carries a significant risk of transforming into a squamous cell carcinoma.

Leukoplakia

Thick, white patches occurring on the tongue, lips and other areas covered with mucous membranes. The hyperplasia (increase in growth of cells) in the patch sometimes denotes cancerous change.

Mumps

Mumps is an acute inflammatory condition of the salivary glands, especially the parotids. The illness mainly affects children and is caused by the mumps virus, one of the parainfluenza group (paramyxoviruses). Fever and headache develop, and the parotid glands on one or both sides swell causing pain on swallowing. The virus is inhaled in infected droplets, and in the 18- to 21-day incubation period, the viruses multiply elsewhere in the body before spreading to the salivary glands. Serious complications are uncommon but can include pancreatitis, orchitis in males after puberty and meningitis. One attack of mumps confers lifelong immunity to the virus. A safe and effective mumps vaccine is available in combination with measles and rubella vaccines (MMR vaccine).

Nasal polyp

A nasal polyp is a benign growth that projects, usually on a stalk (or peduncle), from the mucous membrane lining of the nose. Polyps can cause nasal obstruction and may need to be removed.

Oral cancer

Also known as mouth cancer; this is a condition characterized by the growth of a tumour (Am. tumor) on the tongue, mouth, lips or gums. Less commonly, tumours can develop in the salivary glands, tonsils or pharynx. Squamous cell carcinoma is the most common type, but malignant melanoma and adenocarcinomas can also occur. Risk factors for developing oral cancer include smoking, drinking alcohol and infection with human papilloma virus (HPV). Initially the condition is painless, but as the tumour grows, pain begins, and the patient has difficulty swallowing and speaking. Leukoplakia and erythroplakia are precancerous lesions that may develop into mouth cancer over time. Treatment is with surgery, chemotherapy and radiotherapy.

Oral candidiasis (thrush)

Thrush is the common name for an acute fungal infection of the epithelium of the mouth (or vagina) caused by the yeast *Candida albicans*. The organism is normally present in the mouth and vagina, but it is usually kept under control by the presence of bacteria and other microorganisms. Candida proliferates in adults who are debilitated in some way, for example, in those whose immune system is suppressed by HIV, steroids, antibiotics or cytotoxic drugs. Sore, whitish-yellow raised patches in the mouth characterize the condition.

Vincent disease (acute gingivitis)

Acute gingivitis is an acute infection of the gums with severe necrotizing ulceration. It is caused by two commensal organisms acting together: *Borellia vincenti* and a fusiform bacillus. These organisms occur naturally in the mouth but because of poor dental hygiene, malnutrition or injury may cause serious gum disease.

Associated words

Bolus a rounded mass of food in the mouth ready to swallow

Bruxism the condition of grinding teeth and clenching the jaw, particularly during sleep

Dam a barrier of latex to obstruct the flow of water or other fluid, eg, a dental dam

Deciduous teeth commonly called baby teeth or primary teeth; the first set of (usually) 20 teeth

Deglutition the act of swallowing

Dens a tooth

Dentes teeth; plural of dens

Dysgeusia condition of a bad taste in the mouth (synonym parageusia)

Edentulous pertaining to having no teeth

Epistaxis bleeding from the nose

Eruption the emergence of a tooth from its position in the jaw

Fauces the passage between the throat and pharynx

Gustatory relating to taste

Halitosis condition of having bad breath

Lallation a babbling, an infantile form of speech; pronunciation of /r/as/l/

Lingual frenulum a membrane that attaches the tongue to the floor of the mouth

Malocclusion misalignment of the teeth or jaws; 'a bad bite'

Mastication the chewing of food

Occlusion the relationship of the upper and lower teeth when the mouth is closed

Oral pertaining to the mouth, taken or applied in the mouth

Ostium an opening; eg, an opening into a paranasal sinus

Papillae small, raised, nipple-shaped structures on the tongue associated with taste buds

Parageusia condition of a bad taste in the mouth (synonym dysgeusia)

Permanent teeth the teeth (usually 32) that replace the deciduous or primary teeth

Plaque a colourless, sticky film composed of undigested food particles mixed with saliva and bacteria that constantly forms on the teeth (Am. colorless)

Polyp a growth or mass protruding from a mucous membrane, eg, a nasal polyp

Salivation the process of producing saliva

Septum a division or partition, eg, the nasal septum that separates the nasal cavities

Tartar a common term for dental calculus, a hard deposit that adheres to teeth

Xerostomia condition of having a dry mouth

NOW TRY THE WORD CHECK

WORD CHECK

This self-check exercise lists all the word components used in this unit. First, write down the meaning of as many word components as you can. Then, check your answers using the Exercise Guide and Quick Reference box or the Glossary of Word Components (pp. 383–410).

Prefixes

a-	
dys-	
endo-	
intra-	
macro-	
ortho-	
peri-	
poly-	
post-	
prosth-	
sub-	

Combining forms of word roots

aden/o	
aer/o	
angi/o	
antr/o	
bronch/o	
bucc/o	
cheil/o	
dynam/o	
faci/o	
gingiv/o	
gloss/o	
gnath/o	
labi/o	
laryng/o	
lingu/o	
man/o	

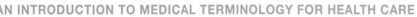

myc/o	
nas/o	
odont/o	
or/o	
ot/o	
palat/o	
phag/o	
pharyng/o	
ptyal/o	
rhin/o	
sial/o	
sin/o, sinus-	
stomat/o	
trich/o	
tympan/o	
uvul/o	

Suffixes

-agogue	
-al	
-algia	
-cele	
-dynia	
-eal	
-ectomy	
-genic	
-gram	
-graphy	
-ia	

-ic	
-ics	
-ist	
-itis	
-lalia	
-lith	
-logy	
-meter	
-metry	
-osis	
-pathy	
-phagia	
-phasia	
-phonia	
-phyma	
-plasty	
-plegia	
-rrhagia	
-rrhoea (Am. -rrhea)	
-schisis	
-scope	
-scopy	
-stomy	
-tomy	
-us	

NOW TRY THE SELF-ASSESSMENT

SELF-ASSESSMENT

Test 12A

Next are some combining forms that refer to the anatomy of the nose and mouth. Indicate which part of the system they refer to by putting a number from the diagrams (Figs 75 and 76) next to each word.

(a) gloss/o

(b) stomat/o

(c) cheil/o

(d) gingiv/o

(e) uvul/o

(f) rhin/o

(g) odont/o

(h) faci/o

Score

8

Test 12B

Prefixes and suffixes

Match each meaning in Column C with a prefix or suffix in Column A by inserting the appropriate number in Column B.

Column A	Column B	Column C
(a) -agogue		1. condition of voice
(b) -cele		2. splitting
(c) -dynia		3. suturing/stitching
(d) -ectomy		4. inflammation
(e) endo-		5. condition of speech
(f) -itis		6. condition of paralysis
(g) -logy		7. straight
(h) -metry		8. measurement
(i) ortho-		9. disease
(j) -pathy		10. condition of excessive flow (of blood)
(k) peri-		11. many
(l) -phasia		12. surgical repair

Column A	Column B	Column C
(m) -phonia		13. condition of pain
(n) -plasty		14. hernia/protrusion/swelling
(o) -plegia		15. removal of
(p) poly-		16. inside/within
(q) prosth-		17. study of
(r) -rrhagia		18. around
(s) -rrhaphy		19. agent that induces/promotes
(t) -schisis		20. addition of artificial part

Score

20

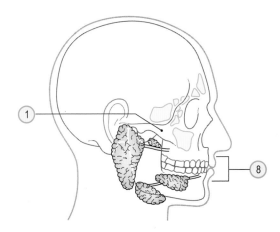

Figure 75   Section of the head showing the sinuses and salivary glands.

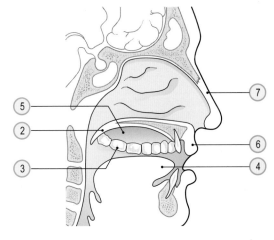

Figure 76   Sagittal section of the nasal cavity and mouth.

Test 12C

Combining forms of word roots

Match each meaning in Column C with a combining form of a word root in Column A by inserting the appropriate number in Column B.

Column A	Column B	Column C
(a) antr/o		1. gum
(b) bucc/o		2. tooth
(c) cheil/o		3. sinus
(d) dynam/o		4. pressure
(e) faci/o		5. larynx
(f) gingiv/o		6. uvula
(g) gloss/o		7. tongue
(h) gnath/o		8. nose
(i) labi/o		9. maxillary sinus / antrum of Highmore
(j) laryng/o		10. hair
(k) man/o		11. mouth
(l) odont/o		12. jaw
(m) palat/o		13. cheek / inside mouth
(n) ptyal/o		14. palate
(o) rhin/o		15. lip (i)
(p) sial/o		16. lip (ii)
(q) sin/o		17. force
(r) stomat/o		18. face
(s) trich/o		19. saliva (i)
(t) uvul/o		20. saliva (ii)

Score [   ] 20

Test 12D

Write the meaning of:

(a) glossodynamom-
    eter
    [   ]

(b) sialometry
    [   ]

(c) stomatoglossitis
    [   ]

(d) gnathopala-
    toschisis
    [   ]

(e) odontogenic
    [   ]

Score [   ] 5

Test 12E

Build words that mean:

(a) incision into a salivary
    gland (use sial/o)
    [   ]

(b) suturing of the palate
    [   ]

(c) condition of fungi in
    the nose
    [   ]

(d) pertaining to the lips
    [   ]

(e) surgical repair of the
    palate
    [   ]

Score [   ] 5

Check answers to Self-Assessment Tests on page 363.

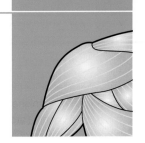

UNIT **13**
THE MUSCULAR SYSTEM

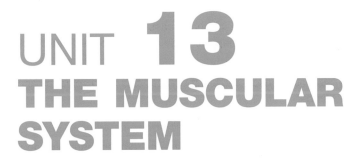

EXERCISE GUIDE

Use this list of word components and their meanings to complete the word exercises in this unit.

Prefixes

dys-	difficult/painful/poor
hyper-	above normal / excessive

Roots / Combining forms

aesthesi/o	sensation (Am. esthesi/o)
cardi/o	heart
electr/o	electrical
esthesi/o (Am.)	sensation
fibr/o	fibre or fibrous tissue (Am. fiber)
neur/o	nerve
paed/o	child (Am. ped/o)
ped/o (Am.)	child
phren/o	diaphragm

Suffixes

-al	pertaining to
-algia	condition of pain
-ar	pertaining to
-genic	pertaining to formation/originating in
-globin	protein
-gram	X-ray/tracing/recording
-graph	usually an instrument that records
-graphy	technique of recording/making an X-ray
-ia	condition of
-ic	pertaining to
-itis	inflammation of
-kymia	condition of involuntary twitching of muscle
-logy	study of
-lysis	breakdown/disintegration
-malacia	condition of softening
-meter	measuring instrument
-oma	tumour/swelling (Am. tumor)
-osis	abnormal condition/disease/abnormal increase
-paresis	slight paralysis
-pathy	disease of
-plasty	surgical repair / reconstruction
-rrhaphy	stitching/suturing
-rrhexis	break/rupture
-sclerosis	condition of hardening
-spasm	involuntary muscle contraction
-tome	cutting instrument
-tomy	incision into
-tonia	condition of tension / tone
-trophy	nourishment/development
-tropic	pertaining to affinity for / stimulating

ANATOMY EXERCISE

When you have finished Word Exercises 1 to 7, look at the word components listed next. Complete Figure 77 by writing the appropriate combining form on each line, more than one component may relate to the same position. (You can check their meanings in the Quick Reference box on p. 194.)

Muscul/o	Tendin/o
My/o	Ten/o

The muscular system

Muscles compose 40% to 50% of the body's weight. The function of muscle is to effect the movement of the body as a whole and to move internal organs involved in the vital processes required to keep the body alive. There are three types of muscles tissue:

- Skeletal muscle moves the vocal chords, diaphragm and limbs.

- Cardiac muscle moves the heart.

- Smooth muscle moves the internal organs, bringing about movement of food through the intestines and urine through the urinary tract. It is also found in the walls of blood vessels, where it acts to maintain blood pressure.

Use the Exercise Guide at the beginning of this unit to complete Word Exercises 1 to 7, unless you are asked to work without it.

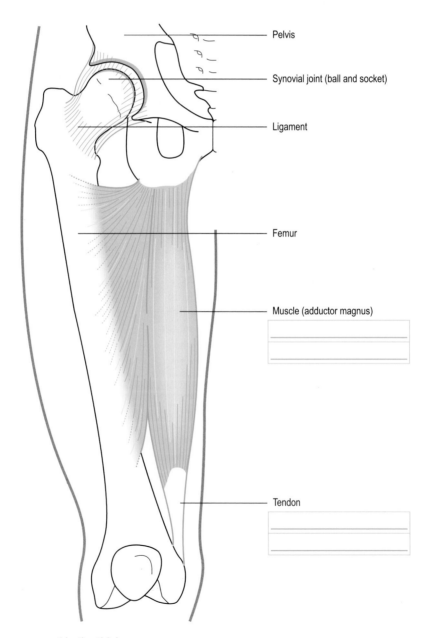

Pelvis

Synovial joint (ball and socket)

Ligament

Femur

Muscle (adductor magnus)

Tendon

Figure 77   A muscle arrangement in the thigh.

Root

My

(*From a Greek word* **mys**, *meaning muscle.*)

Combining forms   My/o, myos

Word Exercise 1

Using your Exercise Guide, find the meaning of:

(a) **my/o**[2]/**neur**[3]/**al**[1]

(b) **my/o**/cardi/o/pathy

(c) **my/o**/dys/trophy

(d) **myos**/itis

(e) **my/o**/fibr/osis

Using your Exercise Guide find the meaning of -globin, -oma, -sclerosis, and -spasm; then build words using my/o that mean:

(f) condition of hardening of a muscle

(g) tumour (Am. tumor) of a muscle

(h) muscle protein

(i) spasm of a muscle

The combining form **lei/o** (from Latin, meaning smooth) is added to myo to give **leiomy/o**, that refers to smooth muscle. A **leiomy**oma is a tumour (Am. tumor) / swelling of smooth muscle.

Using your Exercise Guide, find the meaning of:

(j) **my/o**/kymia

(k) **my/o**/tonia

(l) **my/o**/paresis

(m) **my/o**/rrhexis

(n) **my/o**/malacia

The contraction of a muscle can be measured, using an instrument known as a **myo**graph.

Using your Exercise Guide, find the meaning of electr/o, -gram and -graphy; then beginning with the underlined root, build words that mean:

(o) the technique of recording <u>muscle</u> (contraction)

(p) the technique of recording the <u>electrical</u> currents generated in muscle (contraction)

(q) trace/recording of muscle (made by a myograph)

Root

Rhabd

(*From a Greek word* **rhabdos**, *meaning stripe. Here rhabd/o in combination with my/o it means striped muscle or striated muscle.*)

Combining form   Rhabdomy/o

Word Exercise 2

Without using your Exercise Guide, write the meaning of:

(a) **rhabdomy**/oma

Using your Exercise Guide, find the meaning of:

(b) **rhabdomy/o**/lysis

Root

Muscul

(*From a Latin word* **musculus**, *meaning muscle.*)

Combining form   Muscul/o

Word Exercise 3

Using your Exercise Guide, find the meaning of:

(a) **muscul/o**/tropic

(b) **muscul/o**/phren/ic

Without using your Exercise Guide, write the meaning of:

(c) **muscul**/ar dys/trophy

Note. Loss or impairment of muscular movement due to a lesion in a neuromuscular mechanism is known as a paralysis or palsy (an obsolete term). A paresis is a partial paralysis, and a pseudoparesis is a condition simulating paralysis (*pseud/o-* meaning false). The latter is of hysterical (neurotic) origin and not due to organic disease within a muscle or nerve.

Root

Kine

(*From a Greek word* **kinein**, *meaning movement/motion.*)

Combining forms   Kine/s/i/o, kinet/o

 Word Exercise 4

Using your Exercise Guide, find the meaning of:

(a) **kine**/aesthes/ia
    (Am. **kin**/esthes/ia)

(b) **kine/s/i**/meter

(c) **kinet/o**/genic

(d) hyper/**kines**/ia

Without using your Exercise Guide, build a word using kines/o that means:

(e) condition of disordered movement (involuntary)

A Greek word *taxis* is sometimes used when describing an ordered movement in response to a stimulus. **Ataxia** refers to a disordered movement that is irregular and jerky (*a-* meaning without, ie, condition of without normal movement). There are many types of ataxia, for example, motor ataxia, an inability to control muscles, and Friedreich ataxia, an inherited movement disorder.

Root

Ten

(*From a Greek word* **tenon**, *to stretch. Here ten/o and the combining forms derived from this root all mean tendon. Tendons are the white, fibrous, inelastic cords that attach muscle to bone.*)

Combining forms   Ten/o, tenont/o **(Greek)** tend/o, tendon/o, tendin/o **(Latin).** Note that the combining forms tend/o and tendin/o are derived from Latin tendonis and tendines, meaning tendon.

 Word Exercise 5

Using your Exercise Guide, find the meaning of:

(a) **ten**/algia

(b) **tend/o**/tome

Without using your Exercise Guide, write the meaning of:

(c) **tendin**/itis

(d) **tenont/o**/logy

Using your Exercise Guide and beginning with the underlined root, build words that mean:

(e) repair of a muscle and
    tendon (use ten/o)

(f) incision of a muscle and
    tendon (use ten/o)

A tendon is a fibrous nonelastic cord of connective tissue that is continuous with the fibres of a skeletal muscle; its function is to attach muscle to bone. Tendons must be strong in tension because they are used to pull bones and thereby move the body. If a tendon is wide and thin, it is known as an **aponeurosis**. This word is derived from *apo-* meaning detached/away from, *neur-* meaning tendon (from Greek *neuron*, meaning nerve, sinew, tendon) and *-osis* condition of.

Several words are used with **aponeur/o** meaning an aponeurosis.

Using your Exercise Guide, find the meaning of:

(g) **aponeur/o**/rrhaphy

Without using your Exercise Guide, write the meaning of:

(h) **aponeur**/itis

Root

Orth

(*From a Greek word* **orthos**, *meaning straight. Here orth/o means straight, correct or normal.*)

Combining form   Ortho-, orthot-

 Word Exercise 6

Using your Exercise Guide, find the meaning of:

(a) **ortho**/paed/ic
    (Am. **ortho**/ped/ic)

(Formerly this word applied to the correction of congenital deformities in children. Orthopaedics (Am. orthopedics) is now a branch of surgery dealing with all conditions affecting the locomotor system in children and adults. An orthopaedic surgeon (or orthopaedist) is a medical specialist who deals with problems and injuries that affect the musculoskeletal system.)

Other common words related to this include:

Orthosis
a structure/appliance used to correct a deformity.

Orthotics
the knowledge of use of orthoses.

Medical equipment and clinical procedures

Review the names of all instruments and clinical procedures mentioned in this unit before completing Exercise 7.

 ## Word Exercise 7

Match each description in Column C with a term in Column A by placing the appropriate number in Column B.

Column A	Column B	Column C
(a) myography		1. an appliance used to straighten deformities of the locomotor system
(b) electromyography		2. a recording/trace of muscular movement
(c) myogram		3. a recording of the electrical activity of muscle
(d) kinesimeter		4. technique of recording electrical activity of muscle
(e) orthosis		5. technique of making a recording of muscle (contraction)
(f) electromyogram		6. an instrument used for measuring movement

Other procedures used to investigate the muscular system besides those mentioned in the word exercises include:

Creatine kinase test The enzyme creatine kinase (also known as creatine phosphokinase) is present in all muscle tissue. Any trauma or damage to muscle will result in creatine kinase escaping from cells and subsequently appearing in the plasma. Detection of increased levels in the plasma is an indication that muscle damage has occurred. Increased levels of creatine kinase occur in myositis, muscular dystrophy, muscle trauma and rhabdomyolysis.

Muscle biopsy A small piece of muscle can be removed through an incision or with a hollow needle. Analysis of the tissue sample for cellular and protein abnormalities can distinguish muscular dystrophies from other muscle diseases.
Nerve conduction studies (NCS) Nerve conduction studies measure how quickly a nerve impulse travels along a nerve. If the nerve is trapped, damaged or diseased, then these signals will be altered. The studies help confirm a lesion is in a muscle rather than in the nerve or neuromuscular junction. NCS are typically normal in patients with myopathy.

ANATOMY EXERCISE

Now complete the Anatomy Exercise on page 190.

 ## CASE HISTORY 13

The object of this exercise is to understand words associated with a patient's medical history.

To complete the exercise:

* Read through the passage on Duchenne muscular dystrophy; unfamiliar words are underlined, and you can find their meaning using the Word Help.

* Write the meaning of the medical terms shown in bold print on the lines that follow the Word Help.

Duchenne muscular dystrophy (DMD)

Miss M, a single parent, consulted her GP about her 4-year-old son R, who appeared to have difficulty in climbing the stairs and running. Her son had been slow to sit up and walk and seemed less able than his peers. Her GP observed the child to have a 'waddling' gait and to stand up by 'climbing up his legs' using his hands against his ankles, knees and thighs (Gowers sign). His calf muscles appeared to be bulky and lacking strength. He was referred to the Paediatric (Am. Pediatric) Hospital with suspected muscular **dystrophy**.

Detailed examination revealed R to have proximal weakness in his limbs and **pseudohypertrophy** of his calf muscles. A muscle biopsy showed **dystrophic** changes with muscle fibre necrosis and their replacement with fat. Immunochemical staining detected an absence of dystrophin. His serum creatine phosphokinase levels were grossly elevated. **Electromyography** indicated a **myopathic** pattern with short polyphasic action potentials.

R's mother was also investigated and also found to have raised serum creatine phosphokinase levels and an abnormal **electromyogram**. R was diagnosed as having Duchenne muscular dystrophy, a fatal sex-linked condition inherited from his mother. DMD is due to a mutant gene located on the X-chromosome, and as there appeared to be no previous incidence of this condition in the family, it was likely this was a spontaneous mutation. Miss M was advised by the genetics counsellor that she was a carrier of DMD, and if she produced another boy there was a 50% chance that he would also have DMD.

By the age of 10, R was severely disabled and receiving daily passive physiotherapy to help prevent contractures of his muscles. At 14, he was unable to move his arms and legs and his limb bones were long and thin (disuse **atrophy**). He died at the age of 16 from **myocardial** involvement and pulmonary infection.

Now write the meaning of the following words from the Case History without using your dictionary lists:

(a) dystrophy

(b) pseudohypertrophy

(c) dystrophic

(d) electromyography

(e) myopathic

(f) electromyogram

(g) atrophy

(h) myocardial

(Answers to the Case History exercise are given in the Answers to Word Exercises on page 190.)

Word Help

action potential an electrochemical impulse generated by a muscle or nerve

biopsy removal and examination of living tissue

contractures abnormal shortening/contraction of muscle

dystrophin an essential structural protein found in muscle fibres

gait manner of walking

GP general practitioner (family doctor)

immunochemical pertaining to chemical basis of immunity

mutant a gene that has changed from normal form resulting in a change to the organism inheriting it

mutation a sudden change in the genetic material of cells (in this case, in the mother's sex cells)

necrosis condition of localized death of tissue

passive not produced by the active effort of (the patient)

physiotherapy treatment using physical means to maintain or build physique or correct deformities due to injury or disease (Am. physical therapy)

polyphasic pertaining to many phases (here electrical potentials out of phase)

proximal near to origin/point of attachment

pulmonary pertaining to the lungs

serum a clear fluid separated from blood when it is allowed to clot

sex-linked a gene linked to a sex chromosome (may result in increased frequency of certain disorders in one particular sex, eg, DMD affects boys only)

X-chromosome one of a pair of sex chromosomes that determine the sex of an individual

Quick Reference

Combining forms relating to the muscular system:

Aponeur/o	aponeurosis
Fibr/o	fibre (Am. fiber)
Kinesi/o	movement
Lei/o	smooth (muscle)
Muscul/o	muscle
My/o	muscle
Paed/o	child (Am. ped/o)
Ped/o (Am.)	child
Rhabd/o	striated (muscle)
Tax/o	ordered movement
Tendin/o	tendon
Tend/o	tendon
Ten/o	tendon
Tenont/o	tendon

Abbreviations

Some common abbreviations related to the muscular system are listed next. Note that some are not standard, and their meaning may vary from one healthcare setting to another. There is a more extensive list for reference on page 369.

DTR	deep tendon reflex
EMG	electromyogram/electromyography
i.m.	intramuscular
MAMC	mid-arm muscle circumference
MAP	muscle action potential
MD	muscular dystrophy
MFT	muscle function test
MS	muscle shortening / strength / musculoskeletal
Ortho	orthopaedics (Am. orthopedics)
OT	occupational therapy
PT	physical therapy
ROM	range of movement
TJ	triceps jerk

Pathology notes

Crush injury

Severe trauma or sustained pressure to a skeletal muscle may reduce blood supply and cause ischaemia (Am. ischemia) and massive muscle necrosis. Crush injuries greatly damage the affected muscle tissue, and when the circulation is restored, the muscle pigment myoglobin and other necrotic products are released from the damaged area into the blood. This material is highly toxic to the kidneys, and life-threatening acute renal failure may develop.

Hernia

Weakness of abdominal muscles can lead to protrusion of an abdominal organ (commonly the small intestine) through an opening in the abdominal wall; this is called a hernia. There are several types; the most common, *inguinal hernia*, occurs when the intestine extends through the inguinal canal into the scrotum or labia. Males experience this most often, and it can occur at any age. Some women may experience *femoral hernia* because of changes during pregnancy. Hernia is referred to as reducible when the organ is manipulated back into the abdominal cavity either naturally by lying down or by manual reduction through a surgical opening into the abdomen. A *strangulated hernia* occurs when the mass is not reducible, and blood flow to the affected organ is stopped. When this occurs, pain and vomiting are usually experienced, and emergency surgical intervention is required.

Muscular dystrophy

Muscular dystrophy is not a single disorder but a group of genetic diseases characterized by atrophy (wasting of skeletal muscle tissues). Some but not all forms of muscular dystrophy can be fatal.

The common form of muscular dystrophy is Duchenne muscular dystrophy (DMD) in which formation of excessive amounts of fat and fibrous tissue (pseudohypertrophy) masks the atrophy of muscle. DMD is characterized by mild leg muscle weakness that progresses rapidly to the shoulder muscles. The first signs are apparent at about 3 years of age, and the stricken child is usually severely affected within 5 to 10 years. Death from respiratory or cardiac muscle weakness often occurs before the age of 21. DMD is caused by a mutation in the X-chromosome, and as boys have only one X-chromosome inherited from their mother, they are affected with the disease.

Myasthenia gravis

Myasthenia gravis is a chronic disease characterized by muscle weakness, especially in the face and throat. Most forms of the disease begin with mild weakness and chronic muscle fatigue in the face, and then progress to wider muscle involvement with severe weakness. When severe muscle weakness causes immobility in all four limbs, a myasthenic crisis is said to have occurred; a person in this condition is in danger of dying from respiratory failure because of weakness in the respiratory muscles. Myasthenia gravis is an autoimmune disease in which the immune system attacks muscle cells at the neuromuscular junction. Nerve impulses are then unable to fully stimulate the affected muscle.

Polymyositis

Polymyositis and dermatomyositis are chronic inflammatory diseases affecting many muscles. Although dermatomyositis affects muscle and skin, it can affect other parts of the body such as the oesophagus (Am. esophagus) and lungs. Their exact cause is unknown, but they are autoimmune diseases, and viral infection has been implicated in their development. Symptoms include pain, with marked weakness and/or loss of muscle mass in the muscles of the head, neck, torso and upper arms and legs.

Torticollis

A spasmodic contraction of several superficial and deep muscles of the neck that produces twisting of the neck and an unnatural position of the head (also called wryneck).

Trichinosis

A myositis caused by infection with the parasitic nematode worm *Trichinella spiralis* that encysts in the muscles of humans, pigs and rats. Infection results from eating inadequately cooked pork; symptoms include nausea, diarrhoea (Am. diarrhea) and fever that lead to painful swelling of the muscles and oedema (Am. edema).

Associated words

Atonic pertaining to without tone, lacking normal muscle tone

Contracture a permanent shortening of muscle tissue rendering the muscle highly resistant to passive stretching

Contusion a muscle bruise caused by minor trauma such as a blow to a limb in which there is local internal bleeding and inflammation

Cramp a painful muscle spasm (involuntary twitch), a symptom of irritation that may be due to an ion or water imbalance within a muscle

Dystonia condition of poor tone; abnormal muscle tone that causes impairment of voluntary muscle movement

Extension the movement of a limb that increases the angle between two bones at a joint; the straightening of a limb at a joint

Fasciculation a condition in which there are small, local, involuntary contractions of muscle fibres that are visible under the skin (Am. fibers). The contractions may occur regularly and are not associated with movement of the affected muscle

Fibrillation a small, local, involuntary muscle contraction due to activation of single muscle fibres (Am. fibers)

Flexion the movement of a limb that decreases the angle between two bones at a joint; the bending of a limb at a joint

Hyperextension the forcible extension of a limb beyond its normal limit at a joint

Hypotonia condition of reduced tone in a muscle

Insertion the point of attachment of a muscle to the bone that it moves

Irritability the ability to react to a stimulus, eg, the ability of a muscle to receive and respond to stimulation

Myoclonus a sudden, involuntary contraction of a muscle or group of muscles

Origin the point of attachment of a muscle (to a bone)

Paralysis loss or impairment of movement and/or sensory function in some part of the body; it results from a lesion of nervous or muscle origin

Rigidity a sustained muscle tension causing the affected part to become stiff and inflexible

Spasm a sudden, violent, involuntary contraction of a large group of muscles

Strain overuse or stretching of a muscle or tendon

Tetany increased excitability of nerves and muscles due to low levels of calcium; it results in involuntary muscle contraction and painful spasms in the hands and feet

Tic a spasmodic, compulsive, repetitive and involuntary movement made by muscles that are usually under voluntary control; tics are often seen in the face and shoulders

Tone the normal degree of tension in a muscle that maintains posture and normal movements

Tremor a rhythmic, involuntary, purposeless contraction of antagonistic muscles

NOW TRY THE WORD CHECK

WORD CHECK

This self-check exercise lists all the word components used in this unit. First, write down the meaning of as many word components as you can. Then, check your answers using the Exercise Guide and Quick Reference box or the Glossary of Word Components (pp. 383–410).

Prefixes

a-

dys-

hyper-

Combining forms of word roots

aesthesi/o (Am. esthesi/o)

aponeur/o

cardi/o

electr/o

fibr/o

kinesi/o

lei/o

muscul/o

My/o

neur/o

ortho-

paed/o (Am. ped/o)

phren/o

pseud/o

rhabd/o

tax/o

tendin/o

tend/o

ten/o

tenont/o

Suffixes

-al

-algia

-genic

-globin

-gram

-graph

-graphy

-ic

-itis

-kymia

-logy

-lysis

-meter

-oma

-osis

-paresis

-pathy

-rrhaphy

-rrhexis

-sclerosis

-spasm

-taxia

-tome

-tonia

-trophy

-tropic

NOW TRY THE SELF-ASSESSMENT

SELF-ASSESSMENT

Test 13A

Prefixes, suffixes and combining forms of word roots

Match each meaning in Column C with a word component in Column A by inserting the appropriate number in Column B.

Column A	Column B	Column C
(a) aesthesi/o (Am. esthesi/o)		1. child
(b) cardi/o		2. movement
(c) electr/o		3. tumour (Am. tumor) / swelling
(d) fibr/o		4. diaphragm
(e) -globin		5. slight paralysis/ weakness
(f) kinesi/o		6. rupture/break
(g) muscul/o		7. condition of hardening
(h) my/o		8. electrical
(i) -oma		9. protein
(j) ortho-		10. involuntary contraction of muscle
(k) paed/o (Am. ped/o)		11. condition of continuous slight contrac-tion of muscle
(l) -paresis		12. nourishment
(m) phren/o		13. fibre (Am. fiber)
(n) -rrhexis		14. pertaining to affinity for/ acting on
(o) -sclerosis		15. heart
(p) -spasm		16. muscle (i)
(q) ten/o		17. muscle (ii)
(r) -tonia		18. sensation
(s) -trophy		19. straight
(t) -tropic		20. tendon

Score

20

Test 13B

Write the meaning of:

(a) electromyography

(b) kinesiology

(c) myotenotomy

(d) myoatrophy

(e) musculoaponeurotic

Score

5

Test 13C

Build words that mean:

(a) condition of softening of muscle

(b) pertaining to originating in muscle

(c) disease of muscle

(d) suturing of a tendon (use ten/o)

(e) cutting of a tendon (use ten/o)

Score

15

Check answers to Self-Assessment Tests on pages 363–364.

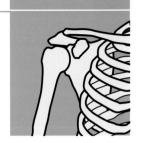

UNIT **14**
THE SKELETAL SYSTEM

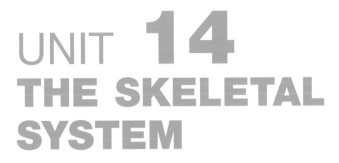

Once you have completed Unit 14, you should be able to do the following:

- understand the meaning of medical words relating to the skeletal system
- build medical words relating to the skeletal system
- associate medical terms with their anatomical position
- understand common medical abbreviations relating to the skeletal system

EXERCISE GUIDE

Use this list of word components and their meanings to complete the word exercises in this unit.

Prefixes

dys-	bad/difficult/painful
endo-	within/inside
inter-	between
poly-	many

Roots / Combining forms

calcin/o	calcium
cost/o	rib
fibr/o	fibre (Am. fiber)
my/o	muscle
petr/o	stone/rock/brittle
por/o	pore
py/o	pus

Suffixes

-al	pertaining to
-algia	condition of pain
-blast	cell that forms/immature germ cell
-centesis	puncture to remove fluid
-clasis	breaking
-clast	a cell that breaks
-desis	fixation/bind together by surgery

-eal	pertaining to
-ectomy	removal of
-genesis	capable of causing/forming
-genic	pertaining to formation / originating in
-gram	X-ray/tracing/recording
-graphy	technique of recording/making an X-ray
-ic	pertaining to
-itis	inflammation of
-lith	stone
-logist	specialist who studies…
-lysis	break down / disintegration
-lytic	pertaining to breaking down/disintegration
-malacia	condition of softening
-oid	resembling
-olisthesis	slipping / forward displacement
-oma	tumour/swelling (Am. tumor)
-osis	abnormal condition/disease/abnormal increase
-ous	pertaining to / of the nature of
-pathy	disease of
-phyte	a plant / a pathological growth
-plasty	surgical repair/reconstruction
-scope	an instrument used to view/examine
-scopy	technique of viewing/examining
-tome	cutting instrument
-trophy	nourishment/development

ANATOMY EXERCISE

When you have finished Word Exercises 1 to 10, look at the word components listed below. Complete Figure 78 by writing the appropriate combining form on each line. (You can check their meanings in the Quick Reference box on p. 207.)

Arthr/o	Myel/o	Spondyl/o
Chondr/o	Oste/o	Synovi/o
Disc/o		

The skeletal system

The supporting structure of the body consisting of 206 bones is known as the skeletal system. This system has five main functions:

- it supports all tissues

- it protects vital organs and soft tissues

- it manufactures blood cells

- it stores minerals that can be released into the blood

- it assists in movement

Cartilage is found at the ends of bones and functions to form a smooth surface for the movement of one bone over another at a joint.

Freely moveable joints are called synovial joints, such as the ball-and-socket type at the shoulder and hip and the hinge type at the elbow, knee and ankle (See Fig. 78(a)). A joint capsule composed of fibrous tissue surrounds the ends of bones in a synovial joint. The synovial membrane underneath the capsule secretes synovial fluid into the small synovial cavity between the bones; the fluid acts as a lubricant and reduces friction between the articular cartilages. To the outside of the capsule lie tough connective tissues

called ligaments; these prevent the joint from separating and provide joint stability. The primary function of ligaments is to join bone to bone and prevent movement that may damage the joint.

Some joints are immovable such as the suture joints between the skull bones. Others such as those between the vertebrae are partially moveable (See Fig. 78(b)).

Use the Exercise Guide at the beginning of this unit to complete Word Exercises 1 to 10, unless you are asked to work without it.

Root

Oste

(*From a Greek word* **osteon**, *meaning bone.*)

Combining form   Oste/o

 Word Exercise 1

Using your Exercise Guide, find the meaning of:

(a) **oste/o**/phyte (refers to a bony outgrowth at joint surface)

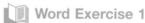

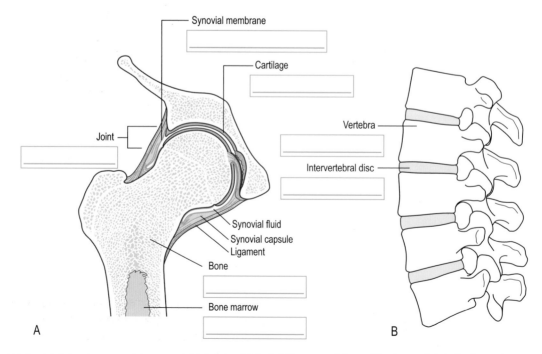

Figure 78   Joints. (a) A freely moveable synovial joint, and (b) slightly moveable cartilaginous joints in the spine.

(b) **oste/o**/por/osis (refers to loss of calcium/phosphorus/bone density)

(c) **oste/o**/malacia (a condition caused by lack of vitamin D in adults)

(d) **oste/o**/petr/osis (refers to spotty calcification of bone, which becomes brittle)

(e) **oste/o**/clasis

(f) **oste/o**/clast (a type of cell, compare with osteoblast)

(g) **oste/o**/dys/trophy

Using your Exercise Guide, look up the meaning of -blast, -logist, -lytic, and -tome; then build words that mean:

(h) a cell that forms bone

(i) pertaining to breaking down of bone

(j) instrument to cut bone

(k) specialist who studies bones

(*Osseus* is a Latin word meaning of bone. The combining form oss/e/o is used in **osse**ous, meaning pertaining to bone or of the nature of bone, and **oss**ification, means to form bone.)

disturbance of connective tissues, especially those associated with joints). See the Pathology Notes on pages 207–209.

(e) **arthr/o**/desis

(Also known as an artificial **ankylosis** (from Greek *agkyloun* meaning to stiffen). An arthrodesis is achieved by surgery; see Fig. 79.)

Without using your Exercise Guide, write the meaning of:

(f) **arthr/o**/clasis

Using your Exercise Guide, look up the meaning of -centesis, -gram, -lith, -pathy, -plasty and -scopy; then build words that mean:

(g) technique of viewing a joint

(h) puncture of a joint to remove fluid

(i) X-ray picture of a joint

(j) disease of a joint

(k) stony material in a joint

(l) surgical repair of a joint

(This operation includes the formation of artificial joints, eg, in a hip replacement where the natural joint is replaced with a metallic prosthesis; Fig. 80.)

Root

Arthr

(*From a Greek word* **arthron**, *meaning joint or articulation, ie, the point where two or more bones meet.*)

Combining form   Arthr/o

Word Exercise 2

Using your Exercise Guide, find the meaning of:

(a) **arthr/o**/scope

(b) **arthr/o**/py/osis

(c) **arthr/o**/graphy

(d) poly/**arthr**/itis

Rheumatoid arthritis refers to a polyarthritis accompanied by general ill health and varying degrees of crippling joint deformities, pain and stiffness (*rheumat/o* refers to rheumatism, a condition marked by inflammation, degeneration and metabolic

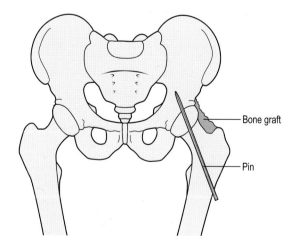

Figure 79   Arthrodesis of the hip.

Root

Synovi

(*From a New Latin word* **synovia**, *meaning the fluid secreted by the synovial membrane that lines the cavity of a joint. Here synovi/o means synovial membrane.*)

Combining forms   Synov/i/o

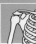
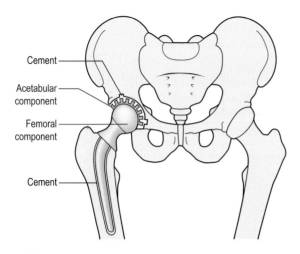

Cement

Acetabular
component

Femoral
component

Cement

Figure 80   Arthroplasty.

 Word Exercise 3

Without using your Exercise Guide, write the meaning of:

(a) arthr/o²/**synov**³/itis¹

Using your Exercise Guide, find the meaning of:

(b) **synov**/ectomy

(c) **synov/i**/oma

Bursae are sacs of synovial fluid surrounded by a synovial membrane; they are found between tendons, ligaments and bones. Inflammation due to pressure, injury or infection results in **burs**itis (from Latin *bursa,* meaning purse).

Root

Chondr

(*From a Greek word* **chondros***, meaning cartilage, the plastic-like connective tissue found at the ends of bones, eg, in joints where it forms a smooth surface for movement of a joint.*)

Combining form   Chondr/o

 Word Exercise 4

Without using your Exercise Guide, write the meaning of:

(a) **chondr/o**/phyte

(b) **chondr**/osse/ous

(c) **chondr/o**/por/osis

(d) **chondr/o**/dys/trophy

(e) **chondr/o**/malacia

Using your Exercise Guide, find the meaning of:

(f) **chondr/o**/cost/al

(g) endo/**chondr**/al

Using your Exercise Guide, find the meaning of -algia, -genesis and -lysis; then build words that mean:

(h) condition of pain in a cartilage

(i) formation of cartilage

(j) breakdown of cartilage

Using your Exercise Guide, find the meaning of:

(k) **chondr/o**/calcin/osis

A cartilage that is often damaged and removed is the crescent-shaped cartilage in the knee joint. The operation to remove this is known as **menisc**ectomy (from Latin *meniscus,* meaning crescent; combining form **menisc/o**).

Root

Spondyl

(*From Greek word* **spondylos***, meaning vertebra, one of the irregular bones that make up the vertebral column or spine.*)

Combining form   Spondyl/o

 Word Exercise 5

Without using your Exercise Guide, write the meaning of:

(a) **spondyl**/algia

(b) **spondyl/o**/py/osis

Without using your Exercise Guide, build words that mean:

(c) breakdown/disintegration of vertebrae

(d) any disease of vertebrae

(e) inflammation of vertebrae

Using your Exercise Guide, find the meaning of:

(f) **spondyl**/olisthesis (this applies to lumbar vertebrae)

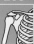

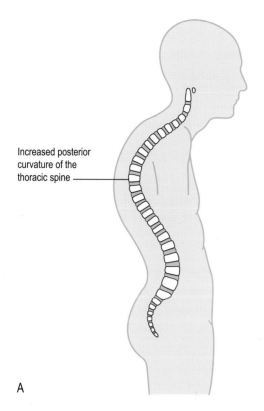

Increased posterior
curvature of the
thoracic spine

A

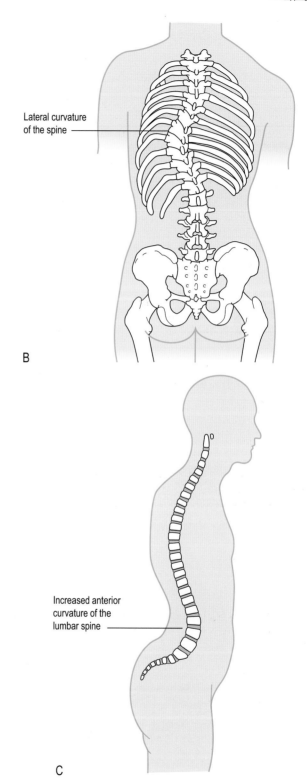

Lateral curvature
of the spine

B

Increased anterior
curvature of the
lumbar spine

C

Figure 81   (a) Kyphosis, (b) scoliosis, and (c) lordosis.

Here we need to mention three other conditions of the vertebrae:

Kyphosis

A condition of increased posterior curvature of the thoracic spine (as viewed from the side), commonly called hunchback or dowager's hump. (**Kyph/o** is from Greek *kyphos*, meaning crooked/hump.) See Figure 81(a).

Scoliosis

A condition of lateral curvature of the spine. (**Scoli/o** is from a Greek word *scoli*, meaning crooked/twisted.) See Figure 81(b).

Lordosis

A condition of anterior curvature of the spine in the lumbar region. (**Lord-** is from a Greek word *lordos*, meaning to bend the body forward). See Figure 81(c).

These words can be combined as in:

Scoliokyphosis
Kyphoscoliosis   ⊢   both conditions show lateral and posterior curvature of the spine

Figure 81, cont'd

▌Root

Disc

(*From a Latin word* **diskus**, *meaning disc. Here disc/o means an intervertebral disc, a pad of connective tissue that acts as a shock absorber between vertebrae.*)

Combining forms   Disc/o, disk/o *(Am.)*

 Word Exercise 6

Using your Exercise Guide, find the meaning of:

(a) **disc**/oid

(b) **disc**/o/genic

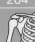

Without using your Exercise Guide, build words that mean:

(c) technique of making an X-ray of an intervertebral disc

(d) removal of an intervertebral disc

The excision of degenerated intervertebral discs requires the removal of a thin layer of bone from the vertebral arch. This operation is termed a **lamin**ectomy (from Latin *lamina*, meaning thin plate; combining form **lamin/o**).

Note. Abnormal protrusion (herniation) of the inner portion (nucleus pulposus) of an intervertebral disc into the spinal cord or spinal nerve is commonly called a slipped disc. It is also known as a prolapsed disc or spinal disc herniation. The condition is due to age-related degeneration of the outer fibrous layer of the disc (annulus fibrosus), trauma or a lifting injury. It often results in low back pain and sciatica (leg pain) when a disc protrudes onto a spinal nerve in the lumbar spine, and neck and arm pain occur when it protrudes onto a nerve in the cervical spine. (See Fig. 82.)

Root

Myel

(*From a Greek word* **myelos**, *meaning marrow. Here myel/o means bone marrow, but it is also used to mean spinal cord and myelocyte, a type of blood cell that forms in bone marrow.*)

Combining form   Myel/o

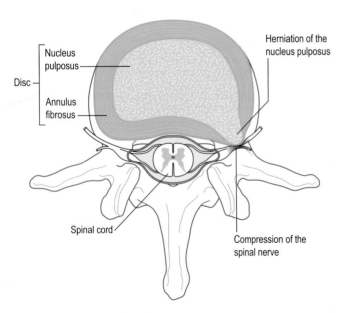

Figure 82   Herniation of an intervertebral disc. (Adapted from Chabner D-E, The Language of Medicine, 10th Edition, 2013, Saunders.)

Word Exercise 7

Without using your Exercise Guide, write the meaning of:

(a) osteo/**myel**/itis

(b) **myel/o**/fibr/osis

Medical equipment and clinical procedures

Review the names of all instruments and clinical procedures mentioned in this unit, and then try Exercise 8.

Word Exercise 8

Match each description in Column C with a term in Column A by placing the appropriate number in Column B.

Column A	Column B	Column C
(a) osteotome		1. puncture of a joint to withdraw synovial fluid
(b) arthrodesis		2. technique of making an X-ray of a joint
(c) replacement arthroplasty		3. fixation of a joint by surgery
(d) arthrocentesis		4. a chisel-like instrument used to cut bone
(e) arthrography		5. insertion of a metallic prosthesis to replace a joint

Other procedures used to investigate the skeletal system besides those mentioned in the word exercises include:

Bone density scan Dual energy X-ray absorptiometry (DEXA or DXA) is a test that measures the density of bones. A DEXA scan passes low-energy X-rays from two different sources through the bone being tested. An X-ray detector then measures how well the X-rays penetrate the bone; the more dense it is, the less X-rays get through. Areas of decreased density indicate the presence of osteopenia and osteoporosis.

Bone scan Also called a radionuclide scan or scintigram, this procedure uses radionuclides to create images of bones. Radionuclides are chemicals that emit gamma rays that can be detected with a scanner called a gamma camera. The tiny amount of radionuclide injected into the bloodstream collects in areas where there is a lot of bone activity (breakdown or new bone formation). The scan shows up areas of infection, stress fractures and tumour formation; these are known as hot spots on the scan (Am. tumor).

Computed tomography (CT) The technique of recording a series of X-rays showing bones, muscles and joints in multiple cross-sectional views.

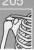

Discography An invasive diagnostic procedure for evaluating intervertebral disc disease. It is used to confirm a suspected disc as the source of pain where other tests have failed. Each disc is injected with a contrast medium using X-rays to guide the needle, and pain responses are noted.

Erythrocyte sedimentation rate (ESR) This is the measurement of the time it takes red blood cells to settle to the bottom of a test tube. Elevated times are associated with inflammatory disorders such as rheumatoid arthritis, tumours and infections of bone and soft tissues.

Magnetic resonance imaging (MRI) This is the technique of using strong magnetic fields and radio waves to create detailed images in three planes; here, it is used to diagnose primary tumours and metastases of bone and image muscles and ligaments (Am. tumor).

Radiography Bone is a dense tissue that shows up clearly on an X-ray. Radiography therefore is very useful for diagnosis of fractures, scoliosis, tumours, osteoporosis and osteomyelitis (Am. tumor).

The skeleton

There are many terms that refer to specific bones within the skeleton. Look at the diagram (Fig. 83), and then complete Exercises 9 and 10.

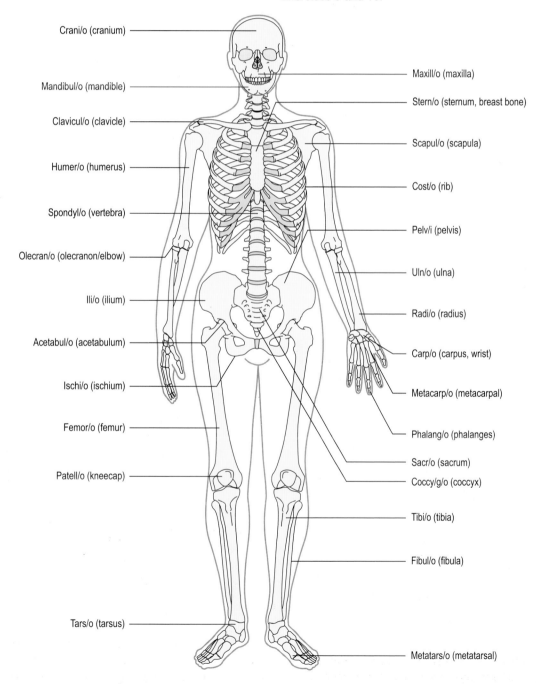

Crani/o (cranium)
Mandibul/o (mandible)
Clavicul/o (clavicle)
Humer/o (humerus)
Spondyl/o (vertebra)
Olecran/o (olecranon/elbow)
Ili/o (ilium)
Acetabul/o (acetabulum)
Ischi/o (ischium)
Femor/o (femur)
Patell/o (kneecap)
Tars/o (tarsus)

Maxill/o (maxilla)
Stern/o (sternum, breast bone)
Scapul/o (scapula)
Cost/o (rib)
Pelv/i (pelvis)
Uln/o (ulna)
Radi/o (radius)
Carp/o (carpus, wrist)
Metacarp/o (metacarpal)
Phalang/o (phalanges)
Sacr/o (sacrum)
Coccy/g/o (coccyx)
Tibi/o (tibia)
Fibul/o (fibula)
Metatars/o (metatarsal)

Figure 83   The skeleton.

Word Exercise 9

Using your Exercise Guide and beginning with the underlined word, build words that mean:

(a) surgical repair/reconstruction of the clavicle (collar bone)

(b) condition of softening of the cranium

(c) pertaining to between the ribs

(d) removal of a finger bone

(e) pertaining to the pelvis

(f) inflammation of an elbow joint

(g) pertaining to the femur and tibia

(h) surgical fixation of the scapula (shoulder blade)

(i) condition of pain in the metatarsal region

(j) surgical operation to reconstruct the hip socket

(k) surgical repair of the lower jaw

(l) inflammation of the upper jaw

(m) pertaining to the ribs and sternum

(n) pertaining to the coccyx and ischium (use -eal)

(h) **patell**/o/**femor**/al

(i) **ili**/o/**sacr**/al

(j) **tibi**/o/**fibul**/ar

ANATOMY EXERCISE

Now complete the Anatomy Exercise on page 200.

 CASE HISTORY 14

The object of this exercise is to understand words associated with a patient's medical history.

To complete the exercise:

- Read through the passage on rheumatoid arthritis; unfamiliar words are underlined, and you can find their meaning using the Word Help.

- Write the meaning of the medical terms shown in bold print on the lines that follow the Word Help.

Rheumatoid arthritis

Mrs N, a 58-year-old female, was referred to the **rheumatologist** by her GP with a generalized **arthralgia** and aggravating symptoms in her left shoulder. Her GP prescribed NSAIDs for 7 weeks, bringing some relief. Five years previously, she had a **bursitis** in the same shoulder that had been successfully treated. There was no history of rheumatoid arthritis in her family.

Examination revealed a widespread symmetrical **polyarthritis** with swelling and tenderness in her **metacarpophalangeal** joints, proximal **interphalangeal** joints and **metatarsophalangeal** joints. Both wrists were swollen and tender, and all metatarsal heads were painful on compression. There were signs of small muscle wasting in both hands. Her back was not affected, and those joints that were seemed to be stiff in the mornings for several hours. She complained of recurrent fatigue.

Mrs N had diminished movement of the chest with dullness on percussion; breath sounds were absent at the right base.

Joint radiography indicated an erosion in the 3rd metatarsophalangeal joint, and a CXR confirmed a right-sided pleural effusion. Haematology (Am. hematology) reported a high rheumatoid factor. A diagnosis of erosive rheumatoid arthritis with pleural effusion was made. Initial treatment of her inflammatory **arthropathy** was enteric-coated aspirin 4 g/day; she was advised of possible side effects.

Word Exercise 10

Using your Exercise Guide and Figure 83, find the meaning of:

(a) inter/**phalang**/eal

(b) **metatars**/algia

(c) tarso/**metatars**/al

(d) **metacarp**/al

(e) **humer**/o/**radi**/al

(f) **uln**/o/**carp**/al

(g) **coccyg**/algia

Word Help

aggravating making worse

base here it refers to the base/lower part of the right lung

compression pressing

CXR chest X-ray

effusion a fluid discharge into a part/escape of fluid into an enclosed space

enteric pertaining to the intestine, here refers to a coating on a pill or tablet that allows it to pass to the intestine without being affected in the stomach

erosion destruction (here of a piece of bone)

GP general practitioner (family doctor)

haematology the study of blood, here refers to the department that analyses blood (Am. hematology)

NSAID a nonsteroidal antiinflammatory drug

percussion striking the body to produce a sound (here striking the thoracic wall)

pleural pertaining to the pleura (membranes that surround the lungs)

proximal near to origin/point of attachment

radiography technique of making an X-ray/recording

rheumatoid resembling rheumatism (a painful condition marked by inflammation and degeneration of connective tissues especially around joints)

rheumatoid factor type of antibody found in the sera of patients with rheumatoid arthritis

symmetrical correspondence on opposite sides of the body/ equality of parts on either side of the midline of the body

Now, write the meaning of the following words from the Case History without using your dictionary lists:

(a) rheumatologist

(b) arthralgia

(c) bursitis

(d) polyarthritis

(e) metacarpophalangeal

(f) interphalangeal

(g) metatarsophalangeal

(h) arthropathy

(Answers to the Case History exercise are given in the Answers to Word Exercises on page 350.)

Quick Reference

Combining forms relating to the skeletal system:

Ankyl/o	fusion/adhesion/bent
Arthro	joint
Burs/o	bursa
Calcin/o	calcium
Chondr/o	cartilage
Cost/o	rib
Disc/o	intervertebral disc
Fibr/o	fibre (Am. fiber)
Kyph/o	crooked/humped
Lamin/o	lamina/part of vertebral arch
Lord/o	bend forward
Menisc/o	meniscus
Myel/o	bone marrow
Osse/o	bone
Oste/o	bone
Petr/o	stone/rock
Por/o	passage/pore
Scoli/o	crooked/twisted
Spondyl/o	vertebra
Synovi/o	synovial fluid / synovial membrane

Abbreviations

Some common abbreviations related to the skeletal system are listed next. Note that some are not standard, and their meaning may vary from one healthcare setting to another. There is a more extensive list for reference on page 369.

ACL	anterior cruciate ligament (of the knee)
BM(T)	bone marrow trephine
C 1–7	cervical vertebrae 1–7
CDH	congenital dislocation of the hip
CTS	carpal tunnel syndrome
Fx	fracture
L 1–5	lumbar vertebrae 1–5
OA	osteoarthritis
Ortho	orthopaedics (Am. orthopedics)
PID	prolapsed intervertebral disc
RA	rheumatoid arthritis
RF (RhF)	rheumatoid factor
T 1–12	thoracic vertebrae 1–12
THR	total hip replacement
TKR	total knee replacement
TMJ	temporomandibular joint

Pathology notes

Bone fracture

A bone fracture is defined as a partial or complete break in the continuity of a bone that occurs under mechanical stress. The most common cause of a fracture is traumatic injury. Bone cancer or metabolic bone disorders can also cause fractures by weakening a bone to the point that it fractures under very little stress. An *open fracture*, also known as a *compound fracture*, is one in which the broken bone projects through surrounding tissue and skin, inviting the possibility of infection. A *closed fracture*, also known as a *simple fracture*, does not produce a break in the skin and therefore does not pose an immediate danger of bone infection. Fractures are also classified as complete or incomplete. A complete fracture involves a break across an entire section of bone; whereas an incomplete fracture involves only a partial break in which bone fragments are still partially joined. Treatment usually involves reduction (realignment) of the bone, immobilization and restoring function through rehabilitation.

Carpal tunnel syndrome (CTS)

The carpal tunnel is a narrow passage in the wrist made up of the carpal bones and the transverse carpal ligament. Within the tunnel are the tendons that move the fingers and the median nerve. When the tendons become inflamed or swollen, the median nerve is compressed causing pain, numbness, paraesthesia (pins and needles, Am. paresthesia) and weakness of the thumb. Treatment is by immobilization of the wrist, antiinflammatory drugs or surgery to sever the transverse carpal ligament.

Ewing sarcoma

Named after James Ewing (1866–1943), this is the second most common primary sarcoma in children and young people. Although it can occur at any age, it is less common after the age of 30. The sarcoma can develop anywhere but is usually found in the pelvis, tibia or femur. In a very few cases, the sarcoma will start in the soft tissues that surround the bone or the joint, rather than the bone itself; this is called an extraosseous Ewing sarcoma. While the cause of Ewing sarcoma is not known, it is thought to relate to the stress placed on bones during times of rapid growth.

Gout

Gout is a type of arthritis more prevalent in males than females. It is a metabolic disorder in which blood levels of uric acid are raised leading to the deposition of sodium urate crystals in the synovial fluid of joints. The crystals are also deposited in soft tissues around joints, where they form hard swellings called tophi; the crystals trigger the chronic inflammation and tissue damage seen with the disease. In many cases, only one joint is involved (monoarthritis) and is typically swollen, hot and painful. The sites most commonly affected are the metatarsophalangeal joint of the big toe and the joints at the wrists, elbows, ankles and knees. A drug for the treatment of gout called allopurinol acts to inhibit the formation of uric acid.

Osteoarthritis (OA)

Osteoarthritis, also known as degenerative joint disease (DJD), is the most common noninflammatory disorder of moveable joints. It is characterized by 'wear and tear' deterioration, atrophy of articular cartilage, formation of new bone at joint surfaces and calcification of ligaments. Osteoarthritis occurs most often in the weight-bearing joints, such as the hips, lumbar spine and knees. Symptoms include stiffness, pain on movement and limited joint motion; there is also frequent involvement of the joints in the fingers. The cause of osteoarthritis is unknown, and no treatment is available to stop degeneration of the joints. Nonsteroidal antiinflammatory drugs (NSAIDs) are used to alleviate symptoms of pain and inflammation.

Osteomalacia and rickets

Osteomalacia is a condition seen in adults characterized by painful softening of bones caused by vitamin D deficiency. In children the condition is called rickets, and the deficiency results in a failure to absorb calcium and phosphorus from the small intestine. As a consequence, there is poor calcification of bone, and when the child walks, the weight of the body causes the legs to bow. The condition may develop because of lack of vitamin D in the diet, lack of exposure of the skin to UV light, malabsorption of vitamin D or intake of drugs and other agents that result in the breakdown of vitamin D.

Osteoporosis

Osteoporosis is an age-related disorder characterized by a reduced mass of bone tissue. The condition develops when bone deposition does not keep pace with bone absorption. Peak bone mass occurs around the age of 35 years and then gradually declines in both sexes. Lowered levels of oestrogen (Am. estrogen) after the menopause are associated with a period of accelerated bone loss in women. Common features of the condition include skeletal deformity, gradual loss of height with age due to compression of vertebrae and a hunched back. Fractures of the wrist, vertebrae and hip at the neck of the femur are frequent.

A range of environmental factors and diseases are implicated in the development of osteoporosis. These include a diet low in calcium and vitamin D, lack of exercise, smoking, early menopause and thin body build in females.

Osteosarcoma (osteogenic sarcoma)

This is the most common type of primary bone cancer found in children and adolescents. Osteosarcoma usually develops from abnormal cells (possibly osteoblasts or undifferentiated mesenchymal stem cells) in an area where bone is growing quickly, especially at the end of long bones. The aggressive malignant cells spread through the bloodstream to other organs, often affecting the lungs. Surgical resection, chemotherapy and sometimes radiotherapy are the main treatments.

Paget disease

A chronic disease of the skeleton in which osteoclasts reabsorb excess bone, softening the tissue. Overactive osteoblasts then deposit abnormal amounts of new bone that is thickened and structurally weak. This predisposes to deformities and fractures commonly of the pelvis, femur, tibia and skull. Most cases occur after 40 years of age, and the cause is unknown.

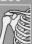

Rheumatism

Rheumatism is a term that refers to any painful state of the supporting structures of the body including bones, ligaments, joints, tendons and muscles. It is characterized by inflammation, degeneration and metabolic derangement of connective tissues accompanied by pain, stiffness and limited motion around joints.

Rheumatoid arthritis (RA)

Rheumatoid arthritis is a chronic progressive autoimmune disease of unknown cause. It is a systemic disease affecting not only joints but organs such as the blood vessels, eyes, lungs and heart. RA is often more severe than other forms of arthritis and is characterized by inflammation of synovial membranes, destruction of cartilage, erosion of bone and progressive crippling deformity. Common signs and symptoms include reduction in joint mobility, pain, nodular swelling and generalized aching and stiffness. As it is a systemic disease, fever, anaemia (Am. anemia), weight loss and profound fatigue are common.

Systemic lupus erythematosus (SLE)

This is a chronic systemic autoimmune disease in which the body's immune system attacks healthy tissue. The condition affects connective tissue including tendons, ligaments, cartilage and bones. Symptoms include joint pain, fever, kidney inflammation and malaise and a scaly red rash over the nose and cheeks (butterfly rash). Treatment is with antiinflammatory drugs, corticosteroids and immunosuppressants.

Associated words

Ankylosing becoming fused or stiff
Articulation a junction of two or more bones
Bunion (hallux valgus) inflammation of the bursa associated with a bony anomaly on the metatarsophalangeal joint of the great toe
Callus the tissue that grows round the fractured ends of bones and develops into new bone
Cancellous having an open, lattice, porous or spongy structure
Cast a stiff dressing or casing usually made of plaster of Paris to immobilize body parts
Clubfoot talipes
Comminute reduced to small pieces
Compression applying pressure, the act of pressing together
Crepitation the grating sound caused by friction of the two ends of a fractured bone
Diaphysis the main (mid) shaft of a long bone
Disimpaction reduction of an impacted fracture
Dislocation the displacement of a bone from its natural position at a joint
Dysostosis abnormal or poor development of bone
Epiphysis the end of a long bone, initially separated from the main section (diaphysis) by cartilage
Exostosis condition of a bony outgrowth from the surface of a bone

Fontanelle a soft membranous space between the cranial bones of an infant
Foramen an opening or perforation in a bone
Fossa a shallow cavity in or on a bone
Ganglion a fluid-filled cyst arising from a joint capsule or tendon, typically in the hand
Greenstick refers to a fracture in which one side of a bone is broken with the other side bent
Immobilization to render incapable of being moved, eg, by surgery, a strapping or cast
Impacted wedged or forced together
Irreducible incapable of being replaced in the normal position
Luxation the dislocation of a joint
Podagra pain caused by gout in the big toe
Popliteal pertaining to the area behind the knee
Reduction to replace a fractured or dislocated bone into the correct position
Resection complete surgical removal of a part
Subluxation partial dislocation of a joint
Sprain wrenching of a joint due to sudden overstretching of surrounding ligaments and tendons but without dislocation and fracture
Suture a type of immoveable joint between bones of the cranium
Symphysis a cartilaginous joint composed of a flat disc of cartilage between two bones
Talipes clubfoot, a deformity due to congenital or acquired contraction of muscles or tendons of the foot
Tophus a stony deposit of sodium urate crystals in the tissues around joints in patients with gout

NOW TRY THE WORD CHECK

WORD CHECK

This self-check exercise lists all the word components used in this unit. First, write down the meaning of as many word components as you can. Then, check your answers using the Exercise Guide and Quick Reference box or the Glossary of Word Components (pp. 383–410).

Prefixes

dys-	
endo-	
inter-	
poly-	

Combining forms of word roots

ankyl/o	
arthro	
burs/o	

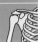
calcin/o

chondr/o

cost/o

disc/o

fibr/o

kyph/o

lamin/o

lord/o

menisc/o

myel/o

osse/o

oste/o

petr/o

phyt/o

por/o

py/o

rheumat/o

scoli/o

spondyl/o

synovi/o

Suffixes

-al

-algia

-blast

-centesis

-clasis

-clast

-desis

-eal

-ectomy

-genesis

-genic

-gram

-graphy

-ic

-itis

-lith

-logist

-lysis

-lytic

-malacia

-oid

-olisthesis

-oma

-osis

-pathy

-plasty

-scope

-scopy

-tome

-trophy

Combining forms referring to specific parts of the skeleton

acetabul/o

carp/o

clavicul/o

cost/o

crani/o

femor/o

fibul/o

humer/o

ili/o

ischi/o

mandibul/o

maxill/o

metacarp/o

metatars/o

olecran/o

patell/o

pelv/i

phalang/o

radi/o

scapul/o

spondyl/o

stern/o

tars/o

tarsometars/o

tibi/o

uln/o

NOW TRY THE SELF-ASSESSMENT

SELF-ASSESSMENT

Test 14A

Below are some combining forms that refer to the anatomy of the skeletal system and its movement. Indicate which part of the system they refer to by putting a number from the diagram (Fig. 84) next to each word.

(a) synovi/o

(b) tendin/o

(c) my/o

(d) arthr/o

(e) oste/o

(f) chondr/o

Score

6

Test 14B

Prefixes and suffixes

Match each meaning in Column C with a prefix or suffix in Column A by inserting the appropriate number in Column B.

Column A	Column B	Column C
(a) -al		1. resembling
(b) -algia		2. tumour (Am. tumor) / swelling
(c) -blast		3. slipping/dislocation
(d) -centesis		4. condition of pain
(e) -clast		5. technique of viewing
(f) -desis		6. surgical repair
(g) dys-		7. cell that breaks down a matrix
(h) -genesis		8. pertaining to destruction/breaking down
(i) -ic		9. condition of softening
(j) inter-		10. instrument used to cut
(k) -itis		11. inflammation of
(l) -lytic		12. puncture to remove fluid
(m) -malacia		13. producing/forming
(n) -oid		14. pertaining to (i)
(o) -olisthesis		15. pertaining to (ii)
(p) -oma		16. instrument to view
(q) -plasty		17. difficult/painful/bad
(r) -scope		18. germ cell
(s) -scopy		19. to bind together
(t) -tome		20. between

Score

20

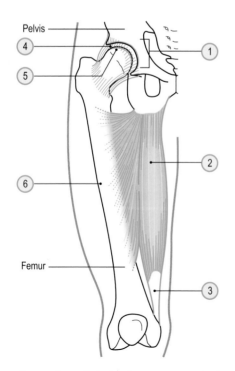

Pelvis

4

5

1

6

2

Femur

3

Figure 84   A muscle and skeletal arrangement in the thigh.

Test 14C

Combining forms of word roots

Match each meaning in Column C with a combining form of a word root in Column A by inserting the appropriate number in Column B.

Column A	Column B	Column C
(a) arthr/o		1. bone
(b) burs/o		2. marrow (of bone)
(c) calcin/o		3. synovia/synovial membrane
(d) chondr/o		4. pus
(e) cost/o		5. joint
(f) disc/o		6. vertebrae
(g) fibr/o		7. bursa/sac of fluid
(h) kyph/o		8. stone/rock
(i) lamin/o		9. calcium
(j) lord/o		10. crescent-shaped/a meniscus
(k) menisc/o		11. bend forward
(l) myel/o		12. cartilage
(m) oste/o		13. crooked
(n) petr/o		14. fibre (Am. Fiber)
(o) phyt/o		15. hunchback
(p) por/o		16. thin plate of a vertebra
(q) py/o		17. rib
(r) scoli/o		18. passage/pore
(s) spondyl/o		19. plant-like growth
(t) synovi/o		20. intervertebral disc

Score

20

Test 14D

Write the meaning of:

(a) arthrochondritis

(b) bursolith

(c) spondylodesis

(d) chondroclast

(e) kyphotic

Score

5

Test 14E

Build words that mean:

(a) condition of pain in a joint

(b) inflammation of bones and synovia

(c) condition of softening of vertebrae

(d) disease of bones and joints

(e) pertaining to synovia/synovial membrane

Score

5

Check answers to Self-Assessment Tests on page 364.

UNIT 15
THE MALE REPRODUCTIVE SYSTEM

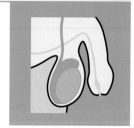

OBJECTIVES

Once you have completed Unit 15, you should be able to do the following:

- understand the meaning of medical words relating to the male reproductive system
- build medical words relating to the male reproductive system
- associate medical terms with their anatomical position
- understand common medical abbreviations relating to the male reproductive system

EXERCISE GUIDE

Use this list of word components and their meanings to complete the word exercises in this unit.

Prefixes

a-	without
crypt-	hidden
oligo-	deficiency/few
trans-	across/through

Roots / Combining forms

cyst/o	bladder
fer/o	to carry
posth/o	prepuce/foreskin
phren/o	diaphragm

Suffixes

-al	pertaining to
-algia	condition of pain
-campsis	curvature/bending
-cele	swelling/protrusion/hernia
-cide	something that kills / killing
-ectomy	removal of
-genesis	forming / capable of causing
-graphy	technique of recording / making an X-ray
-ia	condition of
-ic	pertaining to
-ism	state or condition of
-itis	inflammation of
-lysis	breakdown/disintegration
-megaly	enlargement
-meter	measuring instrument
-oma	tumour/swelling (Am. tumor)
-ous	pertaining to / of the nature of
-pathia	condition of disease
-pathy	disease of
-pexy	surgical fixation / fix in place
-plasty	surgical repair / reconstruction
-rrhagia	condition of bursting forth / discharge
-rrhaphy	stitching/suturing
-rrhea (Am.)	excessive flow / discharge
-rrhoea	excessive flow / discharge (Am. rrhea)
-sect(ion)	cut/cutting/excision
-stomy	opening into
-tomy	incision into
-uria	condition of urine

ANATOMY EXERCISE

When you have finished Word Exercises 1 to 11, look at the word components listed next. Complete Figure 85 by writing the appropriate combining form on each line. (You can check their meanings in the Quick Reference box on p. 223.)

Balan/o	Phall/o	Vas/o
Epididym/o	Prostat/o	Vesicul/o
Orchi/o	Scrot/o	

The male reproductive system

The male possesses paired reproductive organs known as the testes (synonymous with testicles). These are held in position outside the main cavities of the body by a sac known as the scrotum. Each testis produces millions of sperm cells (spermatozoa) that carry the male's genetic information. Once mature, sperms are mixed with glandular secretions to form a liquid known as semen. Semen containing active swimming sperms is ejaculated from the penis during sexual intercourse. Sperms swim along the reproductive tract of the female to the oviducts where a single sperm may fuse with an egg in the process of fertilization.

Andrology (from Greek **andros** meaning man) is the medical specialty concerned with male health, particularly problems relating to the male reproductive system and associated urinary system.

Use the Exercise Guide at the beginning of this unit to complete Word Exercises 1 to 11, unless you are asked to work without it.

Root

Orch

(*From a Greek word* **orchi**, *meaning testis (or testicle). The testis is the male reproductive organ that produces the male sex cells called spermatozoa and the hormone testosterone.*)

Combining forms   Orch/i/o, orchid/o

Word Exercise 1

Using your Exercise Guide, find the meaning of:

(a) **orchi/o**/pathy _____

(b) **orchi/o**/cele _____

(synonymous with scrotal hernia/scrotocele)

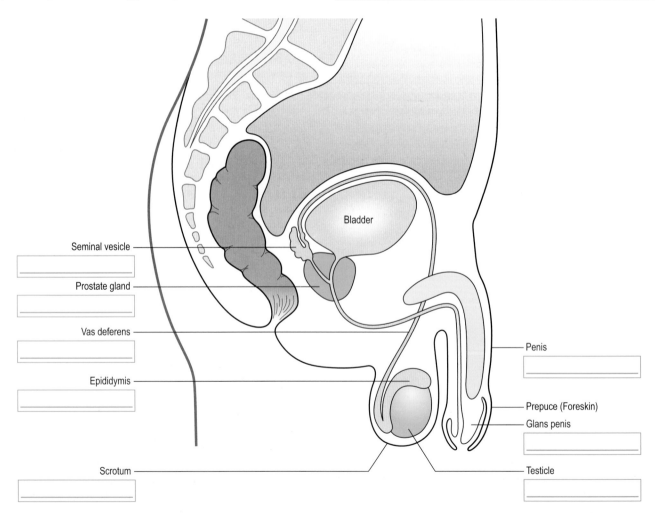

Seminal vesicle _____

Prostate gland _____

Vas deferens _____

Epididymis _____

Scrotum _____

Bladder

Penis _____

Prepuce (Foreskin)

Glans penis _____

Testicle _____

Figure 85   Section through the male showing the reproductive system.

(c) crypt[2]/**orch**[3]/ism[1] _____

Early in fetal life the testes are located in the abdominal cavity near the kidneys but normally descend into the scrotum about two months before birth. Occasionally, a baby is born with undescended testes, a condition called **cryptorchism**, which is readily observed by palpation of the scrotum at delivery. Failure of the testes to descend may be caused by hormonal imbalances in the developing fetus or by a physical deficiency or obstruction. As the higher temperature inside the body inhibits spermatogenesis (sperm formation), measures must be taken to bring the testes down into the scrotum to prevent permanent sterility. Early treatment of this condition by surgery (orchidopexy/ orchiopexy) or injection of testosterone to stimulate the testes to descend results in normal testicular and sexual development.

(d) **orchi/o**/pexy _____
(**orchid/o**/pexy)

Using your Exercise Guide, find the meaning of -algia, -ectomy, -plasty and -tomy; then build words (using **orch/i/o** or **orchid/o**) that mean:

(e) incision into a testicle _____

(f) surgical repair of a testicle _____

(g) removal of a testicle _____

(h) condition of pain in a testicle _____

Without using your Exercise Guide, write the meaning of:

(i) crypt[2]/**orchid/o**[3]/ pexy[1] _____
(synonymous with **orchi/o**/pexy)

Note. The word testicle comes from the Latin *testiculus* meaning testis or male gonad (reproductive organ). The combining form **test/icul/o** is used in several common medical terms, eg, **testo**sterone (-sterone meaning steroid hormone) and intra/**testicul**/ar (intra- meaning within, -ar meaning pertaining to).

Root

Scrot

(*From a Latin word meaning scrotum, the pouch containing the testicles.*)

Combining form   Scrot/o

Word Exercise 2

Without using your Exercise Guide, build words that mean:

(a) removal of the scrotum _____

(b) plastic surgery/repair of the scrotum _____

(c) hernia/protrusion of the scrotum _____

(synonymous with **orchiocele**)

Using your Exercise Guide, find the meaning of:

(d) trans/**-scrot**/al _____

Two other conditions can result in a swelling of the testis:

Hydrocele
a swelling/protrusion/hernia due to an accumulation of fluid within the scrotum.

Varicocele
a swelling/protrusion/hernia of veins of the spermatic cords supplying the testis (from Latin *varicosus,* meaning varicose vein). Varicoceles need to be removed as they lead to pain and infertility.

Root

Phall

(*From a Greek word* **phallo**, *meaning penis, the male copulatory organ. Here phall/o means the penis, the male organ through which urine leaves the body via the urethra. When erect, the penis transfers semen into the female reproductive system at orgasm.*)

Combining form   Phall/o

Word Exercise 3

Using your Exercise Guide, find the meaning of -ic, and -campsis; then build words that mean:

(a) curvature of the penis (when erect) _____

(b) pertaining to the penis _____

Without using your Exercise Guide, build a word that means:

(c) removal of the penis _____

Pen/o is a combining form from *penis*, a Latin word also meaning the male organ of copulation. **Pen**ile is synonymous with (b) in Word Exercise 3, and **pen**itis is an inflammation of the penis. An abnormally enlarged penis is known as a megalo**pen**is or macro**pen**is and is caused by exposure to a high level of testosterone in childhood, eg, from a testicular tumour (Am. tumor).

Several abnormalities of the penis have been noted at birth. The urethra sometimes opens on to the dorsal (upper) surface of the penis. This is known as an **epispadia** (*epi*- meaning above, and -*spadia* condition of drawing out). Sometimes the urethra opens on to the posterior (lower) surface. This is a **hypospadia** (condition of drawing out below).

The swelling of the penis during erotic stimulation is known as **tumescence** (from Latin *tumescere*, meaning to swell). The subsidence of the swelling is known as **detumescence** (*de* meaning lack of). Once erect, the penis can be inserted into the vagina in the act of sex. Words used synonymously with sex include:

Coitus

from Latin *coire*, meaning to come together.

Intercourse

from Latin *intercurrere*, meaning to run between.

Copulation

from Latin *copulare*, meaning to bind together.

The failure to produce an erection and perform the sexual act is known as **impotence** (from Latin *impotentia*, meaning inability). See erectile dysfunction on page 223.

Root

Balan

(*From a Greek word* **balanos**, *meaning acorn. Here balan/o means the glans penis, the sensitive, swollen end of the penis that is covered with the prepuce or foreskin.*)

Combining form   Balan/o

Word Exercise 4

Without using your Exercise Guide, build a word that means:

(a) inflammation of
     the glans penis

Using your Exercise Guide, find the meaning of:

(b) **balan/o**/rrhagia

(c) **balan/o**/posth/itis

The **prepuce**, or covering foreskin of the glans penis, sometimes needs to be cut, a process known as **preputiotomy**. This is performed to relieve **phimosis**, a condition in which the foreskin is too tight and cannot retract.

The prepuce is removed in the process of **circumcision** (ie, cutting around). This is often performed for religious rather than medical reasons.

Root

Epididym

(*Derived from Greek words* **epi-** *on,* **didymos-** *twins (the testicles). Here epididym/o means the epididymis, a coiled tube that forms the first part of the duct system of each testis. The epididymes store sperm.*)

Combining form   Epididym/o

Word Exercise 5

Without using your Exercise Guide, build words that mean:

(a) inflammation of the
     epididymis

(b) removal of the
     epididymis

Without using your Exercise Guide, write the meaning of:

(c) **epididym/o**/-orch/itis

Root

Vas

(*A Latin word meaning vessel or duct. Here vas/o means the vas deferens, the main secretory duct of each testis along which mature sperms move towards the penis.*)

Combining form   Vas/o

Word Exercise 6

Without using your Exercise Guide, write the meaning of:

(a) **vas**/ectomy

(This operation (Fig. 86) is performed to sterilize the male, ie, to make him incapable of reproduction. The cut ends of a section of the vas are tied off, a procedure known as bilateral ligation (from Latin *ligare*, meaning to bind). Following vasectomy, a reduced volume of semen is produced that contains no sperm.)

Using your Exercise Guide, find the meaning of:

(b) **vas/o**/epididym/o/
     stomy

(c) **vas/o**/epididym/o/
     graphy

(d) **vas/o**/section

(e) **vas/o**/rrhaphy

Without using your Exercise Guide, write the meaning of:

(f) **vas/o/**-orchid/o/
stomy

(g) **vas/o/vas/o/**stomy

(h) **vas/o/**tomy

Root

Vesicul

(From a Latin word **vesicula**, *meaning vesicle/little bladder. Here vesicul/o means the seminal vesicles, small pouches lying near the base of the bladder which secrete a nutrient fluid that becomes a component of semen.)*

Combining form Vesicul/o

Word Exercise 7

Without using your Exercise Guide, build words that mean:

(a) technique of mak-
ing an X-ray of the
seminal vesicles

(b) incision into a
seminal vesicle

Without using your Exercise Guide, write the meaning of:

(c) vas/o/**vesicul**/ectomy

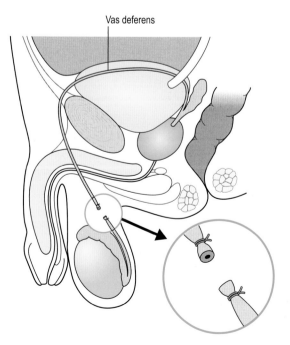

Vas deferens

Figure 86 **Vasectomy.**

Root

Prostat

(From Greek **prostates**, *meaning one who stands before. Here prostat/o means the prostate gland that surrounds the neck of the bladder and urethra in males. Secretions from the prostate gland are added to the semen just before ejaculation.)*

Combining form Prostat/o

Word Exercise 8

Using your Exercise Guide, find the meaning of:

(a) **prostat/o/**cyst/o/tomy

(b) **prostat/o/**megaly

Without using your Exercise Guide, write the meaning of:

(c) **prostat/**ectomy

Benign prostatic hyperplasia (BPH) occurs in 75% of men over the age of 50. An enlargement or hypertrophy of the prostate gland tissue characterizes the condition. As the prostate enlarges, it squeezes the urethra, frequently closing it so completely that urination becomes very difficult or even impossible. In such cases, surgical removal (prostatectomy) of the entire gland or part of it may become necessary. The cause of BPH is not clear, but it may be associated with a decline in androgen secretion in later life that changes the androgen/oestrogen balance.

To alleviate this condition, part or the entire gland can be removed by transurethral resection of the prostate (TURP, *trans*, meaning across and *resection,* meaning removal/excision). TURP involves inserting a resectoscope, a type of endoscope, into the urethra and using it to view and cut out pieces of prostate gland (see Fig. 87).

(d) **prostat/o/**vesicul/
ectomy

Root

Semin

(From a Latin word **seminis**, *meaning seed. Here semin/i means semen, the liquid secretion of the testicles. Note, in a few words, semin- means testicle.)*

Combining form Semin/i

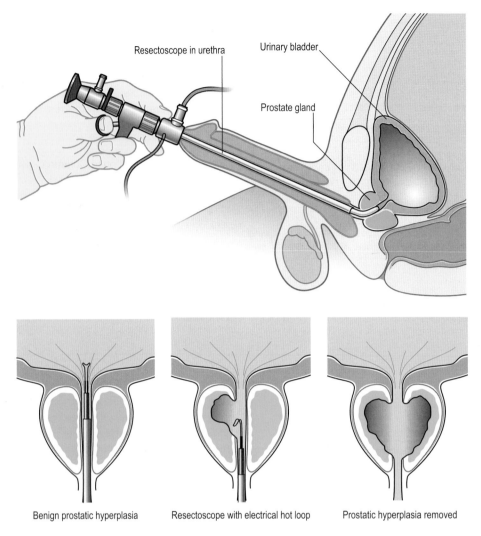

Resectoscope in urethra

Urinary bladder

Prostate gland

Benign prostatic hyperplasia

Resectoscope with electrical hot loop

Prostatic hyperplasia removed

Figure 87   Transurethral resection of the prostate gland (TURP). (Adapted from Chabner D-E, The Language of Medicine, 10th Edition, 2013, Saunders.)

Word Exercise 9

Using your Exercise Guide, find the meaning of:

(a) **semin/i**/fer/ous

(Spermatozoa flow along seminiferous tubules of the testis.)

(b) **semin**/uria

(c) **semin**/oma

(A malignancy of the testis. A change in size and shape of the testes is a symptom of this condition; their size can be measured with an **orchidometer**. When a testis is removed, it can be replaced with a prosthesis.)

In**semina**tion refers to the deposition of semen in the female reproductive tract (from Latin *seminare,* meaning to sow). Artificial insemination (AI) refers to the insertion of semen into the uterus via a cannula (tube) instead of by coitus. This procedure is also known as intrauterine insemination (IUI). The sperm used can be from two sources:

- AI by husband (AIH). In this procedure, semen from the patient's husband/partner is inseminated. This technique is used when there is difficulty in conceiving because of physical and/or psychological problems.

- AI by donor (AID). In this procedure, semen from a male other than the female's partner is used. Artificial insemination by donor sperm is used when the female is fertile and the male partner is sterile. A child produced in this way will be genetically related to the male donor.

Root

Sperm

(*From a Greek word* **sperma***, eaning seed. Here sperm/o means sperm cells or spermatozoa (singular spermatozoon). Sperm are ejaculated in the semen during the peak of sexual excitement known as orgasm.*)

Combining forms   Sperm/o, spermat/o, also sperm/i
                        (from New Latin spermium)

Word Exercise 10

Using your Exercise Guide, find the meaning of:

(a) a/**sperm**/ia

(b) oligo/**sperm**/ia

(c) **sperm/i**/cide

(often used as a cream in conjunction with condoms and other contraceptives)

Using your Exercise Guide look up -genesis, -lysis, -pathia and -rrhoea (Am. rrhea), and then build words using spermat/o that mean:

(d) condition of disease of sperm (abnormal sperm)

(e) formation of sperm

(f) breakdown/disinte-gration of sperm

(g) flow of sperm (abnor-mal, without orgasm)

Sperm counts are performed to estimate the number of sperms, the percentage of abnormal sperms and their mobility. The actual number of sperms is important in deter-mining the fertility of the male; a sperm count of 15 million sperms per millilitre is considered to be normal. A sperm count of less results in decreased fertility, even though only one sperm is required to fertilize an egg.

Oligospermia results from reduced sperm production by the seminiferous tubules of the testes. If the *sperm count* is too low, infertility may result. A large number of sperm is needed to ensure that sufficient will reach the ovum and one will bring about fertilization. Oligospermia can result from factors such as infection, fever, radiation, malnutri-tion and the high temperature of undescended testes. The condition can be temporary, as in some acute infections, or permanent as in untreated cryptorchism. Total absence of sperm production (*aspermia*) always results in *sterility*.

Semen containing sperms can be preserved at very low temperatures in a cryostat. Once thawed, the sperm are capable of fertilizing eggs and are used for artificial insemination.

The process known as IVF or in vitro fertilization was developed in the 1970s, and it became possible to fertil-ize eggs outside the body in laboratory glassware (in *vitro* meaning in glass). Once fertilized, eggs are left to develop for several days in a culture dish, and then healthy looking embryos are selected and transferred into the uterus to initi-ate pregnancy.

Medical equipment and clinical procedures

Review the names of all instruments and clinical procedures mentioned in this unit and then try Exercise 11.

Word Exercise 11

Match each description in Column C with a term in Column A by placing the appropriate number in Column B.

Column A	Column B	Column C
(a) sperm count		1. fusion of an egg and sperm in labo-ratory glassware
(b) transurethral resection		2. material used to tie a cut vas
(c) vasectomy		3. a device used to measure the size of a testicle
(d) orchidometer		4. removal of pros-tate tissue through the urethra
(e) in vitro fertilization		5. an estimate of numbers of sper-matozoa in 1 ml semen
(f) vasoligature		6. the cutting and removal of a section of the sperm duct

Other procedures used to investigate the male reproductive system besides those mentioned in the word exercises include:

Digital rectal examination The physician's gloved, lubricated finger is inserted through the anal canal and rectum to palpate the prostate gland. The gland is felt to estimate its size and check for hard, lumpy or abnormal areas.

Prostate specific antigen test (PSA) This test measures the blood level of prostate specific antigen, a protein pro-duced only by the prostate gland. A blood sample is sent to a laboratory for analysis, and the results are usually reported as nanograms of PSA per millilitre (ng/ml) of blood. Although PSA is often elevated in men with prostate cancer, other conditions can cause a man's PSA level to rise, eg, prostatitis and benign prostatic hyperplasia (BPH).

ANATOMY EXERCISE

Now complete the Anatomy Exercise on page 216.

CASE HISTORY 15

The object of this exercise is to understand words associated with a patient's medical history.

To complete the exercise:

- Read through the passage on seminoma; unfamiliar words are underlined, and you can find their meaning using the Word Help.

- Write the meaning of the medical terms shown in bold print on the lines that follow the Word Help.

Seminoma

Mr O, a 32-year-old father of two children, consulted his GP about a severe back pain. Although a regular football player, he could not recall any recent injury that could account for his condition. During his consultation, he mentioned that several months ago he had noticed his right testicle was swollen. It felt heavy and sometimes uncomfortable, but he had ignored it, assuming it would resolve. When his early medical record was checked, it revealed a history of **cryptorchism** of the right testicle that had been rectified by **orchidopexy** at the age of 5 years.

Palpation showed the right testicle to be hard, smooth and swollen. It was easily separated from the epididymis and did not transilluminate. Mr O had not felt any pain and otherwise appeared in good health. There was no evidence of **orchitis**, epididymitis or torsion. He was counselled by his GP who referred him to the Urology department with suspected cancer of the testis.

Ultrasonography determined the presence of an **intratesticular** mass in the right testicle. A chest X-ray was negative for lung metastases, but a CT scan of his abdominopelvic region revealed retroperitoneal and para-aortic lymphadenopathy. He had elevated levels of the serum tumour (Am. tumor) markers bHCG and lactate dehydrogenase.

Mr O was advised of the need for surgical **orchidectomy**, and the consultant explained the procedure to him.

Mr O's scrotal contents were examined and his right testicle removed through an inguinal approach with early clamping of the **spermatic** cord and its vessels. (Note, **trans-scrotal** biopsy is contraindicated as a means of evaluating scrotal masses as it causes tumour cell shedding and spread of the tumour.)

Histopathological analysis confirmed the presence of a malignant **seminoma** in the right testicle; the contralateral testis was biopsied at the same time and found to be normal.

Mr O's condition was assessed as Stage IIC, and he was given chemotherapy with follow up chest X-ray, abdominopelvic CT scan and serum tumour marker determination every 3 months. At 6 months the residual retroperitoneal mass has shrunk and calcified, and he remains progression free.

Word Help

bHCG a serum tumour marker (beta human chorionic gonadotropin) (Am. tumor)

calcified referring to deposition of calcium salts into a tissue

chemotherapy treatment using drugs (here cytotoxic drugs that destroy cancer cells)

contralateral pertaining to the opposite side

CT computed tomography

epididymis the first part of the duct system that leaves the testis and stores maturing sperm

epididymitis inflammation of the epididymis

GP general practitioner (family doctor)

histopathological pertaining to disease of a tissue

inguinal pertaining to the groin

lactate dehydrogenase a serum tumour marker (Am. tumor)

lymphadenopathy disease of lymph nodes (lymph glands)

malignant dangerous, capable of spreading

metastases parts of a tumour that have spread from one site to another

palpation act of feeling with the fingers using light pressure

para-aortic pertaining to beside the aorta

progression advancing, moving forward of a disease

retroperitoneal pertaining to behind the peritoneum

serum tumour marker certain chemicals are elevated to higher than normal levels in blood serum when tumours are present; they act as signs or markers of the presence of disease

Stage IIC staging is a system of classifying malignant disease that will influence its treatment; this patient is at Stage IIC

torsion act of twisting/rotation

transilluminate shine a bright light through (note, a solid tumour will prevent transmission of light)

ultrasonography technique of recording (an image) using high-frequency sound waves

urology study of the urinary tract (here department that diagnoses and treats disease and disorders of the urinary tract)

Now write the meaning of the following words from the Case History without using your dictionary lists:

(a) cryptorchism

(b) orchidopexy

(c) orchitis

(d) intratesticular

(e) orchidectomy

(f) spermatic

(g) trans-scrotal

(h) seminoma

(Answers to the Case History exercise are given in the Answers to Word Exercises on page 351.)

Quick Reference

Combining forms relating to the male reproductive system:

Balan/o	glans penis
Cyst/o	bladder
Epididym/o	epididymis
Orchi/o	testis
Phall/o	penis
Posth/o	prepuce/foreskin
Prostat/o	prostate
Scrot/o	scrotum
Semin/i	semen/testis
Sperm/i	spermatozoa/sperm
Varic/o	varicose vein
Vas/o	vas deferens/vessel
Vesicul/o	seminal vesicle

Abbreviations

Some common abbreviations related to the male reproductive system are listed next. Note that some are not standard, and their meaning may vary from one healthcare setting to another. There is a more extensive list for reference on page 369.

BPH	benign prostatic hyperplasia or benign prostatic hypertrophy
DRE	digital rectal examination
ED	erectile dysfunction
GU	genitourinary
NSU	nonspecific urethritis
PIN	prostatic intraepithelial neoplasia, a precursor of prostate cancer
PSA	prostate specific antigen
RPR	rapid plasma reagin; a test for syphilis
SPP	suprapubic prostatectomy
STD	sexually transmitted disease
TRUS	transrectal ultrasound (examination of the prostate gland)
TURB	transurethral resection of the bladder
TURP	transurethral resection of the prostate gland

Pathology notes

Carcinoma of the prostate

Malignant tumours (Am. tumors) called adenocarcinomas are a relatively common cause of death in men over 50. Changes in the androgen/oestrogen (Am. estrogen) balance are thought to be significant and, in some cases, viral infection may be involved. Invasion of local tissues is widespread before malignant cells spread in the lymph and blood to distant sites. Metastases appear in lymph nodes and bone, and bone formation rather than bone destruction is a feature. Treatment can include prostatectomy, radiation therapy, brachytherapy, chemotherapy and hormonal treatment to reduce the levels of androgens in the blood.

Erectile dysfunction

Failure to achieve an erection of the penis is called erectile dysfunction or impotence. Although erectile dysfunction does not affect sperm production, it may cause infertility because normal intercourse may not be possible. Anxiety and psychological stress are often cited as causes of this condition, but it may also result from an abnormality in the erectile tissues of the penis or a failure of nerve reflexes that control erection. Drugs and alcohol can cause temporary erectile dysfunction by interfering with the functioning of nerves and blood vessels involved in erection.

Hydrocele

A common cause of scrotal swelling is an accumulation of fluid called a hydrocele. Hydroceles may be congenital, resulting from structural abnormalities present at birth. In adults the condition often occurs when fluid produced by the serous membrane (tunica vaginalis) lining the scrotum is not absorbed properly. The onset may be acute and painful or chronic; in some cases the cause of hydrocele can be linked to trauma or infection.

Inguinal hernia

An inguinal hernia forms when the intestines push through the weak area of the abdominal wall that separates the abdominopelvic cavity from the scrotum. If the intestines push into the scrotum, the digestive tract may become obstructed, resulting in death. Inguinal hernias may be congenital but more often are a result of lifting a heavy object; they are repaired by laparoscopic surgery or open surgery.

Peyronie disease

A condition characterized by an abnormal curvature of the erect penis (phallocampsis) due to the formation of fibrous tissue (plaques) in the tunica albuginea. The tunica albuginea forms the fibrous envelope of the erectile tissue or corpora cavernosum of the penis. The underlying cause is unknown, but it may be an unusual response to minor injury received during sexual activity. Named after French surgeon Francois Gigot de la Peyronie (1678–1747).

Phimosis

Phimosis is a structural abnormality in which the foreskin fits so tightly over the glans that it cannot retract. The usual treatment for this condition is circumcision, a procedure in which the foreskin is cut along the base of the glans and removed. Severe phimosis can obstruct the flow of urine, possibly causing the death of an infant born with this condition. Milder phimosis can result in accumulation of dirt and organic matter under the foreskin, causing severe infection.

Sexually transmitted diseases

These are also known as sexually transmitted infections (STIs) or venereal diseases (from Latin Venus, the goddess of love). They include specific infections that are transmitted by sexual or other genital contact. The most common sexually transmitted diseases caused by bacterial infection include chlamydia, gonorrhoea (Am. gonorrhea) and syphilis.

Note that inflammation of the glans penis and prepuce may be also be caused by a nonspecific infection unrelated to sexual contact. For example, the glans penis and foreskin may become infected with microorganisms due to lack of personal hygiene, especially if phimosis is present. This type of infection may spread to the bladder and other areas from the urethra or be introduced by surgical procedures such as catheterization.

The most common sexually transmitted diseases caused by viral infection include genital herpes due to herpes simplex virus Type 1 or 2, genital warts due to human papilloma virus (HPV) and AIDS caused by human immunodeficiency virus (HIV).

Testicular torsion

The spermatic cord carries blood vessels, nerves, lymphatics and a sperm duct to the testis. When this becomes twisted (torsion) the blood supply to the testis is cut off, leading to acute swelling and severe pain. Emergency surgery is required within 6 to 10 hours to restore the blood circulation and function of the testis.

Testicular tumours

Most testicular tumours (Am. tumors) arise from the sperm-producing cells of the seminiferous tubules. Malignancies of the testes are most common among men 20 to 35 years old. A testicular tumour tends to remain localised for a considerable time but eventually spreads in lymph to pelvic and abdominal nodes, and more widely in the blood. Besides age, this type of cancer is associated with genetic predisposition, trauma or infection of the testis and cryptorchism. Treatment of testicular cancer is most effective when diagnosis is made early in the development of the tumour.

Associated words

Androgen one of a group of steroid hormones produced by the testes and adrenal cortex that promote the development of male secondary sexual characteristics

Azoospermia condition of absence of sperm in the semen

Bulbourethral glands paired, small, bulb-shaped glands opening into the urethra that secrete an alkaline mucus into the urethra before ejaculation; they are also known as Cowper glands (after William Cowper, 1666–1709, English surgeon)

Ejaculation the sudden expulsion of semen from the male urethra as a result of sexual stimulation

Emasculation the removal of the penis or testicles; castration

Emission involuntary ejection of semen

Erogenous pertaining to arousing erotic feelings

Castration the surgical removal of the testicles or their destruction by radiation or infection

Chancre a primary sore of syphilis commonly found on the penis or cervix in women

Chordee downward curvature of the penis caused by a congenital abnormality

Fertility the capacity to induce conception

Flaccid soft; lacking rigidity

Hypogonadism in a male, the condition of having underactive testes that produce little or no testosterone; it results in retarded growth and sexual development

Impotence an outdated term for erectile dysfunction meaning an inability to initiate and maintain an erection until ejaculation

Infertility the inability of the male to bring about conception (pregnancy) or of a female to conceive

Insemination the introduction of semen into the vagina; the fertilization of an egg by a sperm

Libido sexual desire or drive

Masturbation the production of sexual excitement by rubbing the genitals

Orgasm the climax of sexual excitement

Paraphimosis retraction of the prepuce behind the glans penis with inability to restore it to its natural position; it produces a painful constriction

Perineum in the male the area between the thighs bounded by the anus and scrotum

Potency the ability of the male to perform coitus

Precocious puberty puberty occurring at an unusually early age

Priapism persistent erection without sexual stimulation; it may be caused by local or spinal cord injury

Satyriasis abnormal excessive sexual appetite in men
Semen analysis microscopic examination of a semen sample to determine the number of sperm present, their shape and motility (movement); the analysis is used to evaluate male fertility
Smegma the secretion of the sebaceous glands of the prepuce
Sterility the inability of a male to produce potent spermatozoa or the female to produce eggs
Sterilization a procedure that results in a patient becoming incapable of reproduction
Testosterone a hormone secreted by the testes that controls the development of secondary sexual characteristics and the development of sperm; the main androgenic hormone

NOW TRY THE WORD CHECK

WORD CHECK

This self-check exercise lists all the word components used in this unit. First, write down the meaning of as many word components as you can. Then, check your answers using the Exercise Guide and Quick Reference box or the Glossary of Word Components (pp. 383–410).

Prefixes

a-

crypt-

epi-

hypo-

intra-

oligo-

trans-

Combining forms of word roots

balan/o

cyst/o

epididym/o

fer/o

hydr/o

megal/o

orchi/o

phall/o

posth/o

prostat/o

scrot/o

semin/i

sperm/i

varic/o

vas/o

vesicul/o

Suffixes

-al

-algia

-ar

-campsis

-cele

-cide

-ectomy

-genesis

-graphy

-ia

-ic

-ism

-itis

-ligation

-lysis

-oma

-ous

-pathia

-pexy

-plasty

-rrhagia

-rrhaphy

-rrhoea
(Am. -rrhea)

-sect(ion)

-spadia

-stomy

-tomy

-uria

NOW TRY THE SELF-ASSESSMENT

SELF-ASSESSMENT

Test 15A

Next are some combining forms that refer to the anatomy of the male reproductive system. Indicate which part of the system they refer to by putting a number from the diagram (Fig. 88) next to each word.

(a) scrot/o

(b) orchid/o

(c) phall/o

(d) balan/o

(e) vas/o

(f) prostat/o

(g) vesicul/o

(h) epididym/o

Score

8

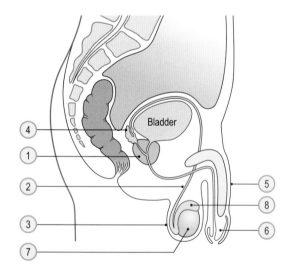

Figure 88   Section through the male showing the reproductive system.

Test 15B

Prefixes and suffixes

Match each meaning in Column C with a prefix or suffix in Column A by inserting the appropriate number in Column B.

Column A	Column B	Column C
(a) -cele		1. fixation
(b) -cide		2. condition of drawing out
(c) crypt-		3. hidden
(d) epi-		4. condition of urine/urination
(e) -genesis		5. opening into
(f) -ia		6. across
(g) -ic		7. back
(h) -ism		8. suturing
(i) oligo-		9. on/above/upon
(j) -ous		10. condition of bursting forth (of blood)
(k) -pexy		11. pertaining to (i)
(l) re-		12. pertaining to (ii)
(m) -rrhagia		13. process of
(n) -rrhaphy		14. excessive flow/ discharge
(o) -rrhoea (Am. -rrhea)		15. producing/ forming
(p) -sect		16. hernia/protrusion/swelling
(q) -spadia		17. condition of
(r) -stomy		18. to kill
(s) trans-		19. cut
(t) -uria		20. little/scanty/few

Score

20

Test 15C

Combining forms of word roots

Match each meaning in Column C with a combining form of a word root in Column A by inserting the appropriate number in Column B.

Column A	Column B	Column C
(a) balan/o		1. to carry
(b) cyst/o		2. testis
(c) epididym/o		3. penis
(d) fer/o		4. glans penis
(e) hydr/o		5. prostate gland
(f) megal/o		6. prepuce
(g) orchid/o		7. semen
(h) phall/o		8. epididymis
(i) posth/o		9. varicose vein
(j) prostat/o		10. vessel
(k) scrot/o		11. vesicle (seminal)
(l) semin/i		12. water
(m) varic/o		13. scrotum
(n) vas/o		14. bladder
(o) vesicul/o		15. abnormal enlargement

Score ☐ 15

Test 15D

Write the meaning of:

(a) orchidoepididymectomy ☐

(b) phallorrhoea (Am. phallorrhea) ☐

(c) epididymovasectomy ☐

(d) vasoligation ☐

(e) spermaturia ☐

Score ☐ 5

Test 15E

Build words that mean:

(a) stitching/suturing of the testis ☐

(b) condition of pain in the prostate ☐

(c) formation of an opening between the epididymis and vas ☐

(d) inflammation of the scrotum ☐

(e) excessive flow/ discharge from the prostate ☐

Score ☐ 5

Check answers to Self-Assessment Tests on page 364.

Test your recall of the meanings of word components in Units 11 to 15 by completing the appropriate self-assessment tests in Unit 22 on page 329.

UNIT 16
THE FEMALE REPRODUCTIVE SYSTEM

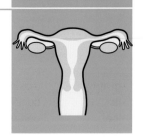

OBJECTIVES

Once you have completed Unit 16, you should be able to do the following:

- understand the meaning of medical words relating to the female reproductive system

- build medical words relating to the female reproductive system

- associate medical terms with their anatomical position

- understand common medical abbreviations relating to the female reproductive system

EXERCISE GUIDE

Use this list of word components and their meanings to complete the word exercises in this unit.

Prefixes

a-	without
-a	a word ending, no meaning
ante-	before
dys-	difficult/painful
endo-	within/inside
eu-	good
micro-	small
multi-	many
neo-	new
nulli-	none
oligo-	deficiency/little/infrequent
peri-	around
pre-	before / in front of
primi-	first
pro-	before
secundi-	second

Roots / Combining forms

cyst/o	bladder (cyst)
cyt/e	cell
fer/o	to carry
haem/o	blood (Am. hem/o)
hem/o (Am.)	blood
myc/o	fungus
perine/o	perineum
periton/e/o	peritoneum
phleb/o	vein
placent/o	placenta
rect/o	rectum
trachel/o	neck
vesic/o	bladder

Suffixes

-a	noun ending / a name, eg, of a condition
-agogue	agent that induces/promotes
-al	pertaining to
-algia	condition of pain
-arche	beginning
-blast	cell that forms…immature germ cell
-cele	swelling/protrusion/hernia
-centesis	puncture to remove fluid
-dynia	condition of pain
-ectomy	removal of
-fuge	agent that suppresses/removes
-genesis	formation of
-genic	pertaining to formation
-gram	X-ray/tracing/recording

-graphy	making an X-ray / technique of recording	**-ptosis**	falling/drooping/displacement/prolapse
-ia	condition of	**-rrhagic**	pertaining to bursting forth (of blood)
-ical	pertaining to dealing with / pertaining to	**-rrhaphy**	suturing/stitching
-ischia	condition of reducing / holding back	**-rrhexis**	breaking/rupturing
-itis	inflammation of	**-rrhea (Am.)**	excessive discharge/flow
-lithiasis	condition of stones	**-rrhoea**	excessive discharge/flow (Am. -rrhea)
-logy	study of	**-sclerosis**	condition of hardening
-malacia	condition of softening	**-scope**	instrument used to view/examine
-meter	measuring instrument	**-scopy**	technique of viewing/examining
-metry	process of measuring	**-staxis**	dripping
-oma	tumour/swelling (Am. tumor)	**-stenosis**	condition of narrowing
-osis	abnormal condition / disease of	**-stomy**	formation of an opening / an opening
-ous	pertaining to / of the nature of	**-tic**	pertaining to
-pathia	condition of disease	**-tome**	cutting instrument
-pathy	disease of	**-tomy**	incision into
-pause	stopping	**-toxic**	pertaining to poisoning
-pexy	surgical fixation / fix in place	**-trophin**	hormone that stimulates/nourishes
-plasty	surgical repair/reconstruction	**-tropic**	pertaining to stimulating / affinity for
-poiesis	formation	**-tubal**	pertaining to a tube

ANATOMY EXERCISE

When you have finished Word Exercises 1 to 14, look at the word components listed next. Complete Figures 89 and 90 by writing the appropriate combining form on each line; more than one component may relate to the same position. (You can check their meanings in the Quick Reference box on p. 245.)

Cervic/o	Hyster/o	Salping/o
Colp/o	Metr/o	Uter/o
Culd/o	Oophor/o	Vagin/o
Endometr/i	Ovari/o	Vulv/o

The female reproductive system

The female possesses paired reproductive organs known as ovaries; these are located in the upper pelvic cavity on either side of the uterus. The function of the ovaries is to produce reproductive cells known as ova (eggs). The ovaries pass through a regular ovarian cycle in which one egg is released (ovulation) every 28 days. The egg passes into the oviduct where it may be fertilized by sperms ejaculated into the female reproductive tract by the male. Should an egg be fertilized, it will divide and grow into a new individual after implanting into the uterus. If the egg is not fertilized, it will disintegrate and may pass out of the body at menstruation.

The study of the female reproductive system in its nonpregnant state is known as gynaecology (Am. gynecology); it is usually studied with obstetrics, the branch of medicine dealing with pregnancy, labour (Am. labor) and the puerperium. The specialties are often abbreviated as OB-GYN or Obs & Gyn.

Use the Exercise Guide at the beginning of this unit to complete Word Exercises 1 to 26, unless you are asked to work without it.

Gynaecology (Am. gynecology)

Gynaecology deals with the health of the female reproductive system including the ovaries, oviducts, cervix, uterus, vagina and vulva. We begin our study with the female reproductive cells and the ovary.

Root

Oo

(*From a Greek word* **oon**, *meaning egg.*)

Combining form　　Oo-

Word Exercise 1

Using your Exercise Guide, find the meaning of:

(a) **oo/blast**

(b) **oo/cyte**

(c) **oo/genesis**

Root

Oophor

(*From a Greek word* **oophoron**, *derived from oion -egg, pherein -to bear. Here oophor/o means an ovary, one of the paired egg-bearing glands in the female.*)

Combining form　　Oophor/o

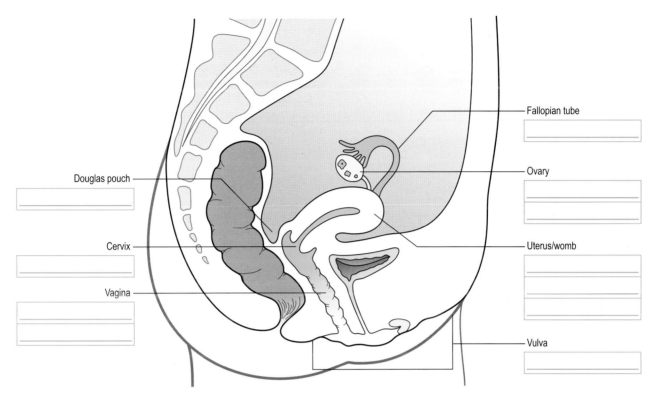

Figure 89   Sagittal section through the female showing the reproductive system.

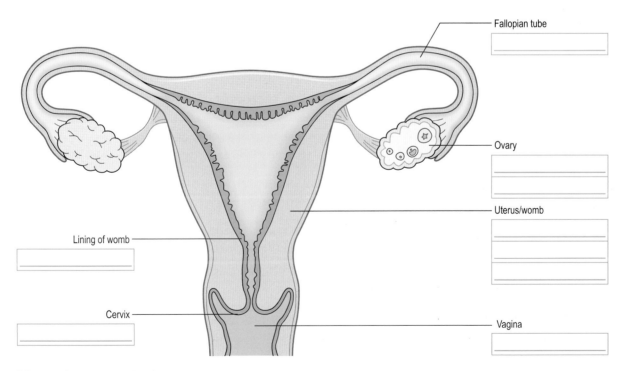

Figure 90   The female reproductive system.

Word Exercise 2

Using your Exercise Guide, find the meaning of -ectomy, -pexy and -tomy; then build words that mean:

(a) removal of an ovary

(b) fixation of an ovary

(c) incision of an ovary

Using your Exercise Guide, find the meaning of:

(d) **oophor/o**[2]/cyst[3]/ ectomy[1] (cyst refers to a bladder-like growth in the ovary)

(e) **oophor/o**/stomy

Root

Ovari

(*From a New Latin word* **ovarium**, *meaning ovary, derived from ova, meaning egg.*)

Combining form   Ovari/o

Word Exercise 3

Without using your Exercise Guide, build words that mean:

(a) removal of an ovary (synonymous with oophorectomy)

(b) incision into an ovary (often used to mean the removal of an ovarian cyst)

Using your Exercise Guide, find the meaning of:

(c) **ovari/o**/rrhexis

(d) **ovari/o**/tubal (refers to an oviduct)

(e) **ovari/o**/centesis

Approximately every 28 days an egg (or ovum) is released from one of the ovaries. This process is known as **ovulation**. Once released, the oviduct picks up the egg, and it moves towards the uterus. An ovary that fails to release eggs is described as **anovular**, meaning pertaining to without eggs.

Root

Salping

(*From Greek* **salpig**. *meaning trumpet tube. Here salping/o means fallopian tube (after Gabriele Fallopio, Italian anatomist, b. 1523), a structure also known as the oviduct or uterine tube. There are two trumpet-shaped uterine tubes; their function is to collect eggs ovulated from the ovaries and transport them to the uterus.*)

Combining form   Salping/o

Word Exercise 4

Without using your Exercise Guide, write the meaning of:

(a) **salping/o**/-oophor/ ectomy

(b) ovari/o/**salping**/ectomy

(c) **salping/o**/pexy

Using your Exercise Guide, find the meaning of:

(d) **salping/o**/cele

(e) **salping/o**/-oophor/itis

Using your Exercise Guide, find the meaning of -graphy, -lithiais and -plasty; then build words that mean:

(f) technique of making an X-ray of the oviduct (follows an injection of opaque dye)

(g) condition of stones in an oviduct

(h) surgical repair of an oviduct

Root

Uter

(*From a Latin word* **uterus**, *meaning womb. Here uter/o means the uterus, the chamber in which a blastocyst develops into a fetus.*)

Combining form   Uter/o

Word Exercise 5

Using your Exercise Guide, find the meaning of -algia and -sclerosis; then build words that mean:

(a) condition of pain in the uterus

(b) hardening of the uterus

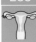

Without using your Exercise Guide, write the meaning of:

(c) **uter/o**/tubal

(d) **uter/o**/salping/o/
graphy

Using your Exercise Guide, find the meaning of:

(e) **uter/o**/vesic/al

(f) **uter/o**/rect/al

(g) **uter/o**/placent/al (the
placenta is a disc-
shaped structure that
attaches the fetus to
the lining of the uterus)

Root

Hyster

(*From Greek word* **hystera**, *meaning womb. Here hyster/o means the uterus, the chamber in which a blastocyst develops into a fetus.*)

Combining form   Hyster/o

Word Exercise 6

Using your Exercise Guide, find the meaning of -gram, -ptosis and -scope; then build words that mean:

(a) instrument to view the
uterus

(b) condition of a falling/
displaced uterus (also
known as a prolapse)

(c) X-ray picture of the uterus

Without using your Exercise Guide, write the meaning of:

(d) **hyster/o**/salping/o/gra-
phy

(e) **hyster/o**/salping/o/
stomy

(f) **hyster/o**/salping/o/-
oophor/ectomy

Using your Exercise Guide, find the meaning of:

(g) **hyster/o**/trachel/o/
rrhaphy

(h) **hyster/o**/trachel/o/tomy

Root

Metr

(*From a Greek word* **metra**, *meaning womb. Here metr/o means the uterus, the chamber in which a blastocyst develops into a fetus.*)

Combining form   Metr/a/i/o

Word Exercise 7

Using your Exercise Guide, find the meaning of:

(a) **metr/o**/staxis

(b) **metr/o**/pathia
haem/o/rrhagic/a
(Am. hem/o/rrhagic/a)

(c) **metr/o**/periton/itis

(d) **metr/o**/phleb/itis

(e) **metr/o**/cyst/osis

(f) **metr/o**/ptosis

Using your Exercise Guide, find the meaning of -malacia and -stenosis; then build words that mean:

(g) condition of a
narrowed uterus

(h) condition of softening
of the uterus

Endo**metri**um (*endo-* meaning within) refers to the lining of the uterus. The endometrium grows during the 28-day menstrual cycle and disintegrates when it ends, producing the menstrual flow.

Using your Exercise Guide, find the meaning of:

(i) **endometr**/itis

(j) **endometr/i**/oma

Without using your Exercise Guide, write the meaning of:

(k) **endometr/i**/osis
(refers to the
endometrial tissue in
abnormal locations
outside the uterus;
see the Pathology
Notes on page 237)

Fibroids (leiomyoma, myoma) are common, often multiple, benign tumours (Am. tumors) of the myometrium (the smooth muscle layer of the uterus that lies under the endometrium). They are firm masses of smooth muscle encapsulated in compressed muscle fibres, and they vary greatly in size. They develop during the reproductive period and may be hormone dependent, enlarging during pregnancy and when oral contraceptives are used. Fibroids tend to regress after the menopause, and malignant change is rare. Large tumours cause pelvic discomfort, frequency of micturition, menorrhagia, irregular bleeding, dysmenorrhoea (Am. dysmenorrhea) and reduced fertility. The procedure of **fibroid**ectomy or **myom**ectomy (**myom-** is from myoma, meaning a muscle tumour) removes fibroids.

▌Root

Men

(From a Latin word **mensis**, *meaning month. Here men/o means menstruation, the monthly bleeding from the womb. The bleeding arises from the disintegration of the endometrium.)*

Combining form   Men/o

Word Exercise 8

Without using your Exercise Guide, write the meaning of:

(a) **men/o**/staxis

Using your Exercise Guide, find the meaning of:

(b) **men**/arche

(c) **men/o**/pause

(d) a/**men/o**/rrhoea (Am. a/**men/o**/rrhea)

(e) dys/**men/o**/rrhoea (Am. dys/**men/o**/rrhea)

(f) oligo/**men/o**/rrhoea (Am. oligo/**men/o**/rrhea)

(g) pre/**menstru**/al

Hysteroscopy and biopsy

In this procedure, a narrow endoscope known as a **hysteroscope** is inserted through the cervix to examine the uterus. Modern hysteroscopes are thin telescopes that fit through the cervix with minimal or no dilatation. The standard 4-mm hysteroscope gives a panoramic view of the cervical canal and uterine cavity and is suitable for most purposes. A diagnostic sheath around the main viewing telescope of the instrument allows saline or carbon dioxide to be pumped in, thereby inflating the uterus and improving the field of view.

A **hysteroscopy** is a simple, inexpensive diagnostic technique used to investigate women with abnormal uterine bleeding. It has been particularly valuable in the investigation of postmenopausal bleeding to exclude endometrial cancer. Once positioned, the hysteroscope is used to observe fibroids, polyps and adhesions, and to biopsy the endometrium (ie, remove living suspicious tissue for examination). Benign polyps are usually removed and examined as they are difficult to differentiate from malignant lesions.

A more complex instrument, the **microcolpohysteroscope** has different levels of magnification (1–150×) as well as diagnostic and operative sheaths. It can produce a panoramic view of the endocervix and uterine cavity or be used at close range to examine the cellular and vascular structure of the endometrium. During **operative hysteroscopy**, various instruments including biopsy or grasping forceps, scissors, diathermy probes and laser fibres are passed into the body through the operative sheath. The surgeon controls the instruments whilst viewing the uterine cavity through the telescope component of the device.

Another instrument called a **resectoscope**, used over many years for prostate and bladder surgery, has been modified for use as an operative hysteroscope. It has a built-in wire loop that uses a high-frequency electric current to cut and coagulate the tissues of the endometrium. The resectoscope is used for transcervical resection of the endometrium (TCRE), a technique of ablating (cutting away) the endometrium in women with dysfunctional uterine bleeding (menorrhagia). It can also remove small to medium submucous fibroids and provide biopsy specimens for histological analysis.

Flexible endoscopy using a 3- to 5-mm directional endoscope with an insufflating channel (to blow in gas or fluid) is also proving useful in hysteroscopy and salpingoscopy. The larger endoscopes also have a channel wide enough to accommodate surgical instruments.

Biopsy specimens removed by any of these instruments are sent to the pathology laboratory for processing and histological analysis. (The word biopsy is formed from *bio*-meaning life and *-opsy* meaning process of viewing. A biopsy is the removal and examination of tissue from a living body.)

▌Root

Cervic

(From a Latin word **cervix**, *meaning the neck. Here cervic/o means the cervix or cervix uteri, the neck of the uterus.)*

Combining form   Cervic/o

Word Exercise 9

Without using your Exercise Guide, build words that mean:

(a) inflammation of the cervix

(b) removal of the cervix

Cervical cancer or carcinoma of the cervix occurs most frequently in women between the ages of 30 and 50, and they are therefore advised to have periodic cervical smears. The procedure involves taking a sample of cells from the cervix and subjecting them to cytological examination called a **Pap test**, named after cytologist G. Papanicolaou. Neoplastic cells can be removed in their early stages of growth, thereby preventing the condition. The cancer begins with *cervical intraepithelial neoplasia* (CIN), a change in the shape, growth and number of cells in the deepest layer of the cervical epithelium. CIN may progress to the full thickness of the epithelium and is then called carcinoma-in-situ. The cancer may develop further and spread locally into the vagina, uterine body and other pelvic structures; more widespread metastases occur late in the disease. In a significant proportion of cases, the risk of developing cervical cancer is related to the number of sexual partners and is the result of transmission of the human papilloma virus HPV. Over 150 types of HPV have been identified, and they are referred to by number. HPV types 16, 18, 31, 33 and 45 are called high-risk types, and their presence increases the risk of developing cervical cancer. HPV 16 and 18 cause approximately 70% of all cancers of the cervix. High-risk HPVs also lead to an increased risk of anal, vaginal, vulvar and penile cancer.

Root

Colp

(*From a Greek word* **colpos***, meaning hollow. Here colp/o means the vagina, a hollow musculo-membranous passage extending from the cervix uteri to the vulva. The vagina receives the penis during copulation and allows the passage of a baby during the birth process.*)

Combining form   Colp/o

Word Exercise 10

Using your Exercise Guide, find the meaning of:

(a) **colp/o**/scopy

(b) **colp/o**/micro/scope
(used in situ, ie, to examine the vagina directly)

Without using your Exercise Guide, write the meaning of:

(c) **colp/o**/perine/o/rrhaphy

The perineum is the region between the thighs bounded by the anus and vulva in the female. Perineotomy is used synonymously with episi/o/tomy (*episi-* meaning pubic region). This incision is made during the birth of a child when the vaginal orifice does not stretch sufficiently to allow an easy birth.

(d) **colp/o**/hyster/ec-
tomy

(e) metr/o/**colp/o**/cele

(f)   cervic/o/**colp**/itis

Without using your Exercise Guide and beginning with the underlined root, build words that mean:

(g) surgical repair of the
<u>vagina</u> and perineum

(h) surgical fixation of the
<u>vagina</u>

Root

Vagin

(*From a Latin word* **vagina***, meaning sheath. Here vagin/o means the vagina, a hollow musculo-membranous passage extending from the cervix uteri to the vulva. The vagina receives the penis during copulation and allows the passage of a baby during the birth process.*)

Combining form   Vagin/o

Word Exercise 11

Without using your Exercise Guide, write the meaning of:

(a) **vagin/o**/perine/o/tomy

(b) **vagin/o**/perine/o/rrhaphy

(c) **vagin/o**/vesic/al

Using your Exercise Guide, find the meaning of -mycosis and -pathy; then build words that mean:

(d) condition of fungal infection of the vagina

(e) disease of the vagina

Investigations of disorders of the vagina and cervix usually require the use of a vaginal speculum to hold the walls of the vagina apart. There are many types of vaginal specula, one of which is shown in Figure 91.

Two small glands situated on either side of the external orifice of the vagina are known as the **greater vestibular glands** or **Bartholin glands** (after C. Bartholin, a Danish anatomist, 1655–1738); they produce mucus to lubricate the vagina. A condition called **bartholin**itis develops when the glands become inflamed.

Root

Vulv

(*From a Latin word* **vulva***, meaning wrapper. Here vulv/o means the vulva, also known as the pudendum femina or external genitalia.*)

Combining form   Vulv/o

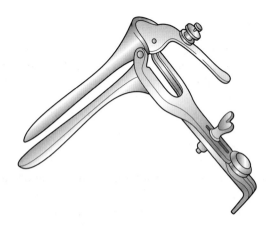

Figure 91   A vaginal speculum.

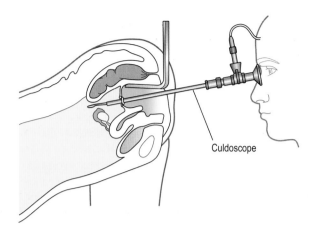

Culdoscope

Figure 92   Culdoscopy.

Word Exercise 12

Without using your Exercise Guide, write the meaning of:

(a) **vulv/o**/vagin/itis

(b) **vulv/o**/vagin/al

Root

Culd

(*From a French word* **cul-de-sac**, *meaning bottom of the bag or sack. Here culd/o means the rectouterine pouch or pouch of Douglas, a blindly ending pouch that lies above the posterior vaginal fornix. Named after James Douglas, 1675–1742, Scottish anatomist.*)

Combining form   Culd/o

Word Exercise 13

Without using your Exercise Guide, write the meaning of:

(a) **culd/o**/scope

(this allows examination of the uterus, oviducts, ovaries and peritoneal cavity; Fig. 92)

(b) **culd/o**/scopy

(c) **culd/o**/centesis

Root

Gynaec

(*From a Greek word* **gyne**, *meaning woman. Here gynaec/o means the female reproductive system.*)

Combining forms   Gynaec/o, (Am. Gynec/o)

Word Exercise 14

Using your Exercise Guide, find the meaning of:

(a) **gynaec/o**/logy (Am. **gynec/o**/logy; refers to diseases peculiar to women, ie, of the female reproductive tract)

(b) **gynaec/o**/log/ical (Am. **gynec/o**/log/ical)

ANATOMY EXERCISE

Now complete the Anatomy Exercise on page 230.

Abbreviations

Some common abbreviations related to the female reproductive system are listed next. Note, however, some are not standard, and their meaning may vary from one healthcare setting to another. There is a more extensive list for reference on page 369.

BSO	bilateral salpingo-oophorectomy
CACX, CaCx	cancer of the cervix
CIN	cervical intraepithelial neoplasia
Cx	cervix
DUB	dysfunctional uterine bleeding
GYN, Gyn	gynaecology (Am. gynecology)
HRT	hormone replacement therapy
IUCD	intrauterine contraceptive device
IUD	intrauterine death, intrauterine device
IUFB	intrauterine foreign body
LMP	last menstrual period
Pap	Papanicolaou smear test
PCOS	polycystic ovary syndrome

PMB	postmenopausal bleeding
PMS	premenstrual syndrome
PV	per vagina, per vaginam (through the vagina)
VE	vaginal examination

Pathology notes

Endometriosis

Endometriosis is a growth of endometrial tissue outside the uterus, most commonly in the ovaries, uterine tubes and other pelvic structures. The ectopic tissue, like the uterine endometrium, is responsive to the fluctuations in sex hormone levels of the menstrual cycle, causing menstrual-type bleeding in the lower abdomen and the formation of chocolate-coloured cysts in the ovaries. There is intermittent pain due to swelling, and recurrent haemorrhage (Am. hemorrhage) causes fibrous tissue formation. Ovarian endometriosis may lead to pelvic inflammation, infertility and extensive pelvic adhesions, involving the ovaries, uterus, uterine ligaments and the bowel. The cause is not clear but may be due to abnormal cell differentiation during fetal development or spread of endometrial cells through the uterine tubes, blood or lymph.

Ovarian cancer

The majority of ovarian tumours (Am. tumors) are benign and usually occur in patients between 20 and 45 years of age. The remainder occur mostly between the ages of 45 and 65 years and are divided between borderline malignancy and malignancy. Three main types of cell form ovarian tumours: epithelial cells, germ cells and hormone-secreting cells.

Epithelial cell tumours are borderline malignant or malignant tumours that vary in size from small to large, and some may be cystic. Large tumours cause pressure on other organs leading to gastrointestinal disturbances, dysuria and formation of ascites. The principal methods of spread are invasion of local and peritoneal structures and through the lymph and blood. The prevalence of this type of cancer is higher in developed societies and in higher socio-economic groups.

Germ cell ovarian tumours occur in children and young adults, and only a few are malignant.

Sex-cord stroma cell tumours develop from cells lining the ovarian follicles, luteal cells or fibrous supporting cells. Mixed tumours can also develop, some of which secrete sex hormones causing precocious sexual development in children.

Ovarian cysts

Ovarian cysts are fluid-filled sacs that are retained within the ovary. They may be benign or malignant and often originate in the ovarian follicles (follicular cysts) or corpus luteum (luteal cysts). If untreated, ovarian cysts can swell to a large size, creating an acute surgical emergency.

Pelvic inflammatory disease (PID)

Pelvic inflammatory disease is an acute inflammatory condition caused by bacterial infection; it can involve the uterus, uterine tubes or ovaries. PID is most commonly caused by gonorrhoea (Am. gonorrhea) and chlamydial infections that spread upward from the vagina. The condition may be accompanied by pain and fever, or there may be no symptoms at all. Early treatment of PID with antibiotics can stop its spread, but delay can lead to serious complications, including ectopic pregnancy, infertility resulting from adhesions and scarring and other damage to the reproductive tract. The infection may also spread to other tissues including the blood where it may cause septic shock and death.

Sexually transmitted disease (STD)

Sexually transmitted diseases or venereal diseases are infections caused by communicable pathogens such as viruses, bacteria, fungi and protozoa. The factor that links all these diseases and gives this disease category is the fact that they can all be transmitted by sexual contact. The term sexual contact refers to sexual intercourse in addition to any contact between the genitals of one person and the body of another. Diseases classified as STDs are not always transmitted sexually; for example, HIV can also be transmitted by blood transfusion or by contact with contaminated needles and syringes. Other common STDs include gonorrhoea (Am. gonorrhea), syphilis, genital herpes and chlamydia.

Associated words

Adhesion the union between two surfaces that are normally separated, usually the result of inflammation

Adnexa appendages or accessory structures of an organ, eg, adnexa uteri associated with the uterus

Ascites accumulation of serous fluid in the abdominal cavity

Areola the pigmented skin around the nipple of the breast

Atony loss of tone in an organ; uterine atony is a lack of contraction of the uterus

Cauterization destruction of a tissue by burning, sometimes used to treat abnormal cervical tissue

Climacteric the period of the menopause

Coitus sexual intercourse

Conization removal of a cone-shaped section of the cervix (a cone biopsy)

Contraception a group of drugs, devices, methods or surgical procedures that is intended to reduce the likelihood or prevent conception.

Copulation sexual intercourse

Disseminated widely dispersed in tissues, organs or systems

Dyspareunia difficult or painful intercourse

Exenteration process of removing internal organs, evisceration

Fimbria a fringe, especially the fimbriae that surround the entrance to the fallopian tube

Frigidity the absence of normal sexual desire

Fundus the base of an organ or the part farthest removed from its opening, eg, the fundus of the uterus (the top of the uterus furthest from the cervix)

Hot flash also called a hot flush, a symptom of the menopause experienced as a feeling of intense heat, sweating and rapid heartbeat that may last for 30 minutes

Hymen a fold of mucous membrane partially enclosing the entrance to the vagina

Infibulation female circumcision performed in some cultures to remove the clitoris and labia, and narrow the vaginal entrance

Insemination the introduction of semen into the vagina, fertilization of an egg by a sperm

Intercourse sexual connection between a male and female via the vagina

Leukorrhoea a white discharge from the vagina (Am. leukorrhea)

Mittelschmerz pain occurring between menses around the time of ovulation

Prolapse downward displacement of an organ, eg, descent of the cervix or whole uterus into the vagina

Thrush infection of mucous membranes, eg, the vagina with the fungus *Candida albicans*

Tubal ligation process of tying off or sealing the fallopian tubes (with sutures, filaments, clips or bands) to prevent fertilization of an egg

Obstetrics

Obstetrics is the branch of medicine that deals with the care of women during pregnancy, childbirth and the recuperative period following birth.

The successful entry of a sperm into an egg at fertilization is known as **conception**, and it is this event that creates a new individual. The fertilized egg then divides and forms into a ball of cells (the blastocyst) that must implant into the lining (endometrium) of the uterus to complete its development. **Pregnancy** begins when implantation is complete.

Occasionally a blastocyst implants and grows outside the uterus (extrauterine development). When this occurs, it is known as an **ectopic** pregnancy (see Fig. 93). The most common site is the fallopian tube, and a pregnancy here is life-threatening to the mother as the tube cannot stretch to accommodate the developing fetus. Eventually, the tube ruptures causing severe haemorrhage (Am. hemorrhage) and a surgical emergency.

Following implantation in a normal pregnancy, a structure known as the **placenta** (from Latin meaning flat cake) forms. This is a vascular structure, developed about the third month of gestation and is attached to the wall of the uterus. Through the placenta the fetus is supplied with oxygen and nutrients, and wastes are removed. The placenta is expelled as the afterbirth, usually within 1 hour of delivery.

After approximately 9 months (**the period of gestation**) a baby is expelled from the mother's body by muscular contractions of the uterus. The onset of uterine contractions is termed labour (Am. labor) or **parturition**. The period immediately following birth is known as the **puerperium**. in which time the

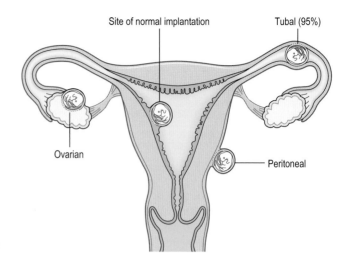

Figure 93 Three types of ectopic pregnancy. (Adapted from Chabner D-E, The Language of Medicine, 10th Edition, 2013, Saunders.)

reproductive organs tend to revert to their original state. The terms **antepartum** and **postpartum** are also used to indicate the periods before and after birth. Antepartum is usually used to mean up to 3 months before birth.

The mammary glands become active in late pregnancy and following the birth of a baby when they produce milk. The process of secreting milk and the period in which milk is produced is called **lactation**.

Root

Gravida

(*From a Latin word* **gravidus**, *meaning heavy or pregnant. Here, -gravida is used to describe a woman in relation to her pregnancies, eg, gravida I (GI), a woman pregnant for the first time.*)

Combining form   -gravida

Word Exercise 15

Using your Exercise Guide, find the meaning of:

(a) primi/**gravida** (gravida I)

(b) secundi/**gravida** (gravida II)

(c) multi/**gravida** (more than twice)

Root

Para

(*From a Latin word* **parere**, *meaning to bear/bring forth. Here, -para is used to mean a woman who has produced a viable child regardless of whether the child was alive at birth or stillborn.*)

Combining form   para

Word Exercise 16

Without using your Exercise Guide, write the meaning of:

(a) primi/**para** (para I)
Syn with uni/para
(uni-, one)

(b) secundi/**para**

(c) multi/**para**

(d) nulli/**para**

Another word that refers to pregnancy is **cyesis** (from Greek *kyesis,* meaning conception). **Pseudocyesis** refers to a false pregnancy, ie, signs and symptoms of early pregnancy, a result of an overwhelming desire to have a child.

Root

Fet

(*From a Latin word* **fetus,** *meaning an unborn baby. Here fet/o means a fetus, the name given to a human embryo at 8 weeks following fertilization, ie, when the organ systems have been laid down.*)

Combining form   Fet/o

> **Note.** Foetus is an alternative spelling of fetus. Once the usual spelling in British English, it is becoming less common.

Word Exercise 17

Without using your Exercise Guide, write the meaning of:

(a) **fet/o**/logy

(b) **fet/o**/scope

(c) **fet/o**/placent/al

Using your Exercise Guide, find the meaning of -toxic and -metry; then build words that mean:

(d) pertaining to poisoning of the fetus

(e) measurement of the fetus

The part of the fetus that lies in the lower part of the uterus is known as the presenting part. In a normal birth the vertex of the skull forms the presenting part, and it enters the birth canal first. If other parts enter first, eg, the buttocks, they are known as **malpresentations.**

Various manoeuvres can be made to turn or change the position of the fetus in the uterus. The term **version** (from Latin *vertere,* meaning to turn) is used for these manoeuvres. Many types have been described, eg:

> **Cephalic version**
>
> changes the position of the fetus from breech (buttocks first) to cephalic (head first) towards the birth canal.
>
> **External version**
>
> changes the position of the fetus by manipulation through the abdominal wall.
>
> **Internal version**
>
> changes the position of the fetus by hand within the uterus.

Root

Amni

(*From a Greek word* **amnia,** *meaning a bowl in which blood is caught. Here amni/o means the amnion, the fetal membrane that retains the amniotic fluid surrounding a developing fetus.*)

Combining form   Amni/o, amnion-

Word Exercise 18

Using your Exercise Guide, find the meaning of:

(a) **amni/o**/tic

(b) **amni/o**/tome

Without using your Exercise Guide, build words that mean:

(c) technique of cutting the amnion

(d) an instrument to visually examine the amnion

Without using your Exercise Guide, write the meaning of:

(e) **amni/o**/centesis

Figure 94 shows the developing amnion and Figure 95 the position of the needle used to withdraw amniotic fluid during amniocentesis.

Various fetal abnormalities can be detected by analysing the amniotic fluid, eg, spina bifida. In this condition the vertebral arches fail to surround the spinal cord, exposing the cord and meninges which may protrude through the defective vertebrae. The disorder can be detected before birth by the presence of increased levels of alpha-fetoprotein (AFP) in the amniotic fluid. AFP is also raised when the fetus is anencephalic (without a brain).

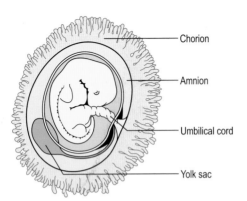

Figure 94   The amnion and related structures in a 5-week embryo.

Genetic disorders can also be identified by analysing the chromosomes present in cells sloughed off the developing fetus into the amniotic fluid, eg, Down syndrome (formerly known as mongolism). In this condition, 47 chromosomes are present instead of the normal 46. Parents can use the information from amniocentesis to decide to continue a pregnancy or abort a Down's fetus.

A new test for Down syndrome is currently being assessed in which samples of the mother's blood are examined for the presence of fetal DNA (genes). The test is able to detect small fragments of the baby's cell-free DNA in the mother's blood. Although not 100% accurate, first indications are that the test reduces the number of false positive results where a healthy baby is wrongly identified as having Down syndrome. Introduction of a reliable blood test should prevent women having an unnecessary amniocentesis, which carries a small risk of causing miscarriage.

The outermost of the fetal membranes is known as the **chorion** (from Greek, meaning outer membrane). It develops extensions, known as villi, that become part of the placenta. The combining form **chori/o** is used to mean chorion (see Fig. 94).

Without using your Exercise Guide, write the meaning of:

(f)   chori/o/**amni/o**/tic

(g)   chori/o/**amnion**/itis

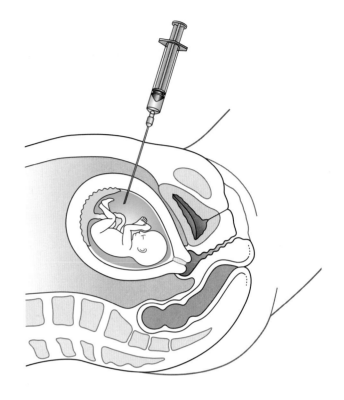

Figure 95   Amniocentesis performed at 15 weeks.

Obstetr- is mainly used in:

Obstetrics

The science dealing with the care of the pregnant woman during all stages of pregnancy and the period following birth.

Obstetrician

A medically qualified person who specializes in obstetrics (*-ician* meaning person associated with).

Obstetrical forceps

Large forceps consisting of two flat blades connected to a handle. They are used to pull on a fetal head or rotate it to facilitate vaginal delivery (Figs 96 and 97) (*-ical* means pertaining to).

Another device used by obstetricians to assist delivery is the **vacuum extractor or ventouse** (from French meaning cupping glass). This suction device is attached to the head as it presents through the birth canal and is used to pull the baby out. The technique is called vacuum-assisted vaginal delivery or vacuum extraction (VE). See Figure 98.

Root

Obstetric

(*From a Latin word* **obstetricare**, *meaning to assist in delivery. Here obstetr- means midwifery or obstetrics, the branch of medicine dealing with childbirth.*)

Combining forms   Obstetr

Root

Placent

(*From a Latin word* **plakoenta**, *meaning a flat cake. Here placent/o means the placenta, the temporary, hormone-secreting, vascular structure that facilitates the exchange of materials between the fetal and maternal blood.*)

Combining form   Placent/o

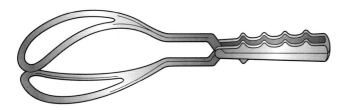

Figure 96   Obstetrical forceps.

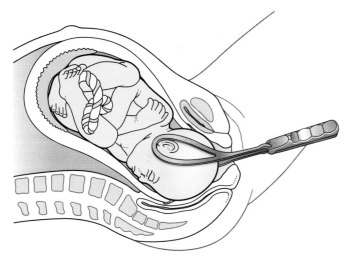

Figure 97   Obstetrical forceps in use.

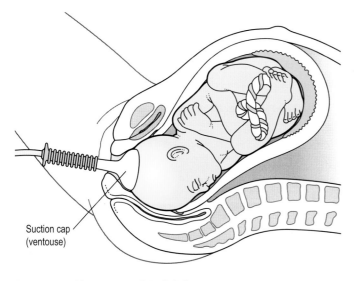

Suction cap
(ventouse)

Figure 98   Vacuum-assisted delivery.

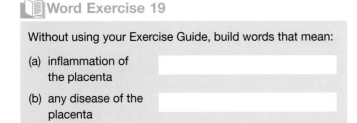

Word Exercise 19

Without using your Exercise Guide, build words that mean:

(a) inflammation of
    the placenta

(b) any disease of the
    placenta

Many abnormalities of the placenta have been noted. Two common disorders are:

Adherent placenta

This placenta is fused to the uterine wall so that separation is slow, and delivery of the placenta is delayed. When the placenta is not expelled after 1 hour, it is known as a retained placenta.

Placenta accreta

This occurs when blood vessels of the placenta grow too deeply into the uterine wall and attach to the myometrium (the muscular layer of the uterine wall). The condition poses a risk of severe haemorrhage (Am. hemorrhage) after delivery (postpartum). Neonatal problems such as premature birth, low birth weight and reduced 5-min Apgar scores are also associated with this condition.

Root

Toc

*(From a Greek word **tokos**, meaning birth. Here toc/o means labour/childbirth (Am. labor).)*

Combining forms   Toc/o, tok/o

Word Exercise 20

Without using your Exercise Guide, write the meaning of:

(a) dys/**toc**/ia

(b) **toco**/logy (synonymous
    with obstetrics)

Using your Exercise Guide, find the meaning of:

(c) eu/**toc**/ia

Labour (Am. labor) can be monitored by recording the force of uterine contractions using a device called a **tocodynamometer** (**Am. tokodynamometer**); the procedure is known as **tocography**. When the fetal heart is monitored with the uterine contractions during delivery, it is known as **cardiotocography**.

If labour is late or slow, the uterus can be induced to produce forcible contractions by the administration of **oxytocin**, a hormone that is produced naturally by the pituitary gland. Various compounds with oxytocin-like activity are available for this purpose.

The period of 6 to 8 weeks following birth is known as the **puerperium** (from Latin *puerperus*, meaning childbearing). This is the time when the reproductive system involutes (reverts) to its state before pregnancy. **Puerperal** fever, also called childbed fever or **puerperal** sepsis, is a serious infection of the genital tract usually diagnosed within 10 days of abortion or childbirth. See the Pathoglogy Notes on page 245.

Root

Nat

(*From a Latin word* **natalis**, *meaning birth*.)

Combining form   Nat/o

Word Exercise 21

Using your Exercise Guide, find the meaning of:

(a) neo/**nat**/al

(b) ante/**nat**/al

(c) peri/**nat**/al

Without using your Exercise Guide, write the meaning of:

(d) pre/**nat**/al

(e) neo/**nat**/o/logy

(A neonate is a newborn baby up to 1 month old.)

Root

Mamm

(*From a Latin word* **mamma**, *meaning breast. Here mamm/o means the breasts (mammary glands), the structures that secrete milk during lactation*.)

Combining form   Mamm/o, mamm/a

Word Exercise 22

Without using your Exercise Guide, write the meaning of:

(a) **mamm/o**/graphy

(b) **mamm/o**/plasty
     (sometimes performed
     for cosmetic reasons
     to increase or decrease
     the size of breasts)

Using your Exercise Guide, find the meaning of:

(c) **mamm/o**/tropic

Root

Mast

(*From a Greek word* **mastos**, *meaning breast. Here mast/o means the breasts (mammary glands), the structures that secrete milk during lactation*.)

Combining form   Mast/o

Word Exercise 23

Without using your Exercise Guide, build words that mean:

(a) condition of pain in the
     breast

(b) falling or drooping of the
     breast

(c) removal of the breast

There are two main forms of this operation for breast cancer:

- Simple mastectomy: removal of the breast tissue and overlying skin

- Radical mastectomy: removal of the breast tissue, overlying skin, underlying muscle and lymphatic tissue

Some patients opt for the removal of a breast tumour (Am. tumor) by a simpler procedure known as a **lumpectomy** (or tylectomy). In this procedure, just the mass of abnormal cells and a minimal margin of normal tissue is removed.

Without using your Exercise Guide, write the meaning of:

(d) **gynaec/o**/mast/ia
     (Am. **gynec/o**/mast/
     ia; seen in males)

Root

Lact

(*From a Latin word* **lactis**, *meaning milk*.)

Combining forms   Lact/i/o

Word Exercise 24

Using your Exercise Guide, find the meaning of:

(a) **lact**/agogue

(b) **lact/i**/fer/ous

(c) **lact/o**/meter (for deter-
     mining specific gravity)

(d) pro/**lact**/in (a hormone
     that acts on breasts)

(e) **lact/i**/fuge

Without using your Exercise Guide, write the meaning of:

(f) **lact/o**/genic

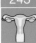

Root

Galact

*(From a Greek word **gala,** meaning milk.)*

Combining form   Galact/o

Word Exercise 25

Without using your Exercise Guide, write the meaning of:

(a) **galact**/agogue

(b) **galact/o**/rrhoea (Am.
galact/o/rrhea; an
abnormal condition)

(c) **galact**/ischia

(d) **galact/o**/poiesis

Medical equipment and clinical procedures

Review the names of all instruments and clinical procedures mentioned in this unit before completing Exercise 26.

Word Exercise 26

Match each description in Column C with a term in Column A by placing the appropriate number in Column B.

Column A	Column B	Column C
(a) vaginal speculum		1. technique of recording uterine contractions
(b) colposcope		2. an instrument used to view the uterus
(c) Pap test		3. technique of examining the peritoneal cavity via the vaginal fornix and rectouterine pouch
(d) culdoscopy		4. an instrument used to cut the amnion
(e) fetoscope		5. an instrument used to view the vagina and cervix
(f) hystero-scope		6. an instrument used to measure the specific gravity of milk

Column A	Column B	Column C
(g) amniotome		7. a procedure used to examine cells from a cervical smear
(h) lactometer		8. an instrument used to assist the passage of a baby through the birth canal
(i) obstetrical forceps		9. an instrument used to hold the walls of the vagina apart
(j) tocography		10. an instrument inserted into the amniotic cavity to visually examine a fetus

Other procedures and treatments not mentioned in the exercises include:

BRCA1 and BRCA2 gene test The <u>BR</u>east <u>CA</u>ncer gene BRCA1 is located on human chromosome 17. The gene normally acts to regulate cell division, repair DNA and restrain the growth of cells in the breast by producing tumour suppressor protein. When the gene mutates (changes), the protein does not function properly, so specific inherited mutations put the patient at increased risk of breast and ovarian cancer. BRCA2 has a similar function to BRCA1, and these were the first genes to be associated with breast cancer. Testing for hereditary mutations is advised for women with a strong family history of breast cancer. The BRCA genes are identified from cells in a blood sample and analyzed for the presence of mutations. The patient is then given an assessment of their risk of developing breast or ovarian cancer. A patient with a significant risk could opt for prophylactic surgery to remove all at-risk tissue, ie, breast, ovaries and fallopian tubes.

Caesarean section (Am. Cesarean) A surgical incision into the abdominal wall and uterine wall to deliver a fetus. The origin of the term is uncertain; it may be named after a law introduced during the time of Julius Caesar requiring a fetus to be removed from a dying or dead mother before burial.

Chorionic villus sampling (CVS) Chorionic villi are finger-shaped projections found in the placenta. The chorion is the principal embryological part of the placenta and has the same genetic material as the fetus. A sample of tissue is removed from the placenta either via a needle inserted into the abdomen (transabdominal CVS) or via a catheter passed into the uterus through the cervix (transcervical CVS). The samples of tissue are checked for chromosome anomalies such as Down syndrome and Edwards syndrome.

Cryopreservation A method of storing of sperm, eggs, embryos and other tissues at very low temperatures.

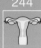
Fetal monitoring The continuous recording of the fetal heart rate and maternal uterine contractions during labour (Am. labor)

Obstetric ultrasonography The technique of producing an image (sonogram or ultrasound scan) of the embryo or fetus in the uterus; it is a standard part of prenatal care. The scan is used to assess movements such as the heartbeat, gestational age, size and growth and the presence of malformations.

Pelvic ultrasonography A technique of producing an image (sonogram) of the pelvic organs using ultrasound. It is a non-invasive procedure used to assess the condition of the uterus, cervix, vagina, fallopian tubes, and ovaries. Doppler ultrasound may also show blood flow in some pelvic organs.

Pregnancy test A test that measures the amount of human chorionic gonadotropin (hCG) in the urine or blood. The hormone is produced by a portion of the placenta and can be detected after implantation, which occurs 6 to 12 days following fertilization.

Triple screen test A screening test that measures serum levels of alpha-fetoprotein, oestriol (Am. estriol) and beta hCG. The patient is then classified as low-risk or high-risk for chromosomal anomalies and neural tube defects, and may be offered further tests, The test is also known as the Kettering test, Bart's test or the multiple-marker screening test.

Tubal ligation A surgical sterilization procedure for women in which the fallopian tubes are blocked, clamped, tied or cut. The purpose of the procedure is to prevent eggs passing down the oviducts where they can be fertilized. Tubal ligation is performed using a hysteroscope inserted via the cervix or through the abdominal wall using a laparoscope; it is a permanent method of female sterilization.

Mrs P's pregnancy progressed normally until 35 weeks of gestation when her BP rose to 150/95 mm Hg. She was admitted to the Obs-Gyn Unit for rest and observation. Serial ultrasound cephalometry was commenced and twice weekly 24-h urine collection for oestrogen excretion estimation.

In addition, daily fetal **cardiotocography** was performed. All these tests were normal, and her BP fell to 124/80 within 2 days of admission. After 5 days, she was allowed home with instructions to rest and was seen weekly at the **antenatal** clinic.

Antenatal investigations continued to be normal with evidence of good fetal growth until 3 days before term, when her blood pressure increased to 155/95, and her urine was protein 11. Over the next 24 hours, her blood pressure was maintained, and she had proteinuria of 3 g/24 h. Vaginal examination showed a long cervix that was not dilated.

Mrs P had developed preeclampsia, increasing the risk of **perinatal** mortality. The **obstetrician** considered performing a lower section Caesarean section (LSCS) since the risk becomes minimal after 24 hours of **puerperium.** Instead, the decision was taken to induce labour. Her cervix was dilated with a catheter left in place for 24 hours and partially ripened by local application of prostaglandin. Labour was induced by artificial rupture of the **amniotic** membranes and an infusion of oxytocin. After 8 hour, she gave birth to a healthy male, and her recovery was uneventful.

👥 CASE HISTORY 16

The object of this exercise is to understand words associated with a patient's medical history.

To complete the exercise:

- Read through the passage on pregnancy-induced hypertension; unfamiliar words are underlined, and you can find their meaning using the Word Help.

- Write the meaning of the medical terms shown in bold print on the lines that follow the Word Help.

Pregnancy-induced hypertension

Mrs P, a **primigravida** aged 25, presented to her GP with 12 weeks of **amenorrhoea** (Am. amenorrhea); examination confirmed the dates of gestation. Her BP was at 120/80, and her urine was sterile and showed no protein on dipstick testing.

Word Help

BP blood pressure

dipstick testing tests using paper sticks coated with indicators that change colour when protein is present

gestation period of pregnancy

GP general practitioner (family doctor)

hypertension high blood pressure

mortality death rate

Obs-Gyn obstetrics and gynaecology (Am. gynecology)

oestrogen a female sex hormone (Am. estrogen)

oxytocin a hormone that stimulates uterine contractions (to induce birth)

preeclampsia condition before or leading to eclampsia

Now write the meaning of the following words from the Case
History without using your dictionary lists:

(a) primigravida

(b) amenorrhoea
    (Am. amenorrhea)

(c) cardiotocography

(d) antenatal

(e) perinatal

(f) obstetrician

(g) puerperium

(h) amniotic

(Answers to the Case History exercise are given in the Answers
to Word Exercises on page 353.)

Quick Reference

Combining forms relating to the female reproductive system:

Amni/o	amnion
Bartholin/o	greater vestibular glands / Bartholin glands of the vagina
Cervic/o	cervix
Chori/o	chorion / outer fetal membrane
Colp/o	vagina
Culd/o	pouch of Douglas / rectouterine pouch
Endometr/i	endometrium / lining of womb / uterus
Fet/o	fetus
Galact/o	milk
-gravida	pregnancy / pregnant woman
Gynaec/o	female gynaecology
Gynec/o (Am.)	female gynaecology
Hyster/o	uterus
Lact/o/i	milk
Mamm/o	breast
Mast/o	breast
Men/o	menses / menstruation / monthly flow
Metr/o	uterus/womb
Nat/o	birth
Obstetr-	pertaining to midwifery or obstetrics
Oo-	egg
Oophor/o	ovary
Ovari/o	ovary
-para	to bear / bring forth offspring
Perine/o	perineum
Placent/o	placenta
Salping/o	fallopian tube
Toc/o	labour (Am. labor) / birth
Trachel/o	neck
Uter/o	uterus
Vagin/o	vagina
Vulv/o	vulva

Abbreviations

Some common abbreviations related to obstetrics
are listed next. Note that some are not standard, and
their meaning may vary from one healthcare setting to
another. There is a more extensive list for reference on
page 369.

AB, ab, abor	abortion
AFP	alpha-fetoprotein
APH	antepartum haemorrhage (Am. hemorrhage)
BBA	born before arrival
CS, C-Section, c/sect	caesarean section (Am. cesarean)
EDD	expected date of delivery
ERPC	evacuation of retained products of conception
FAS	fetal alcohol syndrome
FDIU	fetal death in utero
FHH	fetal heart heard
FHNH	fetal heart not heard
HCG, hCG	human chorionic gonadotropin
LCCS	low segment caesarean section (Am. cesarean)
LGA	large for gestational age
NFTD	normal full-term delivery
PPH	postpartum haemorrhage (Am. hemorrhage)

Pathology notes

Abortion

A *miscarriage* is the loss of an embryo or fetus before the 24th
week of pregnancy. Technically known as a *spontaneous abortion,* the most common cause of such a loss is a structural or
functional defect in the developing offspring. Other causes of
spontaneous abortion include placental abnormalities, hypertension, hormonal imbalance and trauma. After 24 weeks, delivery of a lifeless infant is termed a *stillbirth.*

Induced (nonspontaneous) abortion to intentionally terminate a
pregnancy is brought on by methods such as vacuum aspiration and administration of prostaglandin preparations.

Birth defects

Birth defects, also called *congenital abnormalities,* include any structural or functional abnormality present at birth. Congenital defects may be inherited or may be acquired during gestation or delivery. Acquired defects result from agents called teratogens that disrupt normal embryonic development. Teratogens include chemicals that cross the placental barrier such as alcohol, antibiotics and other drugs; some viruses such as the rubella virus; and exposure to ionizing radiation (X-rays, etc.) that damage the genetic code in embryonic cells.

Breast cancer

Approximately 90% of breast tumours (Am. tumors) are benign (not cancer). Fibroadenomas are the most common type and occur at any time after puberty; incidence peaks in the third decade. Some tumours are cystic, and some solid, and they usually occur in women nearing the menopause. Fibroadenomas do not increase the risk of cancer and are associated with an increased sensitivity to the hormone oestrogen (Am. estrogen).

The most common types of malignant tumour (Am. tumor) usually appear as painless lumps in the upper-outer quadrant of the breast. Breast cancers are often a type of carcinoma called *adenocarcinoma* that starts in the glandular tissue of the breast. The carcinoma can originate in the ducts that transport milk or in the milk-forming lobes. There is usually considerable fibrosis around the tumour that may cause retraction of the nipple and ulceration of the overlying skin. Other types of cancers occur in breast tissue including sarcomas, which originate in the cells of muscle, fat or connective tissue.

Early spread of malignant cells beyond the breast is via the lymph to the axillary and internal mammary nodes. Local invasion involves the pectoral muscles and the pleura. Blood-spread metastases may occur later in many organs and bones, especially lumbar and thoracic vertebrae. The causes of breast cancer are not known, but an important factor appears to be high oestrogen exposure. A genetic component is also likely, with close relatives of cancer sufferers having a significantly elevated risk of developing the disease. One percent of all breast cancer occurs in men.

Endometrial cancer

A type of cancer that develops from a malignant carcinoma in the lining of the uterus. Symptoms include vaginal bleeding not associated with menstruation, pelvic pain and pain on urination. Risk factors for the development of the condition include a family history of endometrial cancer, obesity, excessive oestrogen (Am. estrogen) exposure, diabetes and being postmenopausal. Treatment includes surgery to remove the uterus, fallopian tubes and ovaries (total hysterectomy and bilateral salpingo-oophorectomy), radiotherapy, chemotherapy and hormone therapy.

Erythroblastosis fetalis

A haemolytic (Am. hemolytic) disease of the newborn characterized by an excess of erythroblasts in the blood. The condition is caused by Rh factor incompatibility between the mother and fetus (Mother Rh– and fetus Rh+). The mother produces antibodies that cross the placenta and destroy fetal erythrocytes; the resulting anaemia stimulates the formation of erythroblasts (immature red blood cells). Intrauterine blood transfusion can be given to reduce anaemia, and further transfusions can be administered following birth.

Implantation disorders

Placenta praevia (Am. previa) In this condition the blastocyst implants in the uterine wall near the cervix or over the cervical os (opening). When this occurs, the normal dilation and softening of the cervix that occurs in the third trimester of pregnancy often causes painless bleeding, and the placenta separates from the uterine wall. The massive blood loss that may result can be life-threatening for both mother and offspring.

Abruptio placentae Separation of the placenta from the uterine wall can occur even when implantation takes place in the upper part of the uterus. When this occurs in a pregnancy of 20 weeks or more, the condition is called *abruptio placentae.* Complete separation of the placenta causes immediate death of the fetus. The severe haemorrhaging (Am. hemorrhaging) sometimes hidden in the uterus may cause circulatory shock and death of the mother within minutes. A caesarean (Am. cesarean) section and sometimes hysterectomy must be performed immediately to prevent blood loss and death.

Meconium aspiration syndrome (MAS)

Meconium is the first faecal discharge (Am. fecal) passed by a neonate soon after birth. In this syndrome the fetus passes meconium into the surrounding amniotic fluid whilst still in the uterus. Meconium is taken into the lungs (aspirated) before and during delivery and can block the neonate's airways immediately after birth. There can be prolonged damage to the respiratory system, and cerebral hypoxia may lead to long-term neurological damage or death. The condition is usually secondary to fetal hypoxia that may occur for a variety of reasons, eg, occlusion of the umbilical cord, placental infarction or maternal smoking.

Neonatal respiratory distress syndrome (NRDS)

This serious condition also known as hyaline membrane disease is an acute lung disease usually seen in babies born prematurely. Their lungs are deficient in surfactant, a substance made up of proteins and fats that help keep the lungs inflated. Without surfactant the air sacs (alveoli) may collapse, hyaline forms in spaces within the lungs, and the baby becomes short of oxygen.

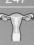

Preeclampsia

It is not uncommon for a woman's blood pressure to rise during pregnancy and remain elevated until the end of pregnancy; this condition is called pregnancy-induced hypertension (PIH). In about 6% to 8% of all pregnancies, PIH may progress to a condition called preeclampsia, formerly known as *toxaemia of pregnancy (Am. toxemia)*. This serious disorder is characterized by the onset of acute hypertension after the 24th week and is accompanied by proteinuria and oedema (Am. edema). The causes of PIH and preeclampsia are largely unknown, but a gene that regulates salt balance may also be involved in raising blood pressure during pregnancy. Preeclampsia can result in complications such as abruptio placentae, stroke, haemorrhage (Am. hemorrhage), fetal malnutrition and low birth weight. The condition can progress to *eclampsia,* a form of PIH that causes severe convulsions, coma, kidney failure and perhaps death of the fetus and mother.

Puerperal fever

Puerperal fever or *childbed fever* is a syndrome of postpartum mothers characterized by a bacterial infection that progresses to septicaemia (Am. septicemia) and possibly death. The infection originates in the birth canal and spreads to the endometrium and other pelvic structures. Modern aseptic techniques prevent most postpartum infections, and those that occur are usually successfully treated with intensive antibiotic therapy.

Associated words

Abortifacient an agent or drug that may induce abortion

Abortion the emptying of the pregnant uterus before the 24th week of gestation; it may be spontaneous (a miscarriage) or therapeutic where a pregnancy is intentionally terminated

Accouchement childbirth, the period of confinement for delivery

Afterbirth a nonmedical term used to describe the placenta, umbilical cord and fetal membranes delivered from the uterus after childbirth

APGAR score a scoring system used in the physical assessment of the newborn 1 and 5 minutes after birth; it checks colour (Am. color), reflexes, muscle tone, heart rate and respiratory effort, devised by Virginia Apgar

Attitude body posture or position particularly in the fetal position as determined by the degree of flexion of the head, eg, flexed

Ballottement using a finger to push sharply against the uterus to detect the presence of a fetus by its return impact

Cerclage also known as a cervical stitch, is a treatment for cervical incompetence when the cervix starts to shorten and open too early during a pregnancy; the cervix is encircled with a suture, band or loop

Chignon a temporary swelling left on an infant's head after a ventouse suction cup has been used for delivery

Colostrum the fluid secreted by the breasts in the first 3 to 4 days following delivery until lactation begins; it is an important source of passive antibody

Conceptus the embryo and its associated membranes (the products of conception)

Congenital pertaining to existing and present at the time of birth, often genetically determined

Contraction a rhythmic shortening of smooth muscle in the upper segment of the uterus that increases in strength, forcing the fetus through the birth canal

Cordocentesis an invasive procedure to remove a blood sample from the umbilical cord of the fetus

Decidua the endometrium of the pregnant uterus that has been thickened and vascularized to enable embryo implantation; it is shed at the end of pregnancy except for its deepest layer

Epidural pertaining to upon the dura mater of the spinal cord, commonly used to mean epidural analgesia, the injection of anaesthetic into the spinal cord to relieve the pain of childbirth (Am. anesthetic)

Episiotomy incision of the perineum during the second stage of labour to prevent tears and facilitate delivery of the fetus (Am. labor)

Fecundation fertilization, impregnation

Fecundity the ability to produce offspring frequently and in large numbers

Fertile possessing the capacity to reproduce

Gas and Air a 50% mixture of nitrous oxide and air inhaled for pain relief during labour (Am. labor); it is commonly marketed as Entonox or Nitronox

Gestation the period of development from fertilization of an ovum to birth, pregnancy

Hydramnios condition of too much amniotic fluid

Impregnation rendering pregnant, insemination

Induction act of initiating something, eg, the artificial starting of labour with the hormone oxytocin (Am. labor)

Intramural pertaining to within the wall of an organ

In vitro in glass, eg, outside the body in a test tube

Involution the process by which the uterus returns to its normal size

Lie the relationship between the longitudinal axis of the fetus with respect to that of the mother, eg, transverse lie

Lochia the discharge of blood and tissue debris from the uterus following childbirth

Meconium the first intestinal discharges of a newborn child

Miscarriage abortion, the spontaneous expulsion of the fetus before the 24th week of pregnancy

Nidation implantation of a conceptus into the endometrium

Oligohydramnios condition of too little amniotic fluid

Orifice an opening

Partus childbirth or labour (Am. labor)

Presentation the portion of the fetal body that is lying closest to the pelvic inlet of the birth canal during labour; it can be cephalic (head), breech (buttocks or feet) or shoulder presentation (Am. labor)

Preterm before term, before the 37th completed week of pregnancy

Procidentia complete prolapse of an organ, eg, prolapse of the uterus so the cervix protrudes through the vagina

Pudendum the external genitalia, especially of women

Quickening the first perceptible fetal movement felt by the mother, usually between the fourth and fifth month of pregnancy

Show the bloodstained discharge that occurs at the onset of labour (Am. labor)

Singleton a fetus that develops alone

Souffle a blowing sound heard on auscultation, eg, uterine souffle due to blood flow in uterine arteries

Stillbirth a baby issued from a mother after the 24th week of pregnancy not showing any signs of life

Striae gravidarum stretch marks, red then white lines that appear on a pregnant abdomen

Teratogenic pertaining to forming a defective embryo (from Greek *teras-*, monster)

Term the end of pregnancy

Trimester a period of three months, eg, the first trimester of pregnancy

Ventouse a vacuum extractor used to facilitate the delivery of a fetus

Vertex the crown of the head, eg, a vertex presentation in which the crown appears in the vagina first

Viable capable of independent life, able to live after birth

Zygote a single, fertilized cell formed from the union of a male and female gamete

NOW TRY THE WORD CHECK

WORD CHECK

This self-check exercise lists all the word components used in this unit. First, write down the meaning of as many word components as you can. Then, check your answers using the Exercise Guide and Quick Reference box or the Glossary of Word Components (pp. 383–410).

Prefixes

a-	
ante-	
dys-	
endo-	
eu-	
extra-	
micro-	
multi-	
neo-	
nulli-	
oligo-	
peri-	
post-	
pre-	
primi-	
pro-	
pseudo-	
secundi-	

Combining forms of word roots

amni/o	
bartholin/o	
cardi/o	
cervic/o	
chori/o	
colp/o	
culd/o	
cyst/o	
cyt/o	
fer/o	
fet/o	
fibr/o	
galact/o	
-gravida	
gynaec/o (Am. gynec/o)	
haem/o (Am. hem/o)	
hyster/o	
lact/o	
mamm/o	
mast/o	
men/o	
metr/o	
myc/o	
nat/o	
obstetr-	

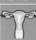

oo-

oophor/o

ovari/o

-para

perine/o

peritone/o

phleb/o

placent/o

rect/o

salping/o

sten/o

toc/o

trachel/o

uter/o

vagin/o

vesic/o

vulv/o

Suffixes

-a

-agogue

-al

-algia

-arche

-blast

-cele

-centesis

-dynia

-ectomy

-fuge

-genesis

-genic

-gram

-graphy

-ia

-ical

-ischia

-itis

-lithiasis

-logy

-malacia

-meter

-metry

-natal

-osis

-ous

-pathia

-pathy

-pause

-pexy

-plasty

-poiesis

-ptosis

-rrhagic

-rrhaphy

-rrhexis

-rrhoea (Am. -rrhea)

-sclerosis

-scope

-scopy

-staxis

-stenosis

-stomy

-tome

-tomy

-toxic

-trophic

-tropic

-tubal

NOW TRY THE SELF-ASSESSMENT

SELF-ASSESSMENT

Test 16A

Next are some combining forms that refer to the anatomy of the female reproductive system. Indicate which part of the system they refer to by putting a number from the diagrams (Figs 99 and 100) next to each word.

(a) oophor/o

(b) salping/o

(c) hyster/o

(d) endometr/o

(e) cervic/o

(f) colp/o

(g) vulv/o

(h) culd/o

Score

8

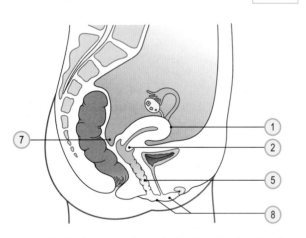

Figure 99   Sagittal section through the female showing the reproductive system.

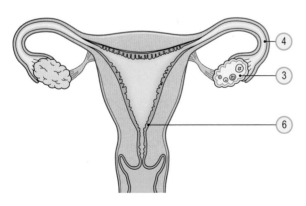

Figure 100   The female reproductive system.

Test 16B

Prefixes and suffixes

Match each meaning in Column C with a prefix or suffix in Column A by inserting the appropriate number in Column B.

Column A	Column B	Column C
(a) -agogue		1. to drip (blood)
(b) ante-		2. pertaining to birth
(c) eu-		3. stop/pause
(d) -ischia		4. new
(e) multi-		5. agent that induces/ promotes
(f) -natal		6. after
(g) neo-		7. few/little
(h) nulli-		8. condition of bursting forth (of blood)
(i) oligo-		9. pertaining to a tube or oviduct
(j) -ous		10. before (i)
(k) -pause		11. before (ii)
(l) -pexy		12. good
(m) post-		13. fixation by surgery
(n) pre-		14. pertaining to stimulating
(o) primi-		15. pertaining to
(p) -rrhagia		16. second
(q) secundi-		17. none
(r) -staxis		18. first
(s) -tropic		19. condition of blocking/holding back
(t) -tubal		20. many

Score

20

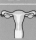

Test 16C

Combining forms of word roots

Match each meaning in Column C with a combining form of a word root in Column A by inserting the appropriate number in Column B.

Column A	Column B	Column C
(a) cervic/o		1. female reproductive system / woman
(b) colp/o		2. breast (i)
(c) culd/o		3. breast (ii)
(d) -gravida		4. menstruation/ monthly
(e) gynaec/o (Am. gynec/o)		5. birth
(f) hyster/o		6. vulva (external genitalia)
(g) lact/o		7. placenta
(h) mamm/o		8. pregnant / pregnant woman
(i) mast/o		9. perineum / area between anus and vulva
(j) men/o		10. midwifery / specialty of obstetrics
(k) metr/o		11. to bear / bring forth baby
(l) nat/o		12. uterus (i)
(m) obstetr-		13. uterus (ii)
(n) oo-		14. uterus (iii)
(o) oophor/o		15. neck (of uterus)
(p) ovari/o		16. Douglas pouch / rectouterine cavity
(q) -para		17. vagina (i)
(r) perine/o		18. vagina (ii)
(s) placent/o		19. egg
(t) salping/o		20. ovary (i)
(u) trachel/o		21. ovary (ii)
(v) uter/o		22. cervix uteri

Column A	Column B	Column C
(w) vagin/o		23. fallopian tube
(x) vesic/o		24. milk
(y) vulv/o		25. bladder

Score

25

Test 16D

Write the meaning of:

(a) tocometer

(b) oophorohysterectomy

(c) mastopexy

(d) hysterorrhexis

(e) metropathy

Score

5

Test 16E

Build words that mean:

(a) surgical repair of the Douglas pouch / rectouterine pouch

(b) formation of an opening into a fallopian tube

(c) rupture of the amnion

(d) displacement / prolapse of the vagina (use colp/o)

(e) study of cells of the vagina (use colp/o)

Score

5

Check answers to Self-Assessment Tests on pages 364–365.

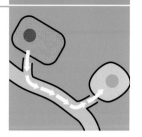

UNIT 17
THE ENDOCRINE SYSTEM

OBJECTIVES

Once you have completed Unit 17, you should be able to do the following:

- understand the meaning of medical words relating to the endocrine system
- build medical words relating to the endocrine system
- associate medical terms with their anatomical position
- understand common medical abbreviations relating to the endocrine system

EXERCISE GUIDE

Use this list of word components and their meanings to complete the word exercises in this unit.

Prefixes

acro-	extremities/point
hyper-	above normal / excessive
hypo-	below normal / deficient
para-	beside/near

Roots / Combining forms

aden/o	gland
blast/o	germ cell / cell that forms…
chondr/o	cartilage
gloss/o	tongue
-gyne	woman
kal/i	potassium
natr/i	sodium

Suffixes

-aemia	condition of blood (Am. -emia)
-al	pertaining to
-ectomy	removal of
-emia (Am.)	condition of blood
-genesis	formation of
-genic	pertaining to formation / originating in
-globulin	protein
-ia	condition of
-ic	pertaining to
-ism	process of / state or condition
-itis	inflammation of
-megaly	enlargement
-micria	condition of small size
-oma	tumour/swelling (Am. tumor)
-osis	abnormal condition/disease of
-plasia	condition of growth / formation of (cells)
-ptosis	falling/displacement/prolapse
-tomy	incision into
-toxic	pertaining to poisoning
-trophic	pertaining to nourishment
-tropic	pertaining to affinity for / stimulating
-uresis	condition of excreting in the urine
-uria	condition of urine

ANATOMY EXERCISE

When you have finished Word Exercises 1 to 6, look at the word components listed next. Complete Fig. 101 by writing the appropriate combining form on each dotted line; more than one component may relate to the same position. (You can check their meanings in the Quick Reference box on p. 260.)

Adren/o	Orchid/o	Parathyroid/o
Adrenocortic/o	Ovari/o	Pituitar-
Hypophys-	Pancreat/o	Thyr/o
Oophor/o		

The endocrine system

The endocrine system is composed of a diverse group of glands that secrete hormones directly into the blood. Once released, the hormones travel in the blood plasma to all parts of the body and act as chemical 'messengers'. Low concentrations of hormones in the blood stimulate specific target tissues and exert a regulatory effect on their cellular processes (metabolism). They do this by attaching to receptors on the surface of target cells or within their cytoplasm, and this action triggers chemical changes within the cell. To summarize their action:

The endocrine gland secretes a hormone directly into the blood	→	The hormone travels around the body in the blood plasma	→	The target tissue responds to the hormone by altering its metabolism

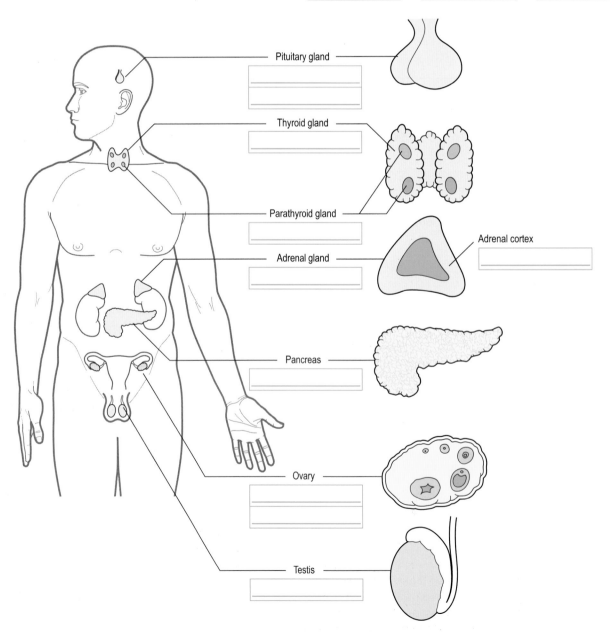

Figure 101   The endocrine system.

The brain and the endocrine glands precisely regulate the concentration of hormones that circulate in the blood. By its actions, the endocrine system plays a major role in regulating homeostasis: by this we mean the maintenance of a relatively constant internal environment of the body. Many endocrine disorders are brought about by changes in the output of hormones. Abnormal levels of hormones produce symptoms that range from minor to severely disabling disease and death.

In this unit, we will examine terms associated with each endocrine gland.

Use the Exercise Guide at the beginning of this unit to complete Word Exercises 1 to 6, unless you are asked to work without it.

The pituitary gland

▌Root

Pituitar

(*From a Latin word* **pituita**, *meaning slime/phlegm. Here -pituitar- means the pituitary gland, a small structure that grows from the base of the brain on a stalk. It is commonly called the 'master' gland of the endocrine system because it releases tropic hormones that regulate other endocrine glands.*)

Combining form   -pituitar-
(-pituitarism is used when referring to the process of pituitary secretion)

📖 Word Exercise 1

Using your Exercise Guide, find the meaning of:

(a) hypo/**pituitar**/ism _____

(b) hyper/**pituitar**/ism _____

One of the hormones produced by the pituitary gland is somatotrophin, also called human growth hormone (HGH) or somatotropin. Underproduction in childhood results in **dwarfism** and overproduction in **giantism**. In adults, underproduction of growth hormone produces **acromicria** and overproduction **acromegaly** (see the Pathology Notes on page 261).

(c) acro/micria _____

(d) acro/megaly _____

Once it was realized that the pituitary gland is not the source of spit and phlegm, scientists renamed the gland the **hypophysis** (*hypo-* below, *physis-* growth, ie, a growth below the brain). Pituitary and hypophysis are now used synonymously. The hypophysis consists of a downgrowth from the brain, known

as the neurohypophysis, and attached to it is a glandular part known as the adenohypophysis.

Removal of the hypophysis is known as **hypophys**/ectomy.

The thyroid gland

▌Root

Thyr

(*From a Greek word* **thyreoidos**, *meaning resembling a shield. Here thyr/o and thyroid/o mean the thyroid gland, the shield-shaped gland that lies above the trachea. It secretes the thyroid hormones triiodothyronine (T₃) and thyroxine (T₄) that control the metabolic rate of all cells.*)

Combining forms   Thyr/o, thyroid/o

📖 Word Exercise 2

Using your Exercise Guide, find the meaning of:

(a) **thyr/o**/gloss/al _____

(b) **thyr/o**/aden/itis _____

(c) **thyr/o**/globulin _____

(d) **thyr/o²**/chondr/o³/tomy¹ _____

(e) **thyr/o**/toxic/osis (also known as Graves disease, now generally replaced by the term hyperthyroidism) _____

A symptom of this disorder is **exophthalmos**, protruding eyes. The extent of this can be measured using a technique known as **exophthalmometry**.

(f) para**thyroid** _____

(This refers to the parathyroid glands that lie on the posterior surface of the thyroid gland (para- meaning beside or near). The parathyroid glands consist of four small glands that secrete parathyroid hormone, PTH.)

(g) **parathyroid**/ectomy _____

Without using your Exercise Guide, write the meaning of:

(h) hyper/**parathyroid**/ism (leads to excess calcium in blood, hyper/calc/aemia; Am. hyper/calc/emia) _____

(i) **thyr/o**/megaly _____

Without using your Exercise Guide, build words that mean:

(j) process of secreting above normal levels of thyroid hormone

(k) process of secreting below normal levels of thyroid hormone

In infants, this results in poor growth and mental retardation and is known as **congenital hypothyroidism** (formerly cretinism). It is caused by deficient secretion of thyroid hormones (T_3 and T_4), and the condition becomes evident within a few weeks or months of birth. Unless treatment begins early in life, the individual remains severely affected.

In adults the condition is known as **hypothyroidism** or **myxoedema** (Am. myxedema), the latter term referring to the accumulation of mucopolysaccharides under the skin. Hypothyroidism is a result of below normal secretion of thyroid hormones T_3 and T_4 in adults; it gives rise to 'puffy' swollen skin, dry hair, weight gain, bradycardia, sensitivity to cold, lethargy and loss of mental and physical vigour (Am. vigor).

Using your Exercise Guide, find the meaning of -genic, -ptosis and -tropic; then build words using thyr/o that mean:

(l) downward displacement of the thyroid

(m) pertaining to affinity for the thyroid gland

(n) pertaining to originating in the thyroid gland

Any enlargement of the thyroid gland is known as **goitre** (Am. **goiter**) and is a feature of several thyroid diseases. There are various types of goitre that have been grouped in different ways, three main types are:

Simple nontoxic goitre (Am. goiter)

A goitre that is not producing the signs and symptoms of hyperthyroidism. Simple goitre is still common in areas of the world where the soil and water contain little iodine. As the diets in these areas are severely deficient in iodine, there is insufficient iodine for synthesis of thyroid hormones (T_3 and T_4).

Toxic nodular goitre (Am. goiter)

A goitre that is producing the signs and symptoms of hyperthyroidism; also known as hyperthyroiditis, exophthalmic goitre and Graves disease.

Malignant goitre (Am. goiter)

A goitre that is the seat of new, malignant growth (carcinoma of the thyroid).

A thyroid scan is used to assess the size, shape and activity of the thyroid gland. The radioiodine (I-123) administered to the patient is taken up by the thyroid gland and used to make thyroid hormones; this makes the gland slightly radioactive. The presence of radioactivity is then detected with a scanner (gamma camera) that creates an image of its distribution. Areas that are very active will take up more radiation and will be visible on the scan as 'hot spots' or 'hot nodules'; these areas secrete more thyroid hormones than normal. Nonfunctioning areas are less radioactive and are known as 'cold spots' or 'cold nodules'.

The recently introduced computerized rectilinear thyroid scan utilizes computer technology to improve the clarity of thyroid scans and enhance thyroid nodules. It measures both thyroid function and thyroid size. The accurate sizing of the thyroid gland aids in the follow-up of nodules to see if they are growing or getting smaller in size. (See Unit 18, page 273 for treatment of hyperthyroidism with radioactive iodine.)

The pancreas

We have already examined the role of the pancreas in digestion in Unit 2; here, we examine its role as an endocrine gland. Among the cells in the pancreas that produce digestive enzymes are small patches of tissue called the **islets of Langerhans**. The islets secrete the hormones **insulin** and **glucagon** directly into the blood; these play a major role in the regulation of blood glucose concentration.

Root

Pancreat

(*Derived from Greek* **pancreas**, *pan- all, kreas- flesh. Here pancreat/o means the pancreas, a large endocrine gland situated below and behind the stomach.*)

Combining form   Pancreat/o

Word Exercise 3

Without using your Exercise Guide, write the meaning of:

(a) **pancreat/o**/tropic (some of the pituitary hormones have such an action)

Insulin (from Latin *insula*, meaning island) is secreted by the islets of Langerhans. Once in the bloodstream, it stimulates the uptake of sugar (glucose) by tissue cells. Blood glucose rises following intake and digestion of carbohydrate, the overall effect of insulin is to lower blood glucose levels in the body after meals. The combining form derived from this **insulin/o** means insulin or the islets of Langerhans.

Using your Exercise Guide, find the meaning of:

(b) **insulin/o**/genesis

(c) **insulin**/oma

Without using your Exercise Guide, write the meaning of:

(d) **insul**/itis

(e) hyper/**insulin**/ism

If the body fails to produce insulin, blood glucose concentration rises, and glucose appears in the urine; this abnormal condition is known as **diabetes mellitus**. The name *diabetes* is derived from a Greek word meaning siphon (to convey liquid through a tube). The name reflects the most obvious symptoms: excessive thirst (**polydipsia**) followed by drinking and excessive urination (**polyuria**), just like the passing of water through a siphon. The second name mellitus is a Latin word meaning honey, the substance originally used as a sweetener instead of sugar. Diabetes mellitus refers to the passing of large quantities of water containing sugar through the body.

(**Polydipsia** is formed from *poly-* meaning too much, *dips/o-* thirst and *-ia* condition of).

There are two main types of diabetes mellitus:

Type I, insulin-dependent diabetes mellitus (IDDM)
This occurs mainly in children and young adults, and the onset is usually sudden. The condition is characterized by deficiency or absence of insulin due to the destruction of the β-islet cells that produce insulin in the pancreas (β = beta). As insulin is required to treat this disorder throughout life, it is called insulin-dependent diabetes mellitus. It is also called *juvenile onset diabetes* because it commonly arises in those under 20 years of age. The cause is unknown, but those affected have a genotype that makes them more susceptible. In many cases, an autoimmune reaction has occurred in which autoantibodies to β-islet cells are present. Without insulin treatment, IDDM is fatal.

Type II, non-insulin-dependent diabetes mellitus (NIDDM)
This is the most common form of diabetes, accounting for about 90% of cases. Type II is also called *adult-onset diabetes* as it tends to develop after the age of 40 in people who are overweight or obese. Recently, the proportion of people diagnosed at a relatively early age has increased markedly. Many type II diabetics secrete sufficient amounts of insulin into the blood, but their cells are less sensitive to the hormone: they are said to be insulin resistant. For this reason, type II diabetes is also known as non-insulin-dependent diabetes and can usually be controlled by dietary changes, exercise and/ or administration of antidiabetic drugs. The cause is unknown and insulin secretion may be above or below normal.

Complications of diabetes mellitus include a tendency to develop cataracts, retinopathy and neuropathy. Blood glucose estimation and glucose tolerance tests are used to diagnose the condition. The latter test involves administering a known quantity of glucose and measuring the amount that appears in the blood in a set time.

Next are terms that can be used to describe sugar (glucose) levels in blood and urine. The combining form **glyc/o/s** is used to mean sugar (from Greek *glykys,* meaning sweet).

Using your Exercise Guide, find the meaning of:

(f) hypo/**glyc**/aemia (Am. hypo/**glyc**/emia)

(g) hyper/**glyc**/aemia (Am. hyper/glyc/emia)

(h) **glycos**/uria

Diabetics may use urine test strips to monitor their condition; the strips contain glucose oxidase and change colour in response to the presence of glucose in the urine. The strips are also used for routine screening in general practice.

Diabetic patients can now estimate their own blood sugar level using a blood sample obtained by lancing a finger to obtain a spot of blood and analyzing the sample with a blood glucose meter, also called a blood glucose monitor.

Untreated diabetes results in the tissue cells using fatty acids as a source of energy instead of glucose. This leads to the release of chemicals known as ketones into the blood and urine. Ketones such as acetone have a toxic effect on the body and produce a condition known as **ketosis**. Accumulation of ketones can lead to an increase acidity of the blood (**ketoacidosis**), and this may be fatal in uncontrolled diabetes. Patients can estimate the concentration of ketones in their urine using test strips that change colour on contact with ketones. If levels rise, they may need to seek medical assistance to bring their blood sugar under control.

Note. Glucagon is a hormone secreted by the α cells in the islets of Langerhans that can raise blood sugar by converting glycogen, a stored carbohydrate found in liver and muscle, into glucose (α = alpha).

The adrenal gland

Root

Adren

(*From Latin* **ad-** *to/near,* **renes-** *kidneys. Here adren/o means the adrenal gland, a small triangle-shaped gland that lies above a kidney. The inner part of the gland called the medulla secretes adrenaline; the outer part called the cortex secretes steroid hormones.*)

Combining form   Adren/o, adrenal-

Word Exercise 4

Without using your Exercise Guide, build words that mean:

(a) an enlarged adrenal gland

(b) removal of the adrenal gland (use adrenal-)

(c) pertaining to stimulating/ acting on the adrenal gland

The adrenal cortex forms the outer layer of the adrenal gland; it produces a variety of steroid hormones (**steroido-genesis**). There are three main types:

Androgens

types of male sex hormone. eg, testosterone

Glucocorticoids

hormones that control glucose, protein and lipid metabolism. eg, cortisol

Mineralocorticoids

hormones that regulate fluid and electrolyte balance.

Aldosterone is an example of a mineralocorticoid. It enables the body to retain sodium and excrete potassium. Abnormal aldosterone production results in the disturbances of sodium and potassium levels named in (d), (e) and (f).

Using your Exercise Guide, find the meaning of:

(d) hyper/natr/aemia (Am. hyper/natr/emia)

(e) hypo/kal/aemia (Am. hypo/kal/emia)

(f) natr/i/uresis

The combining form **adrenocortic/o** is used when referring to the adrenal cortex itself. Adrenocorticoid refers to any steroid hormone of the adrenal cortex.

(g) **adrenocortic/o/ trophic** (ACTH produced by the pituitary has this effect)

(h) **adrenocortic/o/ hyper/plasia**

ACTH adrenocorticotropic hormone is secreted by the anterior hypophysis (anterior pituitary gland). It travels in the blood and stimulates the adrenal cortex to produce glucocorticoids, eg, cortisol. ACTH is produced in response to stressful situations.

Three major endocrine disorders caused by abnormal secretion of hormones from the adrenal cortex include:

Cushing syndrome

This is a rare condition that develops when the level of glucocorticoids in the body (eg, cortisol) is too high. This can be caused by exogenous administration of drugs prescribed by a doctor or from an endogenous source within the body. The excess glucocorticoids raise blood pressure, increase sodium retention and bring about hyperglycaemia (Am. hyperglycemia). Other signs and symptoms include obesity, moon face, muscle wastage, acne, hirsutism and psychotic disturbances. When Cushing syndrome is caused by a pituitary adenoma, high levels of ACTH and cortisol can be detected in the blood, and it is called Cushing disease.

Adrenogenital syndrome

This condition is also called *adrenal virilism* and is due to overproduction of male sex hormones (androgens) by the adrenal gland. When present at birth, there is premature sexual development: the female develops an enlarged clitoris and may be confused with a male. The male child may develop pubic hair and an enlarged penis. In both sexes, there is rapid growth, muscularity and advanced bone age.

Adrenal tumours (Am. tumors) or adrenal hyperplasia (increase in number of cells) can cause this condition to develop in adult women. When this occurs, it is characterized by the appearance of secondary male characteristics (virilism). Symptoms include hirsutism (excessive hair growth in the male pattern on the face and body), amenorrhoea (Am. amenorrhea), acne and deepening of the voice.

Addison disease (chronic adrenal cortex insufficiency)

A condition due to the failure of the adrenal cortex to produce sufficient glucocorticoids and mineralocorticoids. The most common cause of this condition is development of antibodies to cells of the adrenal cortex. It results in loss of sodium and water, and a fall in blood pressure. Treatment is essential to avoid an adrenal crisis (Addisonian crisis). When secretion of adrenocorticoids falls significantly, patients will die within 4 to 14 days unless given hormone replacement therapy.

The ovary and testis

The ovary and the testis are endocrine organs as well as reproductive organs. In their endocrine role, they produce sex hormones that function to control the development of the reproductive system and maintain its activity. Note that we have already used the combining forms for the ovary (oophor/o and ovari/o) and testis (orchid/o) in Units 15 and 16.

First, let us examine the endocrine role of the testis. This gland secretes male sex hormones called **androgens** that stimulate the development of the male reproductive tract and secondary sexual characteristics such as beard growth, a deep voice and the male physique. The main androgen produced by the testis is **testosterone**; it is also produced in small quantities by the adrenal cortex of both men and women. In women, excess secretion leads to virilism (masculinization), one obvious effect being the growth of facial hair (hirsutism).

Root

Andr

(*From a Greek word* **aner**, *meaning man/male.*)

Combining form Andr/o

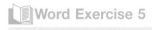 **Word Exercise 5**

Using your Exercise Guide, find the meaning of:

(a) **andr/o**/gyn/ous

(b) **andr/o**/blast/oma

The ovary is also an endocrine gland secreting several types of sex hormone, for example:

Oestrogens (Am. estrogens)

Steroid hormones that regulate the development of the female reproductive tract, menstrual cycle and secondary sexual characteristics, such as the growth of pubic hair and breasts. Compounds that have oestrogen-like actions on the body are described as **oestrogenic** (Am. estrogenic).

Progestogens

Steroid hormones that maintain the receptivity of the uterus to fertilized eggs and stimulate the growth of the uterus during pregnancy.

Medical equipment and clinical procedures

Review the names of medical equipment and clinical procedures mentioned in this unit, and then try Exercise 6. Some imaging techniques used for examining the endocrine system will be studied in Unit 18 as they are similar to those used for other systems.

Word Exercise 6

Match each description in Column C with a term in Column A by placing the appropriate number in Column B.

Column A	Column B	Column C
(a) adrenal function test		1. imaging of the thyroid gland following administration of radioactive iodine
(b) glucose tolerance test		2. a test for hypothyroidism by measuring concentration of iodine in blood
(c) protein-bound iodine test (PBI)		3. a test used to diagnose diabetes mellitus
(d) blood glucose monitor		4. measurement of the 24-h output of adrenocorticoids
(e) thyroid scan		5. a device that measures the amount of sugar in a spot of blood

Other procedures not mentioned in the exercises include:

Computed tomography (CT) Technique of recording a series of X-rays showing structures in multiple cross-sectional views. This can be used to image endocrine glands to assess their size and the extent of tumour infiltration (Am. tumor).

Exophthalmometry The technique of measuring the degree of forward displacement (protrusion) of the eye with an exophthalmometer.

Magnetic resonance imaging The technique of using strong magnetic fields and radio waves to create detailed images in three planes; it is used to image the pituitary gland to locate abnormalities.

Thyroid function test (TFT) This is a blood test used to check the functioning of the thyroid gland and is requested when a patient is suspected of having thyroid disease or conditions linked to it. A TFT could include tests for the presence of TSH (thyroid stimulating hormone), thyroxine (T4) and triiodothyronine (T3).

Ultrasonography This technique of producing an image (sonogram or ultrasound scan) using high-frequency sound waves is used to produce images of the endocrine organs, eg, the thyroid gland can be evaluated and checked for size and abnormalities.

ANATOMY EXERCISE

Now complete the Anatomy Exercise on page 254.

CASE HISTORY 17

The object of this exercise is to understand words associated with a patient's medical history.

To complete the exercise:

• Read through the passage on diabetes mellitus; unfamiliar words are underlined, and you can find their meaning using the Word Help.

• Write the meaning of the medical terms shown in bold print on the lines that follow the Word Help.

Diabetes mellitus

W, a 14-year-old boy on holiday in the locality, was brought into Accident and Emergency by his worried parents. Prior to admission, he had complained of tiredness and <u>insomnia</u>, and his mother had noticed that despite a good appetite he had become thinner. On the morning of admission, he suffered abdominal pain, nausea and vomiting, his breathing had become irregular, and at times, he appeared semiconscious. Further questioning of the parents indicated the patient had recently developed <u>polydipsia</u> and **polyuria**.

On admission, he was conscious and <u>hyperventilating</u>; he was dehydrated, and his breath had the fruity odour of <u>ketones</u>. Blood and urine samples were analyzed and quickly indicated clinically significant levels of **glycosuria, hyperglycaemia** and **ketonaemia**. W's condition was diagnosed as diabetic **ketoacidosis** and emergency treatment was commenced.

Vital signs on admission

Pulse	Oral temp	BP
98 per minute	36.0 °C	110/70
Blood glucose	Urine 3+	Hyperventilating
28 mmol/L	ketones	

He was given an initial intravenous infusion of 6 units of soluble <u>insulin</u>, followed by 6 units hourly. His fluid and <u>electrolyte</u> loss were replaced by an intravenous saline infusion. His blood glucose was monitored hourly and electrolytes two hourly in the initial phase of treatment. When his blood glucose reached its normal value, he was given a saline infusion of 5% dextrose containing 20 mmol/L KCl. The dose of insulin was adjusted according to the hourly blood glucose results.

W's parents were informed their son was suffering from type 1 diabetes mellitus, also known as insulin-dependent diabetes mellitus (IDDM), a <u>chronic</u>, incurable condition brought on by a failure of the **pancreatic** <u>islets</u> to produce insulin.

Once recovered from his acute attack, he was referred to the diabetic <u>clinician</u> for advice on insulin therapy, and his <u>GP</u> was informed. He responded well to advice and now self-administers two daily injections of insulin. His <u>regimen</u> was adjusted to avoid **hypoglycaemia** and give good **glycaemic** (Am. glycemic) control. Both injections consist of a mixture of short- and intermediate-acting insulin, the first before breakfast and the second before his evening meal.

Word Help

clinician an expert on treating and advising patients

chronic lasting/lingering for a long time

electrolyte the ionized salts in the blood (eg, sodium and potassium ions)

GP general practitioner (family doctor)

hyperventilating above normal ventilation rate of the lungs (rapid, deep breathing)

insomnia condition of inability to sleep

insulin a hormone secreted by the pancreas that lowers blood sugar

islets small islands of cells that secrete insulin in the pancreas (islets of Langerhans)

ketones ketone bodies (chemicals formed in diabetes from breakdown of fat)

polydipsia condition of too much/excessive thirst

regimen a regulated scheme (eg, of taking drugs/medication)

Now write the meaning of the following words from the Case History without using your dictionary lists:

(a) polyuria

(b) glycosuria

(c) hyperglycaemia (Am. hyperglycemia)

(d) ketonaemia (Am. ketonemia)

(e) ketoacidosis

(f) pancreatic

(g) hypoglycaemia (Am. hypoglycemia)

(h) glycaemic (Am. glycemic)

(Answers to the Case History exercise are given in the Answers to Word Exercises on page 354.)

Quick Reference

Combining forms relating to the endocrine system:

Aden/o	gland
Adren/o	adrenal gland
Adrenocortic/o	adrenal cortex
Andr/o	male
Cortic/o	cortex
Estr/o (Am.)	estrogen
-globulin	protein
Glyc/o	sugar
Hypophys-	hypophysis / pituitary gland
Insulin/o	insulin/islet of Langerhans
Kal/i	potassium
Ket/o	ketones
Natr/i	sodium
Oestr/o	oestrogen (Am. estr/o)
Oophor/o	ovary

Orchid/o	testis
Ovari/o	ovary
Pancreat/o	pancreas
Parathyroid/o	parathyroid gland
Pituitar-	pituitary
Progest/o	progesterone
Thyr/o	thyroid gland

Abbreviations

Some common abbreviations related to the endocrine system are listed next. Note that some are not standard, and their meaning may vary from one healthcare setting to another. There is a more extensive list for reference on page 369.

ACTH	adrenocorticotropic hormone
FBS	fasting blood sugar
FSH	follicle-stimulating hormone
HGH, hGH	human growth hormone
HRT	hormone replacement therapy
IDDM	insulin-dependent diabetes mellitus
LH	luteinizing hormone
NIDDM	non-insulin-dependent diabetes mellitus
OGTT	oral glucose tolerance test
PRL	prolactin
SIADH	syndrome of inappropriate antidiuretic hormone (secretion)
T_3, T_4	triiodothyronine, tetraiodothyronine (thyroxine)
TSH	thyroid stimulating hormone

Pathology notes

Acromegaly

Hypersecretion of human growth hormone (HGH) after skeletal fusion has occurred in adults results in acromegaly. In this condition, excess HGH causes bones to become abnormally thick and leads to enlargement of the hands, feet, face and jaw.

Acromicria

A condition of smallness of the hands, nose, jaws and feet, probably due to deficiency of human growth hormone from the pituitary gland after puberty.

Chronic thyroiditis (Hashimoto disease)

This is an autoimmune condition in which the body's immune system attacks the thyroid gland; the resulting inflammation leads to an underactive thyroid gland. The condition affects mainly middle-aged women and is the most common form of goitrous hypothyroidism. The cause is unknown, but it tends to run in families, and environmental factors such as overexposure to iodine, ionizing radiation and infection have been implicated as triggers for its development.

Diabetes insipidus

A condition due to undersecretion of antidiuretic hormone (ADH) caused by damage to the pituitary gland or hypothalamus. Lack of ADH results in failure of water reabsorption by the renal tubules of the kidneys, leading to excessive excretion of urine, dehydration, and extreme thirst (polydipsia).

Dwarfism

Hyposecretion of human growth hormone (HGH) during growth years results in stunted body growth known as *pituitary dwarfism.* In this condition the epiphyseal plates of long bones ossify before normal height is reached, and other organs fail to grow to their normal size.

Giantism

Hypersecretion of human growth hormone (HGH) while epiphyseal cartilages of long bones are still growing and before their ossification is complete results in giantism. The bones of the limbs are particularly affected, and individuals may grow to heights of 2.1 to 2.4 m although body proportions remain normal.

Hyperparathyroidism

A condition characterized by excessive secretion of parathyroid hormone (PTH) by the parathyroid glands. Hyperparathyroidism is often caused by the presence of adenoma or by hyperplasia (increase in number of cells) in the parathyroid glands. The action of PTH brings about reabsorption of calcium from bones into the blood. The resulting increase in blood calcium results in *osteitis fibrosa cystica,* a condition characterized by decalcification of bones, bone pain, spontaneous fractures, cyst formation and kidney damage.

Hyperthyroidism (Graves disease)

The term hyperthyroidism refers to any condition that results in an excessive secretion of thyroid hormones. Graves disease (also called exophthalmic goitre or toxic diffuse goitre) accounts for 90% of cases of hyperthyroidism or thyrotoxicosis in which body tissues are exposed to excessive levels of thyroid hormones (T_3 and T_4). The main signs and symptoms are due to an increased basal metabolic rate, and patients may suffer from weight loss, nervousness, increased heart rate and exophthalmos (protruding eyes). In Graves disease, autoantibodies mimic the action of thyroid stimulating hormone (TSH) and stimulate the secretion of high levels of thyroid hormones.

Hypoparathyroidism

A condition characterized by deficient secretion of parathyroid hormone (PTH) by the parathyroid glands. Lack of PTH causes reduced calcium absorption from the small intestine and reduced reabsorption from bones. Abnormally low levels of calcium in the blood result in tetany (strong, painful spasms of muscles), psychiatric disturbances, grand mal epilepsy and paraesthesia (abnormal sensation, Am. paresthesia).

Phaeochromocytoma (Am. pheochromocytoma)

Phaeochromocytoma is a tumour (Am. tumor) that develops in the adrenal medulla; it secretes excessive amounts of adrenaline and noradrenaline into the blood. The symptoms are due to excess of these hormones and include raised BP, excessive metabolic rate, headache and nervousness. The name comes from the fact that the tumour is selectively coloured when stained with chromium salts (phae/o or phe/o meaning dark).

Thyroid tumours (Am. tumors)

Thyroid tumours may be benign or malignant. Adenomas are benign tumours that sometimes secrete sufficient thyroid hormones to cause hyperthyroidism; they have a tendency to become malignant in the elderly.

Malignant cancers (carcinomas) are rare; they vary in their rate of growth and malignancy. Some types grow slowly and can be cured if caught and treated early. Anaplastic thyroid tumours (Am. tumor) are rare but aggressive and metastasize; they have a poor prognosis. A hard, rapidly growing lump in the gland is usually an indication of thyroid cancer.

Benign adenomas are distinguishable from thyroid carcinomas by radionuclide scanning. Adenomas take up large amounts of iodine and form 'hot' nodules. 'Cold' nodules taking up little iodine can be benign or malignant and ultimately need to undergo biopsy.

Associated words

Adenohypophysis the anterior lobe of the pituitary gland
Antithyroid drug a medication that slows down the thyroid gland's ability to produce thyroid hormone
Benign nonmalignant, innocent
Cold nodule a lump in the thyroid gland visible on a scan that does not take up iodine as well as the surrounding thyroid tissue
Cortex the outer layer of an organ or structure
Diffuse widespread, not localized
Feedback a control mechanism that enables the body to maintain homeostasis (constant internal conditions)
Gonadotropin a type of hormone secreted by the anterior pituitary gland that acts on the gonads (reproductive organs), eg, FSH (follicle-stimulating hormone) and LH (luteinizing hormone)
Gynaecomastia condition of female breasts, seen in males (Am. gynecomastia)
Hirsutism condition of having excessive growth of hair, especially in women

Homeostasis the maintenance of a relatively constant internal environment in the tissue fluid around body cells
Hot nodule a lump in the thyroid gland visible on a scan that concentrates iodine more than the normal surrounding thyroid tissue
Hypergonadism condition of increased functional activity of the gonads leading to precocious sexual development
Insulin shock an acute physiological condition resulting from excess insulin in the blood, it leads to low blood sugar, weakness, convulsions, and potential coma
Malignant dangerous, capable of spreading
Medulla the innermost part of an organ
Metabolism the biochemical processes occurring within the cells of an organism
Neoplasm a new growth of cells, a tumour (Am. tumor)
Neurohypophysis the posterior lobe of the pituitary gland
Nodule a lump or growth of cells within the thyroid gland
Multinodular goitre (Am. goiter) an enlargement of the thyroid containing many lumps (nodules)
Steroid a type of hormone related to cholesterol; steroids include the sex hormones and adrenocortical hormones
Tetany increased excitability of nerves and muscles due to low levels of calcium, eg, in hypoparathyroidism
Thyroid scan an image obtained of the thyroid gland after oral administration of radioiodine
Thyroid storm a life-threatening condition that develops in cases of untreated thyrotoxicosis
Torpor a sluggish condition in which response to stimuli is slow or absent
Vasopressin an antidiuretic hormone used to treat diabetes insipidus
Virilism masculine traits exhibited by a female owing to production of excessive amounts of androgenic hormones from the adrenal cortex or an ovarian tumour (Am. tumor)

NOW TRY THE WORD CHECK

WORD CHECK

This self-check exercise lists all the word components used in this unit. First, write down the meaning of as many word components as you can. Then, check your answers using the Exercise Guide and Quick Reference box or the Glossary of Word Components (pp. 383–410).

Prefixes

acro-	
hyper-	
hypo-	
para-	
poly-	

Combining forms of word roots

acid/o	
aden/o	
adren/o	
andr/o	
blast/o	
chondr/o	
cortic/o	
dips/o	
estr/o (Am.)	
-globulin	
gloss/o	
-gyne	
insulin/o	
kal/i	
ket/o/n	
natr/i	
oestr/o (Am. estr/o)	
pancreat/o	
-physis	
pituitar-	
progest/o	
thyr/o	

Suffixes

-aemia (Am. -emia)	
-al	
-ectomy	
-emia (Am.)	
-genesis	
-genic	
-ia	
-ic	
-ism	
-itis	

-megaly	
-micria	
-oid	
-oma	
-osis	
-plasia	
-ptosis	
-tomy	
-toxic	
-trophic	
-tropic	
-uresis	
-uria	

NOW TRY THE SELF-ASSESSMENT

SELF-ASSESSMENT

Test 17A

Next are some combining forms that refer to the anatomy of the endocrine system. Indicate which part of the system they refer to by putting a number from the diagram (Fig. 102) next to each word.

(a) adren/o

(b) parathyroid/o

(c) andr/o

(d) thyroid/o

(e) pancreat/o

(f) ovari/o

(g) pituitar-

(h) adrenocortic/o

Score

8

Test 17B

Prefixes, suffixes and combining forms of word roots

Match each meaning in Column C with a word component in Column A by inserting the appropriate number in Column B.

Column A	Column B	Column C
(a) acro-		1. germ cell
(b) aden/o		2. small
(c) andr/o		3. pancreas
(d) blast/o		4. progesterone
(e) -globin		5. a growth
(f) glyc/o		6. condition of growth (increase of cells)
(g) hyper-		7. oestrogen (Am. estrogen)
(h) hypo-		8. sugar
(i) insulin/o		9. hypophysis
(j) micr/o		10. below/below normal
(k) oestr/o (Am. estr/o)		11. gland
(l) pancreat/o		12. thyroid
(m) para-		13. pertaining to affinity for / acting on
(n) -physis		14. pertaining to nourishment
(o) -plasia		15. insulin/islets of Langerhans
(p) pituitar-		16. extremity/point
(q) progest/o		17. beside/near
(r) thyr/o		18. above / above normal
(s) -trophic		19. protein
(t) -tropic		20. man/male

Score

20

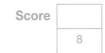

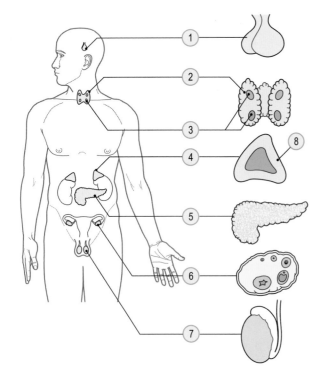

Figure 102   The endocrine system.

Test 17C

Write the meaning of:

(a) thyroparathyroid-
    ectomy

(b) pituicyte

(c) adrenomegaly

(d) glycotropic

(e) hyperketonaemia
    (Am. hyperk-
    etonemia)

Score

5

Test 17D

Build words that mean:

(a) process of producing too
    much insulin

(b) condition of too little
    sodium in the blood

(c) pertaining to nourishing
    the thyroid gland (use
    thyr/o)

(d) pertaining to acting on /
    stimulating the adrenal
    gland

(e) process of producing too
    little parathyroid hormone

Score

5

Check answers to Self-Assessment Tests on page 365.

UNIT 18
RADIOLOGY

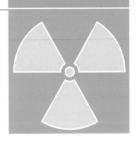

OBJECTIVES

Once you have completed Unit 18, you should be able to do the following:

- understand the meaning of medical words relating to radiology

- build medical words relating to radiology

- understand common medical abbreviations relating to radiology

EXERCISE GUIDE

Use this list of word components and their meanings to complete the word exercises in this unit.

Prefixes

ultra-	beyond

Roots / Combining forms

angi/o	vessel
cardi/o	heart
encephal/o	brain
esophag/o (Am.)	esophagus/gullet
oesophag/o	oesophagus/gullet (Am. esophag/o)

Suffixes

-er	one who
-genic	pertaining to formation / originating in
-gram	X-ray picture/tracing/recording
-graph	usually an instrument that records / an X-ray picture
-graphy	technique of recording/making an X-ray
-ical	pertaining to or referring to
-ist	specialist
-logist	specialist who studies
-logy	study of
-scope	an instrument used to view/examine
-scopy	technique of viewing/examining
-therapy	treatment

Radiology

Radiology (now known as clinical radiology) is the study of the diagnosis of disease by the use of radiant energy (radiation). In the past, this meant the use of X-rays to make an image of the internal components of the body. Today, besides X-rays, other forms of radiation are used, and a radiographer may specialize in diagnostic radiology or therapeutic radiology. Diagnostic radiography employs a range of imaging techniques including digital radiography, fluoroscopy, computed tomography, ultrasonography, magnetic resonance imaging and nuclear medicine. Therapeutic radiographers are qualified to plan and deliver radiotherapy to treat tumours (Am. tumor) using a wide range of technical equipment.

Diagnostic radiography

Before completing the first exercise, review the terms below:

> **-gram**
>
> a recording/picture/tracing/X-ray.
>
> **-graph**
>
> usually refers to an instrument that records by making a picture or tracing, but it is also used here to mean a recording or X-ray picture.
>
> **-graphy**
>
> a technique of making a recording, such as a picture, X-ray, tracing or writing.

Use the Exercise Guide at the beginning of this unit to complete Word Exercises 1 to 10, unless you are asked to work without it.

▌Root

Radi

(*From a Latin word* **radius***, meaning a ray. Here radi/o means X-rays, the invisible rays produced by an X-ray machine. This combining form is also used to mean radiation/radioactivity.*)

Combining form   Radi/o

📖 Word Exercise 1

Using your Exercise Guide, find the meaning of:

(a) **radi/o**/log/ist

(b) **radi/o**/graph
    (refers to an image)

(c) **radi/o**/graphy

(d) **radi/o**/graph/er

(e) **radi/o**/therapy

> **Note.** X-rays are electromagnetic waves of high energy and very short wavelength emitted by electrons outside the nucleus of an atom. X-rays **are** able to pass through many solid materials opaque to light.

X-rays and contrast media

Some radiographic procedures require the use of a contrast medium or agent to improve the quality of the image. Contrast agents are required because there is little difference in the density of the soft parts of the body, and X-rays pass through them without producing a distinct image of individual organs. The contrast medium is administered to the patient, filling a cavity such as the stomach. The X-ray is taken and the outline of the cavity recorded on the radiograph.

An example of a contrast medium is barium sulphate, a radiopaque substance that absorbs X-rays. It shows up on X-ray film as a white area that has not allowed X-rays to pass. This property of barium sulphate makes it particularly useful for outlining the digestive tract where it is administered as:

> **A barium 'meal' (or swallow)**
>
> To outline the upper parts of the digestive system the barium is given as a drink.
>
> **A barium enema**
>
> To outline the lower parts of the digestive system. In this procedure, barium is injected via the anus into the rectum and colon. Sometimes air is also administered with the barium to increase contrast; this is known as a **double contrast radiograph**.

Iodine is another contrast agent that can be added to make various fluids radiopaque. It is often the contrast agent used in angiocardiography, arteriography and venography.

▌Root

Roentgen

(*From the name of Wilhelm C.* **Röntgen***, a German physicist (1845–1923) who discovered X-rays. Here roentgen/o means X-rays/Röntgen rays.*)

Combining form   Roentgen/o

📖 Word Exercise 2

Without using your Exercise Guide, write the meaning of:

(a) **roentgen/o**/graphy

(b) **roentgen/o**/logist
    (synonymous with radiologist)

Using your Exercise Guide, find the meaning of:

(c) **roentgen/o**/gram
(synonymous with
radiograph and rönt-
genogram, radiograph
is in common use)

Fluoroscopy

The movement of internal parts of the body can be observed using a technique known as fluoroscopy. In this procedure, X-rays are directed through the body onto a phosphor screen (a fluorescent screen, ie, one from which light flows). As the X-rays strike the screen, the phosphor emits light, producing an image that is viewed as it is generated. Fluoroscopy is useful for observing movement of organs such as the oesophagus (Am. esophagus), stomach and heart; it is also used to guide instruments and implants into the body at surgery. Modern fluoroscopes couple the phosphor screen to an image intensifier and video camera allowing the images to be recorded and displayed on a computer screen.

Root

Fluor

(*From a Latin word* **fluere***, meaning to flow. Here the fluor/o mean something that is luminous, ie, emitting light or fluorescent*)

Combining form Fluor/o

Word Exercise 3

Using your Exercise Guide, find the meaning of -scope and -ical; then build a word that means:

(a) instrument used for
the direct X-ray exami-
nation of the body by
fluoroscopy

(b) pertaining to fluoroscopy

Without using your Exercise Guide, build a word that means:

(c) technique of recording
a radiographic image
produced by fluoros-
copy

Root

Cine

(*From a Greek word* **kinein***, meaning movement. Here the combining form cine/o means movement or motion. Cinemat/o means a motion picture on film, video or other recording device.*)

Combining forms Cine/o, cinemat/o

Word Exercise 4

Without using your Exercise Guide, write the meaning of:

(a) **cine**/radi/o/graphy

(b) **cine**/radi/o/graph
(refers to an image)

Using your Exercise Guide, find the meaning of:

(c) **cine**[2]/angi/o[3]/cardi/
o[4]/graphy[1]

(d) **cine**/oesophag/o/
gram (Am. **cine**/
esophag/o/gram)

Root

Tom

(*From a Greek word* **tomos***, meaning a slice or section.*)

Combining form Tom/o

Word Exercise 5

Without using your Exercise Guide, write the meaning of:

(a) **tom/o**/gram

(b) **tom/o**/graphy

Computed tomography

A **tomograph** is an instrument that uses X-rays to obtain images of sections through the body. It uses a thin beam of X-rays that rotates around the patient. X-ray photons emitted from the patient are detected and converted into an image by a computer. The images produced by this device show more detail than a simple X-ray. See Figure 103.

The procedure of producing an image in this way is known as computed tomography (a CT scan) or less commonly as computerized axial tomography (a CAT scan). The CT scanner is able to produce multiple cross-sectional images that can detect disease within bone and internal organs. With the use of contrast media, blood vessels and soft tissues can also be outlined. New high-speed CT scanners produce multiple images of tomographic slices through the body that can be used to build high-resolution three-dimensional images of internal organs. These multidetector CT scanners (MDCT) can image the beating heart and detect plaques in the walls of coronary arteries and other blood vessels; the availability of these images is changing the way vascular and cardiac problems are diagnosed.

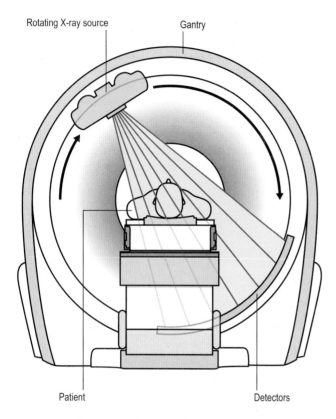

Figure 103   Computed tomography.

Nuclear medicine

This branch of medicine uses **radioisotopes** (also called **radio-nuclides**) to diagnose and treat disease. In some texts, it is called nuclear radiology. Terms used for diagnostic radiology include nuclear imaging and radionuclide imaging.

Radioisotopes are elements that exhibit the property of spontaneous decay, emitting radiation in the process. The radiation is in the form of high-speed particles and energy-containing rays. Elements that emit alpha, beta or gamma radiation are used as diagnostic labels to trace the route and uptake of chemicals administered into the body. The radioisotope behaves like a transmitter, passing radiation from inside to the outside of the body. Ideally, radioisotopes should give off gamma radiation as alpha and beta particles can damage cells. Many different diagnostic techniques have been devised that use radioisotopes; one procedure is described next.

First, the specific isotope or tracer is given to the patient. Once in the body, it continues to emit radiation and is absorbed or excluded from the tissues and organs under investigation. Next a gamma camera is passed over the surface of the body to detect gamma rays emitted by the isotope; this is also known as a **radioisotope scan**. Finally, an image is constructed showing the distribution of radioactivity within the tissues and organs. **Radioisotope scans** are used to image the heart, liver, biliary tract, bones, thyroid and kidney.

Here are some examples of the use of specific radioisotopes:

^{99M}Tc (technetium)

^{99M}Tc is administered to the patient in trace quantities. It is excluded from normal brain tissue but accumulates in some brain tumours (Am. tumors). A tumour can be detected by locating the gamma rays emitted from it.

^{123}I (Iodine)

^{123}I is rapidly taken up by the thyroid gland. A radioisotope scan of the gland will outline the now radioactive gland, and information from this will aid the diagnosis of various thyroid disorders, eg, thyrotoxicosis.

^{57}Co (cobalt)

^{57}Co is used to trace the uptake of vitamin B_{12} by the body, and from this a diagnosis of megaloblastic anaemia can be made.

Radioactive iodine uptake test (RAIU) and thyroid scan
RAIU is one of two types of test used to diagnose thyroid disease; the other is the thyroid scan (see Unit17, page 256). They are usually carried out at the same time. The RAIU test measures the rate at which the thyroid gland absorbs radioactive iodine in a given time; whereas the thyroid scan produces an image of the distribution of radioactive iodine in the thyroid gland.

In the RAIU test a small dose of Iodine-123 or Iodine-131 is administered to the patient in liquid or capsule form. The radioactive iodine is taken up by the thyroid gland and emits gamma radiation. This is measured using a gamma probe placed over the gland at specific time intervals, eg, after 4, 6 or 24 h. The probe measures how much iodine the thyroid has absorbed at the time of the scan. Hypothyroid patients usually take up too little iodine and hyperthyroid patients too much.

Scintigraphy

Scintigraphy is the technique of producing a radioisotope scan. A radioisotope with an affinity for a particular organ or tissue is injected into the body, and the distribution of the radioactivity is followed using an instrument called a **scintillation counter** (**scintiscanner**). This device contains a **scintillator**, a substance that emits light when in contact with ionizing radiation. There is a flash of light for each ionizing event, and the number of flashes (or counts) is related to the radioactivity present in the area being scanned. Scintillation counters can be moved over the outer surface of the body to locate radioisotopes within particular organs and build an image (scintigram/scintiscan) of their distribution. The **gamma camera** mentioned earlier is a scintillation counter.

Root

Scint

(*From a Latin word* **scintillatio**, *meaning spark/emitting sparks/light.*)

Combining forms   Scint/i, scintill/a

Word Exercise 6

Without using your Exercise Guide, write the meaning of:

(a) **scinti**/gram

(b) **scinti**/graphy

Positron emission tomography (PET)

This is another imaging technique that traces the distribution of radioisotopes within the body. **Positron emission tomography** (PET scanning) uses radioisotopes (radionuclides) that emit short-lived particles called positrons (β^+ radiation). Particular tissues take up the isotopes, which are injected intravenously. For example, fluorodeoxyglucose (also called FDG, ^{18}F-FDG or fludeoxyglucose) penetrates the blood–brain barrier and is used by brain cells as a source of energy. Once inside a brain cell the isotope decays, emitting positrons; the more active the cell, the more labelled glucose is taken up, and the more positrons are emitted.

The positrons immediately collide with electrons, yielding gamma ray photons that have sufficient energy to leave the body. These photons are detected by a large array of scintillation detectors that surround the patient. The position of the emerging photons is determined and used to construct a cross-sectional computerized image that shows the distribution of the radioisotopes in the tissues.

PET is used to investigate physiological processes such as the blood perfusion of organs and metabolism. Its medical applications include the study of the brain in patients with neurological deficits caused by strokes and epilepsy, and the detection and staging of cancer.

The half-life of radionuclides used in PET is short-lived, so they cannot be stored and used when required. The technique is dependent on the immediate production of radionuclides in a complex and expensive device called a **cyclotron** and the services of **radiochemical** and **radiopharmaceutical** laboratories. These restrictions have limited the use of PET to special centres with appropriate facilities. Recently, mini-cyclotrons have been designed for on-site production of radionuclides and these are leading to increased use of this imaging technique.

> **Note.** The following two diagnostic techniques do not use X-rays or radiopharmaceuticals.

Ultrasonography

This procedure is also called ultrasonic scanning or ultrasound imaging; it uses high-frequency, inaudible sound waves to produce an image. The waves are transmitted via a transducer or probe placed on or near a surface of the body. The internal organs and masses reflect the sound to different extents and are said to have different echo textures. The echoes bounce back to the transducer and are recorded as a sonogram; this is a composite image of the area being investigated. Ultrasound imaging is used to diagnose a wide variety of conditions that affect the organs and soft tissues of the body, eg, the heart (see Fig. 104), blood vessels, liver, gallbladder, kidneys, prostate, uterus and eyes. Ultrasound imaging of an embryo or fetus in the uterus has become a standard part of antenatal care, enabling early detection of potential problems.

Root

Son

(*From a Latin word* **sonus**, *meaning sound.*)

Combining form   Son/o

Note the next exercise refers to techniques using **ultrasound**, high-frequency sounds beyond human hearing.

Word Exercise 7

Using your Exercise Guide, find the meaning of:

(a) ultra/**son**/o/gram

Without using your Exercise Guide, write the meaning of:

(b) ultra/**son**/o/graphy

(c) ultra/**son**/o/graph

Root

Echo

(*A Greek word meaning sound. Here echo- means an ultrasound echo generated by the reflection of sound waves off an obstacle.*)

Combining form   Echo-

Word Exercise 8

Using your Exercise Guide, find the meaning of:

(a) **echo**/encephalo/gram

Using your Exercise Guide, find the meaning of -genic, and then build a word that means:

(b) pertaining to forming/ generating an echo

Without using your Exercise Guide, build words that mean:

(c) a recording/picture of echoes (synonymous with ultrasonogram)

(d) an instrument that records echoes from the brain

(e) a recording/picture of echoes from the heart

(f) technique of making a picture/tracing/recording using echoes

Magnetic resonance imaging

This diagnostic procedure used in radiology was formerly known as nuclear magnetic resonance imaging (NMRI); it uses magnetic fields and radio waves to form images of the internal structure of the body. The patient is positioned within the MRI scanner that forms a strong magnetic field around the area to be imaged. Each hydrogen atom found in the water molecules of soft tissues contains a proton, a spinning positive charge that acts like a bar magnet. The protons become aligned to the strong magnetic field of the scanner. Radio waves from the scanner then cause the protons to move out of alignment, and when the transmission stops, the protons realign. As the protons realign, they emit radio wave signals which are detected by receivers providing information about the location of protons within the body. Protons in different types of tissue realign at different speeds and produce distinct signals, enabling the construction of a two- or three-dimensional image of the inside of a human body.

MRI imaging demonstrates superior soft tissue contrast compared to CT scans and plain films, making it ideal for examination of the brain, spine, joints and other soft tissue body parts. MRI scans are harmless as the patient is not exposed to ionizing radiation.

Radiotherapy (Radiation therapy)

Radiotherapy is the treatment of disease by X-rays and other forms of radiation. In particular, the radiation is used to destroy malignant cancer cells by exposing them to a lethal dose of radiation.

This branch of medicine is now referred to as clinical oncology (onc/o meaning tumour, Am. tumor).

Teletherapy (external beam radiotherapy)

This is the administration of radiation from an external source at a distance from the body (tele- meaning far away/operating at a distance). Radiotherapy machines generate the radiation used in this form of treatment, and there has been a move towards ever more powerful devices. To maximize the therapeutic advantages of radiotherapy, it is necessary to give a tumouricidal (Am. tumoricidal) dose of radiation to a planned target volume and minimize the dose to surrounding tissue. (Here tumour- means a mass of cancer cells, and -cidal pertains to killing.)

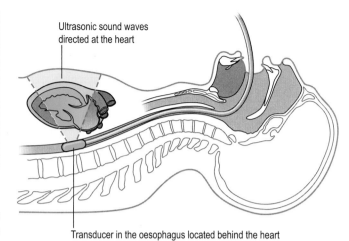

Ultrasonic sound waves directed at the heart

Transducer in the oesophagus located behind the heart

Figure 104 Transoesophageal echocardiography (Am. transesophageal) being used to make images of the heart. (Adapted from Chabner D-E, The Language of Medicine, 10th Edition, 2013, Saunders.)

The first high-energy beams were produced by the decay of radioactive sources. The cobalt 60 (^{60}Co) radiotherapy machine still in use produces radiation at energies of between 1 and 4 MeV (mega-electronvolts, 1 MeV = 1 million electronvolts). At its centre is a cobalt 60 high-energy radiation source that emits gamma (g)-ray photons that are directed at the patient through an opening called a collimator. This machine has been particularly useful for treating tumours of the head, neck and metastases in lymph nodes.

Cobalt 60 machines have been largely superseded by linear accelerators that generate X-ray photons or electron beams at very high energy levels (3 to 35 MeV) and contain no radioactive sources. In electron mode, these complex machines accelerate a beam of electrons to near the speed of light and direct them on to superficial lesions near the surface of the body. In photon mode the beam of electrons is made to collide with a metal target, generating high-energy X-ray photons that can be used to destroy tumours deep within the body (see Fig. 105).

Brachytherapy

The term **brachytherapy** (brachy- meaning short) means the administration of radiation in close proximity to a tumour. It is accomplished by the implantation of radioactive sources into the body. The sealed source has been used to deliver radiation in three main ways: into the surface of the skin, into a cavity (intracavity) and directly into a tissue or tumour (interstitial).

The first sources to be used were needles containing radium (^{226}Ra) and emitting gamma ray photons at 0.2 to 2.4 MeV. A needle consists of a platinum or alloy tube with a sharp (trocar) point at one end and an eyelet for a thread at the other. The radioactive material is loaded into the tube and sealed with gold solder. The needle is then inserted directly into a tumour and left for a fixed time before being withdrawn. Caesium (^{137}Cs)

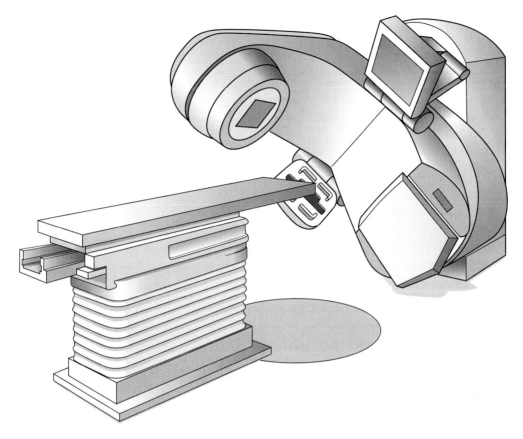

Figure 105   A linear accelerator.

(Am. cesium) has been used as a radium substitute for intracavity and interstitial brachytherapy.

Tubes and seeds are similar to needles, but they have no sharp points; instead, they fit into an applicator for insertion into a body cavity. Radon gas seeds (^{222}Rn) were used as a substitute for radium, and gold (^{198}Au) seeds for interstitial implants have superseded these. Typically, they have a length of 5 mm and a diameter of 1.35 mm, small enough to be inserted into a tumour and left, forming harmless foreign bodies once their radioactivity has decayed to a negligible value (half-life is 3.8 days).

Other sources include palladium(^{103}Pd) seeds and iridium (^{192}Ir) wires, hairpins, seeds and ribbons.

In the 1930s, brachytherapy needles were inserted into the patient manually; this exposed medical and nursing staff to high doses of radiation. The afterloading technique has been developed to reduce the handling times of radioactive sources. In this procedure, nonradioactive needles, tubing and applicators are precisely positioned in the patient before the introduction of the radioactive sources. The sources are only introduced when they can be quickly loaded into the appropriate points in the patient, thereby reducing exposure to medical staff. Improved afterloading machines are now available that further reduce unwanted exposure. This, with the development of new radionuclides, has made brachytherapy a much safer form of treatment.

Radionuclides are also administered to patients in unsealed forms. For example, iodine (^{131}I) emits beta radiation and is used as a treatment for thyrotoxicosis. The iodine is available as an injection, drink or capsule, the latter being safer as it reduces the risk of spillage.

Radioactive iodine therapy (RAI)

This is a form of internal radiotherapy used for the treatment of hyperthyroidism and some thyroid cancers. A high dose of Iodine-131 (^{131}I) is administered to the patient; it travels in the bloodstream and is actively absorbed by the thyroid gland. Radiation in the form of beta particles emitted from the iodine destroys both cancerous and normal thyroid cells with minimal effect on the rest of the body.

The most common use of RAI in cancer treatment is to destroy (ablate) the small amount of normal thyroid that remains after thyroidectomy. Ablation also aims to eliminate any thyroid cancer cells that have spread to other parts of the body.

The role of RAI in the treatment of hyperthyroidism is to destroy sufficient thyroid tissue to render the patient either euthyroid (having normal thyroid function) or hypothyroid. The hypothyroid patient is then given thyroid replacement therapy.

Medical equipment and clinical procedures

Review the names of all instruments and clinical procedures mentioned in this unit before trying Exercise 9.

📖 Word Exercise 9

Match each description in Column C with a term in Column A by placing the appropriate number in Column B.

Column A	Column B	Column C
(a) radiography		1. an instrument that detects gamma rays from radioisotopes
(b) fluoroscopy		2. technique of using ultrasound echoes to image the heart
(c) radionuclide		3. a chemical used to improve the detail of an X-ray
(d) ultrasonograph		4. technique of making an X-ray
(e) computerized tomograph		5. an instrument that makes a tracing/picture using reflected sound
(f) radiotherapy		6. an instrument that uses X-rays to image a slice through the body
(g) cineradiography		7. direct observation of an X-ray picture using a fluorescent screen
(h) gamma camera		8. an element that spontaneously decays and emits radiation
(i) echocardiography		9. the treatment of disorders using radiation
(j) contrast medium		10. technique of using X-rays to make a moving picture

👥 CASE HISTORY 18

The object of this exercise is to understand words associated with a patient's medical history.

To complete the exercise:

- Read through the passage on cancer of the larynx; unfamiliar words are underlined, and you can find their meaning using the Word Help.

- Write the meaning of the medical terms shown in bold print on the lines that follow the Word Help.

Cancer of the larynx

Mr R, age 42, was referred to the ENT clinic with suspected cancer of the larynx. He had been a 15-per-day cigarette smoker for 22 years. His main symptom was hoarseness (dysphonia) that had been present for about 2 months; otherwise, he seemed to be in good health. He was admitted to have his larynx formally assessed.

Direct laryngoscopy under anaesthesia confirmed the presence of a glottic tumour (Am. tumor) affecting both vocal cords. Following biopsy, histological analysis classified the tumour as a squamous cell carcinoma.

A chest **radiograph** excluded the presence of metastatic deposits and bronchial carcinoma. Computed **tomography** excluded lymph node and cartilage involvement with no spread into the hypopharynx.

Following discussion at a joint clinic, the ENT surgeon and clinical oncologist staged Mr R's tumour at $T_2 N_0 M_0$. He was prescribed a course of radical **radiotherapy** to try to conserve his larynx.

Immobilization of Mr R's neck was achieved by a well-fitting Perspex shell reaching from the angle of the jaw down to just below the clavicle. The therapeutic radiographer placed him in the supine position (without a mouth bite) with his neck straight to prevent the spinal cord curving anteriorly. The tumour was localized using CT scanning and the dose distribution outlined on the **tomogram** centring on the proposed target volume.

Mr R was placed in the same Perspex shell and position for radiotherapy. The aim of his treatment was to administer a **tumouricidal** (Am. **tumoricidal**) dose of **radiation** centred on his vocal cords. As he had a short neck, two anterior, oblique beams were used to irradiate the whole larynx. The wedged beams were angled at 90° to give a homogeneous dose to the target volume and to reduce the dose to the skin and spinal cord. He was administered 60 Gy in 25 fractions in 5 weeks (4 to 6 MeV) from a **linear accelerator**.

Mr R was advised of the possibility of side-effects such as difficulty in swallowing, exacerbated hoarseness, <u>desquamation</u> and, rarely, <u>oedema</u> (Am. edema) leading to obstruction. These often peak around the 12th treatment with <u>resolution</u> of the tumour in approximately 2 months.

Mr R made an uneventful recovery, his only complaints being difficulty in swallowing and a sore throat. Recent follow-up examinations by the ENT surgeon and diagnostic **ultrasonography** showed no evidence of tumour recurrence. He appears well, and his voice is showing signs of recovery.

Word Help

anterior front/from the front of the body

biopsy removal and examination of living tissue

carcinoma a malignant growth from epidermal cells

clavicle the collar bone

desquamation the shedding of cells from the epidermis

dysphonia condition of difficulty/pain on speaking

ENT ear, nose and throat

glottic pertaining to the glottis (vocal apparatus of the larynx)

Gy gray (SI unit of absorbed radiation dose)

histological pertaining to histology (here histological analysis for classification and signs of malignancy in the biopsied tissue)

hoarseness rough, grating, discordant voice making speech difficult

homogeneous uniform quality in all parts

hypopharynx the laryngeal part of the pharynx

laryngoscopy technique of viewing the larynx

localized here refers to determination of the position of the target volume in relation to the patient's anatomy and skin reference points

metastatic pertaining to metastases (parts of a tumour that have spread from one site to another)

MeV mega-electronvolt

oblique slanting

oedema (Am. edema) accumulation of fluid in a tissue

oncologist a doctor who has specialized in the study and treatment of tumours, most clinical oncologists were formerly known as radiotherapists

squamous pertaining to scale-like/from squamous epithelium

supine lying on the back so the face is upward

target volume volume of the tumour (Am. tumor)

radical direct to the root or cause (treatment to eliminate disease) extensive

resolution abatement of a pathological process and the return of affected tissues to normal

$T_2 N_0 M_0$ staging symbols: T = tumour, N = node, M = metastasis; T_2 = tumour at stage 2 (the tumour invades the vocal cords without fixation of the larynx), N_0 = no node involvement and M_0 = no metastases

wedge wedge-shaped devices that act as filters to absorb radiation. They are used to adjust the dose received on either side of the body

Now write the meaning of the following words from the Case History without using your dictionary lists:

(a) radiograph

(b) tomography

(c) radiotherapy

(d) tomogram

(e) tumouricidal (Am. tumoricidal)

(f) radiation

(g) linear accelerator

(h) ultrasonography

(Answers to the Case History exercise are given in the Answers to Word Exercises on page 355.)

Quick Reference

Combining forms relating to radiology:

Cine/o	movement/motion (picture)
Ech/o	reflected sound
Fluor/o	fluorescence / fluoroscopy
Radi/o	radiation / X-ray
Roentgen/o	X-ray
Scint/i	spark/flash of light
Son/o	sound
Therm/o	heat
Tom/o	slice/section
Ultrason/o	ultrasound

Abbreviations

Some common abbreviations related to radiology are listed next. Note that some are not standard, and their meaning may vary from one healthcare setting to another. There is a more extensive list for reference on page 369.

AXR	abdominal X-ray
Ba	barium
BE	barium enema
CT	computerized tomography, computed tomography
CXR	chest X-ray
DEXA	dual-energy X-ray absorptiometry
DSA	digital subtraction angiography
DXT	deep X-ray therapy
EUA	examination under anaesthesia (Am. anesthesia)
EUS	endoscopic ultrasound
FMRI	functional magnetic resonance imaging
IMRT	intensity-modulated radiotherapy
MRI	magnetic resonance imaging
NMRI	nuclear magnetic resonance imaging
PET	positron emission tomography
RT	radiation therapy, radiotherapy
US	ultrasound/ultrasonography
XR	X-ray
XRT	X-ray therapy/radiation therapy/radiotherapy

Associated words

Ablation destruction by surgical or radiological means

Electron beam form of low-energy radiation for treatment of skin or surface tumours (Am. tumors)

Field the dimensions of the area that is to be irradiated by a radiotherapy machine

Fractionation the division of the total dose of radiation into small doses administered at intervals

Gamma rays highly energetic, penetrating photons emitted from the nuclei of some radioactive atoms; they are used in tracer studies, diagnostic nuclear medicine and radiotherapy

Gray (Gy) a unit of absorbed radiation dose

Half-life the time required for a radioactive substance to lose half of its radioactivity as it disintegrates; eg, the half-life of ^{123}I used in thyroid investigations is 13 hours

Ionization the process of transforming electrically neutral substances into electrically charged particles, X-rays cause ionization of particles within tissues

Palliative a treatment that relieves symptoms but does not cure

Photon a quantum of electromagnetic radiation

Photon therapy a type of radiotherapy that uses X-rays or gamma rays

Proton therapy a type of radiotherapy that uses a beam of positively charged subatomic particles called protons that can be precisely focused onto a target

Radiodermatitis inflammation of the skin due to radiotherapy

Radioimmunoassay a test that combines antibodies and radioactive substances to detect traces of substances in a patient's blood

Radiolabeling the incorporation of a radioactive element into a compound to investigate its metabolism, fate and utilization; the production of a radiopharmaceutical used in nuclear medicine

Radiolucent allowing the passage of X-rays or other forms of radiation

Radiomimetic pertaining to producing effects similar to those of ionizing radiation

Radionecrosis condition of death of tissue due to exposure to radiant energy

Radiopaque obstructing the passage of X-rays or other forms of radiation

Radiopharmaceutical a radioactive substance made up of a radionuclide and another chemical administered to the body for a diagnostic or therapeutic purpose

Radioresistant refers to tumours (Am. tumors) that require a large doses of radiation to bring about their death

Radiosensitive pertaining to structures that respond to readily to radiation

Radiosensitizer a drug that makes tumour cells more sensitive to radiation (Am. tumor) than normal tissues

Simulation the process of planning radiotherapy by putting the patient into the correct position and making the target area of the body before treatment begins; it sometimes involves use of CT or MRI scanning

Skiagram a picture made of shadows and outlines; a radiograph

Tagging attaching a radionuclide to a chemical and following its path in the body

Transducer a handheld device that sends and receives ultrasound signals

Uptake the rate or act of absorbing and incorporating a radionuclide into an organ or tissue

NOW TRY THE WORD CHECK

WORD CHECK

This self-check exercise lists all the word components used in this unit. First, write down the meaning of as many word components as you can. Then, check your answers using the Exercise Guide and Quick Reference box or the Glossary of Word Components (pp. 383–410).

Prefixes

ultra-

Combining forms of word roots

angi/o

cardi/o

cine/o

ech/o

encephal/o

esophag/o (Am.)

fluor/o

oesophag/o (Am. esophag/o)

radi/o

roentgen/o

scint/i

son/o

tom/o

Suffixes

-cidal

-er

-genic

-gram

-graph

-graphy

-ist

-logy

-scope

-scopy

-therapy

NOW TRY THE SELF-ASSESSMENT

SELF-ASSESSMENT

Test 18A

Prefixes, suffixes and combining forms of word roots

Match each meaning in Column C with a word component in Column A by inserting the appropriate number in Column B.

Column A	Column B	Column C
(a) angi/o		1. radiation
(b) brachy-		2. X-rays
(c) cine/o		3. specialist
(d) ech/o		4. treatment
(e) -er		5. beyond/excess
(f) -fluor/o		6. slice/section/cut
(g) genic		7. sound
(h) -gram		8. short
(i) -graph		9. technique of recording/making a picture X-ray
(j) -graphy		10. technique of visual examination
(k) -ist		11. vessel
(l) radi/o		12. picture / tracing / X-ray picture
(m) roentgen/o		13. movement / motion picture
(n) scint/i		14. pertaining to formation / originating in
(o) -scope		15. reflected sound
(p) -scopy		16. instrument to view
(q) son/o		17. fluoroscope / fluoroscopy
(r) -therapy		18. spark (flash or light)
(s) tom/o		19. instrument that records
(t) ultra-		20. one who

Score ___ 20

Test 18B

Write the meaning of:

(a) tomograph _____

(b) sonographer _____

(c) teletherapy _____

(d) radioisotope _____

(e) ultrasonotomography _____

Score ___ 5

Test 18C

Build words that mean:

(a) the treatment of a tumour by delivery of radiation at a short distance (Am. tumor) _____

(b) will not allow the passage of X-rays/ radiation _____

(c) technique of making a picture of blood vessels using a scintillation counter (use scinti-) _____

(d) technique of using ultrasound echoes to make an image of the heart (use ech/o) _____

(e) technique of using ultrasound echoes to make an image of the brain (use ech/o) _____

Score ___ 5

Check answers to Self-Assessment Tests on page 365.

UNIT 19
ONCOLOGY

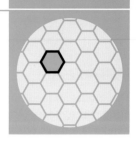

OBJECTIVES

Once you have completed Unit 19, you should be able to do the following:

* understand the meaning of medical words relating to oncology

* build medical words relating to oncology

* understand common medical abbreviations relating to oncology

EXERCISE GUIDE

Use this list of word components and their meanings to complete the word exercises in this unit.

Roots / Combining forms

angi/o	blood vessel
chondr/o	cartilage
bronch/o	bronchus
fibr/o	fibre/fibrous tissue (Am. fiber)
gastr/o	stomach
hepat/o	liver
leiomy/o	smooth muscle
mening/i	meninges (membranes of CNS)
rhabdomy/o	striated muscle

Suffixes

-eal	pertaining to
-genesis	formation of
-genic	pertaining to formation / originating in
-ia	condition of
-ic	pertaining to
-ist	specialist
-logist	specialist who studies
-logy	study of
-lysis	breakdown/disintegration
-oma	tumour/swelling (Am. tumor)
-osis	abnormal condition/disease/abnormal increase
-static	pertaining to stopping/controlling
-tropic	pertaining to stimulating / affinity for

Oncology

This branch of medicine deals with the study and treatment of malignant tumours (Am. tumors) commonly called cancers. A tumour is a mass or swelling forming from dividing cells which appear to be out of control. Benign tumours remain localized and do not threaten life, but malignant tumours spread and may lead to death. Tumours spread when they release cells into the blood and lymph; the tumour cells multiply in new sites forming secondary growths or **metastases** (from Greek *meta histanai*, *meta* meaning changed in form, *histanai* to place/set, ie, a growth in a different position). See Figure 106.

As malignant tumours grow and divide, they consume nutrients, depriving normal cells of essential metabolic components. A clinical feature called **cachexia** is seen in advanced stages of disease (from Greek *kakos* meaning bad and *hexis* meaning state). The body appears to suffer from malnutrition and becomes thin and 'wastes' away.

In this unit, we will examine terms that relate to common types of tumours.

Use the Exercise Guide at the beginning of this unit to complete Word Exercises 1 to 3, unless you are asked to work without it.

▌Root

Onc

(*From a Greek word* **ogkos**, *meaning a swelling. Here onc/o means a tumour (Am. tumor).*)

Combining form   Onc/o

📖 Word Exercise 1

Using your Exercise Guide, find the meaning of:

(a) **onc**/osis

(b) **onc/o**/genesis

(c) **onc/o**/trop/ic

Using your Exercise Guide, find the meaning of -genic, -logist and -lysis; then build words that mean:

(d) pertaining to formation of a tumour

(e) breakdown/disintegration of a tumour

(f) person who specializes in the study and treatment of tumours

The process of tumour formation is also known as **neoplasia** (*neo-* meaning new, *-plas-* forming/growing and *-ia* condition

A

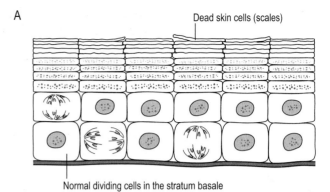

Dead skin cells (scales)

Normal dividing cells in the stratum basale

B

Basement membrane   A malignant cell dividing

C

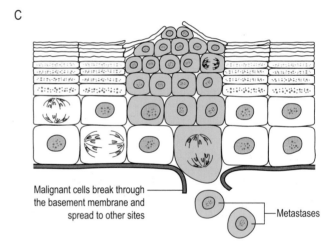

Malignant cells break through the basement membrane and spread to other sites

Metastases

Figure 106   Malignant cells forming and growing in the epidermis. (a) Normal epidermis, (b) a cell becomes malignant, and (c) a primary tumour forming and malignant cells spreading (metastasizing).

of) and the tumour itself as a **neoplasm**. Neoplastic, derived in the same way, is also used to mean pertaining to a new growth.

Before we study the next word root, we need to examine the use of the suffix *-oma*. Used by itself in combination with a tissue type, it indicates a benign tumour, eg, oste**oma**, a benign bone tumour; chondr**oma**, a benign tumour of cartilage.

Malignant tumours may also be designated by **-oma**, but they are usually preceded by the word **malignant**, eg, **malignant melanoma**, a malignant tumour of the pigment cells and **malignant lymphoma**, a malignant tumour of lymphatic tissue.

The suffix *-oma* is also used in **blastoma**, meaning a malignant tumour that forms from embryonic (germ) cells of an organ. Examples include **glioblastoma**, a tumour that contains neuroglia (a type of brain cell or gliacyte), and **retinoblastoma** a tumour that grows from embryonic cells in the retina of the eye.

(To confuse matters, *-oma* is occasionally used for a non-neoplastic condition such as **haematoma** (Am. **hematoma**), which refers to a swelling filled with blood and is not a new growth of cells.)

Two terms that are widely used when referring to malignant tumours are:

Carcinoma

a malignant tumour of epithelial origin. Remember, epithelia cover organs and line cavities and form membranes and glands.

Sarcoma

a malignant tumour of supporting tissues, including all connective tissues and muscle.

These terms are studied in the exercises that follow:

Root

Carcin

(*From a Greek word* **karkinos**, *meaning crab. Here carcin/o means a malignant tumour/cancer.*)

Combining form   Carcin/o

A **carcin**oma is a tumour of an epithelium, and there are numerous types. They are usually named by using the word carcinoma preceded by the histological type and followed by the organ of origin, eg:

Squamous cell carcinoma of the lung

originates in nonglandular epithelium.

Adenocarcinoma of the breast

originates in a glandular epithelium within the breast.

Often carcinomas are more simply named, eg, as carcinoma of the colon or carcinoma of the urinary bladder.

Note. A substance that stimulates the formation of a malignant tumour is known as a **carcinogen**.

Word Exercise 2

Without using your Exercise Guide, write the meaning of:

(a) **carcin/o**/gen/ic [_____]

(b) **carcin/o**/lysis [_____]

Using your Exercise Guide, find the meaning of:

(c) **carcin/o**/stat/ic [_____]

Also from this root, we have the word **cancer**, which is imprecisely used to mean carcinoma or cancer in situ.

Root

Sarc

(*From a Greek word* **sarkoma**, *meaning a fleshy growth. Here sarc/o means a malignant tumour of connective tissue.*)

Combining form   Sarc/o

Sarcomas are malignant tumours of the connective tissues and muscle such as bone, cartilage blood, lymph, glial tissue, smooth muscle and striated muscle. The word **sarcoma** is preceded by the tissue type as in osteo**sarcoma**, a malignant bone tumour. (**Sarcomat/o** is the combining form of sarcoma.)

Word Exercise 3

Using your Exercise Guide, find the meaning of:

(a) chondr/o/**sarcoma** [_____]

(b) leiomy/o/**sarcoma** [_____]

(c) rhabdomy/o/**sarcoma** [_____]

(d) mening/eal **sarcoma** [_____]

(e) angi/o/**sarcoma** [_____]

Without using your Exercise Guide, write the meaning of:

(f) **sarcomat**/osis [_____]

Most malignant tumours arise from epithelial tissues. When malignant cells grow, they sometimes resemble the cells from which they originate and are said to be **well differentiated**. Other malignant cells may be **undifferentiated** and may change their character back to a more primitive or embryonic type. When this occurs, they are described as **anaplastic** (*ana-* meaning backward, *-plast-* to mould or form and *-ic* pertaining to). A characteristic of all malignant cells within a tumour is that they have an increased capacity to divide.

Another form of malignancy is the mixed tissue tumour. This type contains cells that may resemble both epithelial and connective tissue cells.

Diagnosis of malignant tumours (cancers)

Precise classification of malignant tumours is essential for determining their likely growth characteristics. Once a tumour has been classified, appropriate treatment can be planned, and the patient can be given a prognosis (forecast of the probable course of their disease).

The classification of a tumour usually requires the microscopic examination of a sample of its cells; this procedure is called a **biopsy**. The word biopsy is formed from *bio-* meaning life and *-opsy* meaning process of viewing. A biopsy is the removal and examination of tissue from a living body.

A biopsy will determine a tumour's type, whether benign or malignant and whether it has spread to other tissues. Most biopsies are minor procedures, but some require general anaesthesia (Am. anesthesia). There are several types, including:

- a **needle biopsy**: removal of a small sample of cells using a fine, hollow needle
- an **incision biopsy**: removal of a small sample of skin or muscle through an incision
- an **excision** or **resection biopsy**: removal of a whole tumour which is then sent for analysis
- an **open biopsy**: removal of tissue from within the body during an operation
- an **endoscopic biopsy**: removal of tissue using forceps attached to a fibreoptic endoscope.

Cancer classification

Cancers are classified according to:

- **Histological type and origin**: this describes the type of tissue from which the cancer cells begin to develop and their origin, eg, a carcinoma of the lung
- **Grading**: a pathologist grades the tumour cells obtained at biopsy from 1 to 4 according to their appearance under the microscope
- **Staging**: a system of classification that attempts to describe the size and extent of spread of a tumour

We'll examine these in more detail below:

Histological type and origin

Here, the many different types of cancer are grouped into six main categories based on their type and origin:

Carcinoma

A carcinoma is a malignant tumour of epithelial origin. Epithelial tissue consists of epithelial membranes and epithelial glands that form the internal and external linings of the body. Carcinomas are divided into two major subtypes: adenocarcinoma that develops from an epithelial gland, and squamous cell carcinoma that develops from a squamous epithelium. Carcinomas affect glands or organs covered or lined with epithelial membranes that are capable of secretion such as the breast, prostate gland, bronchus and colon.

Sarcoma

Sarcomas are rare malignant tumours derived from cells that have their origin in the middle layer of the embryo called mesoderm. All connective tissues have their origin in mesenchyme cells of this layer, eg, cartilage, areolar tissue, adipose tissue and bone. Muscle tissue such as smooth muscle and striated muscle also develops from cells in the mesoderm. Sarcomas generally occur in young adults as soft tissue sarcomas or more commonly as painful, solid masses called osteosarcomas in bone; sarcomas usually resemble the tissue from which they originate.

Leukaemia (Am. Leukemia)

Leukaemia is a cancer of the blood-forming cells in the bone marrow. The disease affects the immature cells that produce leucocytes (Am. leukocytes), hence the term leuk/aem/ia, meaning a condition of white blood or too many white cells.

Leucocytes normally protect us from disease, but the leukaemic white cells lose their ability to protect us against micro-organisms, leaving the patient prone to infection. Leukaemia can also affect the immature cells that produce erythrocytes, resulting in the symptoms and signs of anaemia (Am. anemia) and interference with blood clotting.

There are many types, eg:

- acute myeloid leukaemia: a malignancy of the myeloid stem cells in bone marrow
- chronic lymphocytic leukaemia: a malignancy of cells that produce lymphocytes

Myeloma

A myeloma is a tumour that originates in the plasma cells of bone marrow. The cancerous cells produce many of the proteins found in blood. For example, in multiple myeloma, plasma cells derived from β lymphocytes produce an abnormal amount of immunoglobulin.

Lymphoma

Lymphoma develops in the nodes and organs of the lymphatic system. A lymphoma is a solid tumour that arises in an organ such as the spleen, tonsil, thymus gland or lymph node. Extranodal lymphomas are also found in other organs such as the stomach or brain. Lymphomas are classified into two subtypes:

- Hodgkin lymphoma
- non-Hodgkin lymphoma

Mixed tumours

In mixed tumours the cells may be of different origins, and they can be grouped into different categories, eg:

- carcinosarcoma: a malignant tumour composed of cells originating in epithelial and connective tissue
- adenosquamous carcinoma: a malignant tumour composed of glandular cells and squamous epithelial cells.

Grading

Cells taken at biopsy are subjected to examination under the microscope and graded according to their appearance and how well they are differentiated (specialized). Cells that are well differentiated and closely resemble cells from the normal parent tissue are classified as low-grade tumours (Grade 1). Cells that appear undifferentiated or anaplastic and are highly abnormal with respect to surrounding cells are classified as high-grade tumours (Grade 4). In the system shown next, tumours are graded from 1 to 4.

Grade 1: well-differentiated cells appear normal (low-grade)

Grade 2: cells are moderately differentiated and slightly abnormal (intermediate-grade)

Grade 3: cells are poorly differentiated and very abnormal (high-grade)

Grade 4: cells are anaplastic, undifferentiated and very abnormal (high-grade)

Grade X: cannot be assessed (undetermined grade)

Staging

Attempts to develop an international language for describing the extent of malignant disease have been made. One of these is in widespread use and is known as the **TNM** system.

T = tumour
categorizes the primary tumour and its size.
N = nodes
defines the number of lymph nodes that have been invaded.
M = metastases
indicates the presence or absence of metastases.

The extent of malignant disease defined by these categories is termed **staging**. Staging defines the size of tumour, its growth and progression at any one point.

Many different staging systems are in use for different cancers. It is not possible to study them here, but we have included a basic system that is outlined next.

T	
T_0	no primary tumour
T_1	primary tumour limited to site of origin
T_{2-4}	progressive increase in size of primary tumour
T_x	primary tumour cannot be assessed
T_{is}	primary tumour in situ

N	
N_0	no evidence of spread to nodes
N_1	spread to a node in the immediate area
N_{2-4}	increasing number of lymph nodes invaded
N_x	lymph nodes cannot be assessed

M	
M_0	no evidence of metastases
M_{1-3}	ascending degrees of metastases

Using this system, we can see the principle of how a cancer is staged. For example, a tumour classified at stage T_2 N_1 M_0 indicates the primary tumour is large (T_2) and has spread to one lymph node draining the area (N_1), and there is no evidence of a distant metastasis (M_0).

Staging is not an exact description of a tumour's progress, but it is a useful way to estimate the course of the disease when planning treatment (therapy). A patient can be re-staged following a period of treatment and assessment of its effect.

Effective treatment can lead to the disappearance of all signs and symptoms of disease; this is known as **remission**. However, if treatment does not completely eradicate the cancerous cells, symptoms of disease will return; this is known as a **relapse**. Sometimes a cancer is described as **refractory**, ie, resistant to treatment, and the patient may never go into remission.

If treatment is deemed to be successful, the patient will be asked to attend the outpatient clinic on a regular basis for assessment by the oncologist. This is known as **follow-up**, and its purpose is to monitor the patient for signs of reoccurrence of the disease.

Medical equipment and clinical procedures

We have already described the main instruments and clinical procedures that are used in the diagnosis and treatment of cancers in Unit 18. Tumours can be detected using radiography, computerized tomography, magnetic resonance imaging, positron emission tomography, ultrasound, etc.

The main types of treatments are:

- radiotherapy: the use of radiation/X-rays by medically qualified radiotherapists to destroy tumour cells
- chemotherapy: the use of chemicals, ie, cytotoxic drugs to poison tumour cells
- excision surgery: the use of surgery to remove a tumour
- immunotherapy: the process of restoring or enhancing the immune system's ability to destroy a tumour; it can involve the administration of synthetic components such as monoclonal antibodies and cytokines

Other types of diagnostic procedure not mentioned in the exercises include:

Tumour marker test

A tumour marker is a substance found in blood, urine, stool and other body fluids or tissues that can be elevated in patients with cancer. Tumour markers are produced by malignant cells or by other body cells in response to the presence of a tumour. Most markers are proteins, and they can be elevated for other benign reasons. Tumour markers are used to aid diagnosis, monitor patients following cancer treatment and in specific cases screen for the presence of disease. Two examples of widely used tumour markers are:

Carcinoembryonic antigen (CEA)

- Associated cancer type: colorectal and breast
- Tissue analyzed: blood
- Use: to check whether colorectal cancer has spread or to look for breast cancer reoccurrence and assess response to treatment

Cancer antigen (CA-125)

- Associated cancer type: ovarian
- Tissue analyzed: blood
- Use: to aid diagnosis, assess response to treatment and evaluate recurrence

Cytogenetics testing

Cancer is a genetic disease, and tumour cells are different from normal cells because of changes in their DNA called mutations. Cytogenetics testing is the process of examining chromosomes and genes found in the nuclei of cells. Mutations can develop when egg and sperm cells are being made, during early fetal development, or after birth in any cell in the body.

Now write the meaning of the following words from the Case History without using your dictionary lists:

 CASE HISTORY 19

The object of this exercise is to understand words associated with a patient's medical history.

To complete the exercise:

- Read through the passage on glioblastoma multiforme; unfamiliar words are underlined, and you can find their meaning using the Word Help.

- Write the meaning of the medical terms shown in bold print on the lines that follow the Word Help.

Glioblastoma multiforme

Mr S, a 59-year-old, male, senior office worker, noticed a loss of verbal fluency and had difficulty in recalling the names of common objects and friends. His employer reprimanded him over a decline in his previously high standard of written work. His condition worsened, and he was persuaded by his colleagues to seek medical advice. He was referred to the neurology unit by his GP.

On examination by the neurologist, he appeared alert and intelligent but made several mistakes when asked to name common objects and spell simple words. He could not remember a simple name and address after 5 minutes.

His optic discs were normal, but there was no venous pulsation. Vision was restricted in the upper temporal visual field in the right eye and upper nasal field in the left eye. There was a mild lower facial weakness and a slight increase in reflexes of the right arm and leg. The right plantar reflex was extensor.

The presence of dysphasia, memory loss, right homonymous field restriction and mild pyramidal signs suggested a lesion affecting the upper temporal lobe of the left cerebral hemisphere.

A CXR excluded a bronchial **neoplasm**, which is the most common cause of cerebral **metastases** in a smoker. A CT scan demonstrated a mixed, high- and low-density intracranial lesion in the left temporal region and excluded **meningioma**. EEG demonstrated a wave abnormality in the left temporal region and a left carotid arteriogram indicated displacement of cerebral branches by a temporal **mass**. The most common cause of lesions presenting in this way is malignant **glioma**.

A case conference was arranged with the clinical **oncologist** to disclose the prognosis to Mr S and his family and to outline the options for treatment. Histological confirmation of the diagnosis was requested before commencing treatment. Mr S was administered dexamethasone to reduce the oedema (Am. edema) around the tumour and improve the symptoms of raised intracranial pressure. A brain biopsy confirmed glioblastoma multiforme.

Mr S underwent neurosurgery, part of the temporal lobe was removed to provide an internal decompression, and the tumour was sucked out. Unfortunately, malignant gliomas infiltrate into brain tissue and are difficult to remove completely. A radical course of cobalt 60 radiotherapy in combination with **chemotherapy** and small doses of steroids followed surgery. His speech defect and writing improved considerably for many months following surgery. Now, a year later, he shows signs of deterioration with a right hemiparesis, dysphasia, occasional grand mal seizures and **cachexia**.

Word Help

arteriogram tracing/X-ray picture of arteries

biopsy removal and examination of living tissue

carotid the carotid artery in the neck

cerebral hemisphere a lateral half of the cerebrum

cobalt 60 (^{60}Co) isotope of cobalt that emits gamma rays that can destroy cancer cells

CT computed tomography

CXR chest X-ray

decompression relief of pressure

dysphasia condition of difficulty in speaking

EEG electroencephalogram/electroencephalography

extensor straightening (here refers to the Babinski reflex, a response in which the toes curl upwards or dorsiflex when the sole of the foot is stroked, instead of the normal plantar flexion in which the toes curl down)

glioblastoma tumour of embryonic/germ cells that contains neuroglia (type of supporting cell found in the brain)

GP general practitioner (family doctor)

grand mal seizure a form of epileptic fit in which consciousness is lost

hemiparesis partial or slight paralysis affecting one side of the body, eg, weakness of a limb

histological pertaining to histology (here histological analysis for classification and signs of malignancy in brain tissue)

intracranial pertaining to within the cranium

homonymous corresponding halves

lesion a pathological change in a tissue

malignant dangerous, capable of spreading

multiforme having many forms (here referring to the fact that the tumour may be derived from different types of cells)

oedema accumulation of fluid in a tissue (Am. edema)

plantar pertaining to the sole of the foot

prognosis a forecast of the probable outcome and course of a disease

pyramidal referring to the pyramidal tract in the brain, an area that initiates voluntary skilled movements of skeletal muscles, especially the fingers

radical direct to the root or cause (treatment to eliminate disease), extensive

steroid a drug used to suppress inflammation and reduce oedema (Am. edema)

temporal pertaining to the temple/temporal bone (the temple is the flat region on either side of the head)

(a) neoplasm

(b) metastases

(c) meningioma

(d) mass

(e) glioma

(f) oncologist

(g) chemotherapy

(h) cachexia

(Answers to the Case History exercise are given in the Answers to Word Exercises on page 355.)

Quick Reference

Combining forms relating to oncology:

Aden/o	gland
Blast/o	embryonic / germ cell
Cancer/o	cancer
Carcin/o	cancerous/malignant tumour
Melan/o	pigment
Onc/o	tumour (Am. tumor)
Sarc/o	connective tissue / fleshy
Sarcomat/o	sarcoma / malignant tumour

Abbreviations

Some common abbreviations related to oncology are listed next. Note that some are not standard, and their meaning may vary from one healthcare setting to another. There is a more extensive list for reference on page 369.

BX, Bx, bx	biopsy
CA, Ca	cancer/carcinoma
CR	complete response, complete remission
FNA	fine needle aspiration
MEN	multiple endocrine neoplasia
Metas, mets	metastasis
NAD	no abnormality detected
N & V	nausea and vomiting
NED	no evidence of disease
O/E	on examination
PR	partial response
Prot.	protocol (a detailed plan)
TNF	tumour necrosis factor (Am. tumor)
TPN	total parenteral nutrition

Associated words

Ablation destruction of tissues and tumours by surgery or radiotherapy

Acute sudden, severe symptoms or signs of short duration

Adjuvant therapy a treatment given in conjunction with another

Alopecia condition of loss of hair, a side effect of some cancer treatments

Analgesia condition of without pain, pain relief

Anaplastic pertaining to cancer cells that grow rapidly and have little or no resemblance to normal cells

Antiemetic a drug that acts to prevent nausea and vomiting

Aspiration the drawing off of fluid from a cavity by suction

Central line a thin, plastic line into a vein in the chest used for the delivery of chemotherapy

Chronic pertaining to of long duration, persisting for a long time

Cytokine a substance secreted by cells of the immune system that can affect other cells, eg, interferon

Differentiated describes a cell that has grown and specialized to perform a specific function

Disseminated scattered or distributed over a large area or range

Dysplastic pertaining to abnormal growth of cells, their size shape and organization (not clearly cancerous)

Excision cutting out

Follow-up periodic visits by a patient to the oncologist to ensure there has been no reoccurrence of disease

Fungating process of producing a fungus-like growth, characteristic of some cancers

Gavage the force-feeding of nutrients via a tube into the oesophagus or stomach (Am. esophagus)

Histopathology the study of diseased tissues using a microscope

Hospice a system of care given to the chronically or terminally ill person and family

Hyperplasia condition of abnormal increase in the number of normal cells in a tissue increasing its volume

Idiopathic pertaining to disease of unknown cause

Infiltrating cancer malignant cells that have spread beyond the layer of tissue in which they developed and into surrounding healthy tissues

Invasive having the ability to infiltrate and destroy surrounding tissue, a characteristic of malignant tumours

Latent condition a condition that is present but not active or temporarily concealed

Metaplastic pertaining to a change in cells to a form that does not occur in the tissue in which they are found (a loss of differentiation)

Mitosis the division of a parent cell into two identical daughter cells

Modality the method of employment of any form of therapeutic agent, eg, chemotherapy

Morbidity the condition of being sick or state of being diseased

Oncogene a gene (piece of DNA) that has the potential to cause a normal cell to become malignant

Palliative treatment a treatment that relieves symptoms but does not cure

Polycythaemia vera a malignancy of red blood cells (Am. polycythemia vera)

Pruritus itching

Radical pertaining to dealing with the root cause of disease

Refractory not responding to treatment

Regression a return to a previous state of health; a decrease in size of a tumour or extent of a cancer in the body (Am. tumor)

Resection excision or surgical removal of a part

Restaging act of staging a patient after a period of treatment to access the response to therapy

Screening checking for disease when there are no symptoms

Terminal disease a disease that cannot be cured and will cause death

Undifferentiated like a primitive cell without any development to a more specialized type

NOW TRY THE WORD CHECK

WORD CHECK

This self-check exercise lists all the word components used in this unit. First, write down the meaning of as many word components as you can. Then, check your answers using the Exercise Guide and Quick Reference box or the Glossary of Word Components (pp. 383–410).

Prefixes

ana-	
meta-	
neo-	

Combining forms of word roots

aden/o	
angi/o	
blast/o	
cancer/o	
carcin/o	
chem/o	
chondr/o	
cyt/o	
gli/a/o	
leiomy/o	

melan/o

meningi/o

onc/o

rhabdomy/o

sarc/o

sarcomat/o

Suffixes

-genic

-genesis

-ia

-ic

-ist

-logy

-lysis

-oma

-osis

-plasia

-plastic

-static

-therapy

-toxic

-tropic

NOW TRY THE SELF-ASSESSMENT

SELF-ASSESSMENT

Test 19A

Prefixes, suffixes and combining forms of word roots

Match each meaning in Column C with a word component in Column A by inserting the appropriate number in Column B.

Column A	Column B	Column C
(a) aden/o		1. pertaining to
(b) ana-		2. change position or form
(c) cancer/o		3. pertaining to formation/originating in
(d) carcin/o		4. membranes of CNS
(e) chondr/o		5. striated muscle
(f) -genic		6. condition of growth (increase of cells)
(g) -ic		7. pertaining to stopping/controlling
(h) -ist		8. pertaining to affinity for/acting on
(i) leiomy/o		9. gland
(j) melan/o		10. cancer (general term)
(k) meningi/o		11. cancer/tumour (combining form)
(l) meta-		12. cartilage
(m) neo-		13. tumour (suffix)
(n) -oma		14. a malignant tumour of epithelium
(o) onc/o		15. a malignant tumour of supporting tissue
(p) -plasia		16. specialist
(q) rhabdomy/o		17. smooth muscle
(r) sarcomat/o		18. black pigment
(s) -static		19. new
(t) -tropic		20. backward

Score

20

Test 19B

Write the meaning of:

(a) fibrosarcoma

(b) gastric adenocarcinoma

(c) hepatocellular carcinoma

(d) anaplastic thyroid carcinoma

(e) bronchogenic carcinoma

Score

5

Test 19C

Build words that mean:

(a) malignant tumour of lymph (use sarc/o)

(b) benign tumour of cartilage

(c) a malignant tumour originating in bone (use sarc/o)

(d) condition of a new growth of cells

(e) the treatment of tumours

Score

5

Check answers to Self-Assessment Tests on pages 365–366.

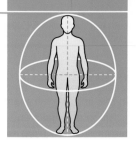

UNIT **20**
ANATOMICAL POSITION

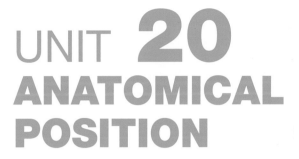

Once you have completed Unit 20, you should be able to do the following:

- understand the meaning of medical words relating to the anatomical position
- build medical words relating to regions and positions in the body
- associate medical terms with their anatomical position

- understand common medical abbreviations relating to anatomical positions
- visualize and name the planes of the body
- visualize and name the cavities of the body

EXERCISE GUIDE

Use this list of word components and their meanings to complete the word exercises in this unit.

Prefixes

epi-	above/upon/on
hypo-	below/under

Roots / Combining forms

bucc/o	cheek
cardi/o	heart
cephal/o	head
chondr/o	cartilage
cost/o	rib
crani/o	cranium/skull
derm/o	skin
faci/o	face
-ganglion	ganglion
gastr/o	stomach
hepat/o	liver
ili/o	hip/ilium/flank

mamm/o	breast / mammary gland
nas/o	nose
or/o	mouth
ot/o	ear
placent/o	placenta
stern/o	sternum
ven/o	vein
vertebr/o	vertebra/spine

Suffixes

-ac	pertaining to
-al	pertaining to
-ary	pertaining to
-ic	pertaining to
-ous	pertaining to / of the nature of
-ver(ted)	turned

Anatomical position

In this unit, we will examine a selection of terms that refer to the position of organs and tissues within the body. Many of these terms are also used to indicate the position of injuries, pain, disease and surgical operations.

The **anatomical position** of the body (Fig. 107) is a reference system that all doctors and medical texts use when describing body components. We always refer to position in the patient's body as if he/she were standing upright with arms at the sides and palms of the hands facing forward, head erect and eyes looking forward.

With the body in the anatomical position, we can draw an imaginary line down the middle of the body (Fig. 107). This is called the **midline** or **median line**, and it bisects the body into right and left sides. Note that right and left refer to the sides of the patient in the anatomical position, not those of the observer.

Directions

We can now see how the imaginary midline can be used to indicate directions when a body is in the anatomical position. Parts that lie nearer to the median line of the body than other parts are described as **medial** to that part. Any part that lies further away is said to be **lateral** to the first part (Fig. 108). To summarize:

Medial   pertaining to towards the median line (or midline)
Lateral   pertaining to away from the median line (or midline)

Other directions can also be seen in Figure 108.

> **Superior**
> towards the head, upper
> **Inferior**
> away from the head, lower
> **Anterior (ventral)**
> front
> **Posterior (dorsal)**
> back
> **Proximal**
> pertaining to near point of attachment or point of origin
> **Distal**
> pertaining to further from point of attachment or origin
> **Superficial**
> pertaining to near the surface of the body
> **Deep**
> away from the surface of the body

 Word Exercise 1

Using the information in Figure 108, complete the following sentences by inserting the correct word in each box.

(a) The eyes are superior/ inferior to the mouth. [   ]

(b) The mouth is superior/ inferior to the nose. [   ]

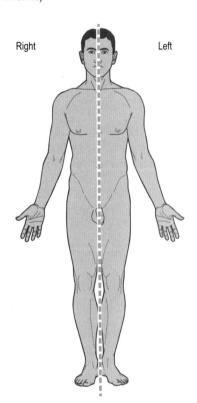

Figure 107   The anatomical position.

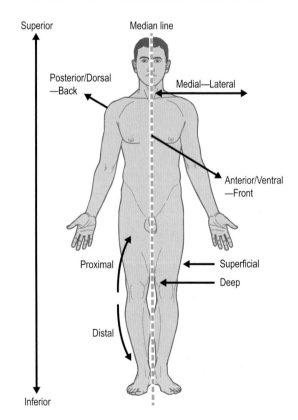

Figure 108   Anatomical directions.

(c) The ear is medial/lateral to the eye.

(d) The nostril is medial/lateral to the eye.

(e) The umbilicus lies on the anterior/posterior surface of the abdomen.

(f) The vertebrae lie close to the dorsal/ventral surface of the body.

(g) The wrist is proximal/distal to the elbow.

(h) The ankles are proximal/distal to the toes.

(i) The ribs are superficial/deep to the lungs.

These terms can also be applied to organ systems and tissues within the body. They too are described as if they are in the anatomical position, eg, the digestive system (Fig. 109).

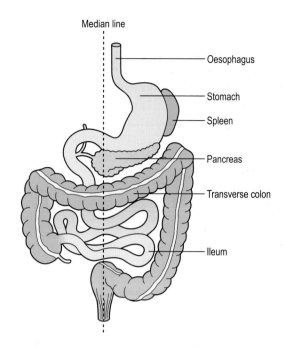

Figure 109   The digestive system in the anatomical position.

📖 Word Exercise 2

Using information from Figure 109, complete the following sentences by inserting the correct word in each box.

(a) The pancreas is superior/inferior to the stomach.

(b) The oesophagus (Am. esophagus) is superior/inferior to the stomach.

(c) The stomach is medial/lateral to the spleen.

(d) The oesophagus (Am. esophagus) is proximal/distal to the stomach.

(e) The transverse colon is anterior/posterior to the ileum.

(f) The ileum is dorsal/ventral to the transverse colon.

Cavities

The term cavity is used to describe a hollow space or a potential space within the body or one of its organs; cavities form another organizational reference system. The body has two major cavities and each is divided into lesser cavities. The internal organs of a cavity are collectively known as viscera.

The main cavities are shown below:

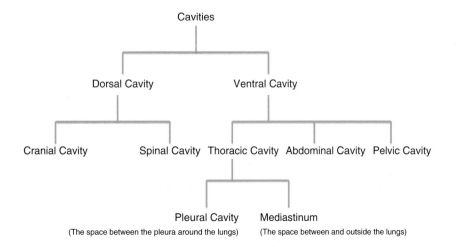

Word Exercise 3

Match a cavity in Column A to a number from Figure 110 in Column B.

Column A	Column B
(a) Cranial cavity	
(b) Abdominal cavity	
(c) Dorsal cavity	
(d) Pelvic cavity	
(e) Spinal cavity	
(f) Ventral cavity	
(g) Thoracic cavity	

Regions

With the body in the anatomical position, it can be divided into the cephalic, thoracic, abdominal and pelvic regions (Fig. 111).

Each of these regions can be subdivided; the simplest example is perhaps the division of the abdominopelvic region into quadrants (Fig. 112).

Doctors and health personnel often use this simple system to describe the position of abdominopelvic pain. Imaginary vertical and horizontal lines through the umbilicus form the quadrants. A more complex method is to divide the abdominopelvic region into nine regions (Fig. 113).

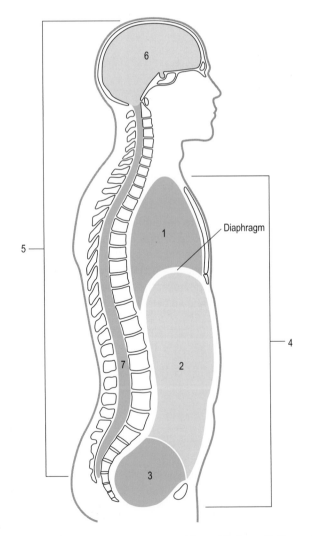

Figure 110　Body cavities. (Adapted from Chabner D-E, The Language of Medicine, 10th Edition, 2013, Saunders.)

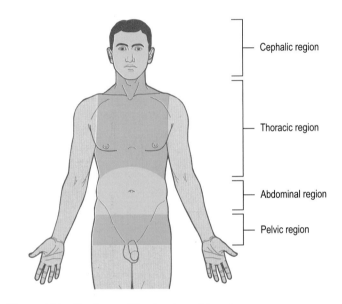

Figure 111　Regions of the trunk and head.

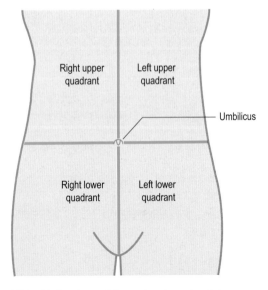

Figure 112　Abdominopelvic region (quadrants).

Word Exercise 4

Using your Exercise Guide, find the meaning of:

(a) hypo/chondr/i/ac region
(the word refers to the
cartilage of the rib cage)

(b) epi/gastr/ic region

(c) ili/ac region

The cephalic regions and the upper and lower extremities can also be subdivided into regions. These are examined in the next two exercises. Use your Exercise Guide to find the meaning of unfamiliar words.

Word Exercise 5

Examine Figure 114 and match the regions listed in Column A with a number from the diagram in Column B.

Column A	Column B
(a) cephalic region	
(b) cranial region	
(c) facial region	
(d) otic region	
(e) oral region	
(f) mammary region	

Column A	Column B
(g) nasal region	
(h) buccal region	

Word Exercise 6

Look at Figures 115 and 116 and label the regions of each limb by selecting an appropriate region from the list below. The first region has been labelled for you.

tarsal region	ankle bones
brachial region	arm
axillary region	armpit
hallux region	great toe
digital/phalangeal region	fingers
pedal region	foot
antebrachial region	forearm
crural region	leg
patellar region	knee
palmar/volar region	palm
femoral region	thigh

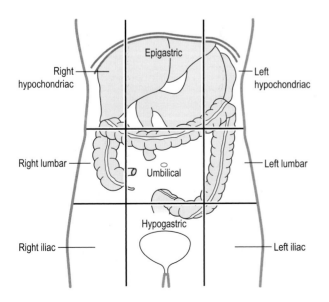

Figure 113   Abdominopelvic region (nine regions).

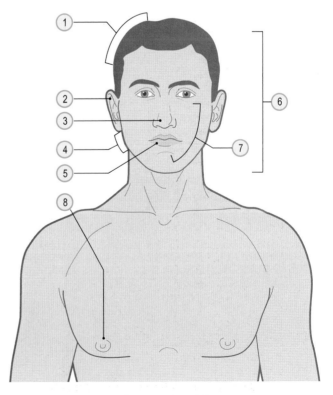

Figure 114   Regions of the head and thorax.

pollex region	thumb
digital/phalangeal region	toes
carpal region	wrist bones

Planes

Planes are imaginary flat surfaces that form a reference system indicating the direction in which organs have been cut, drawn or photographed. When a body structure is studied, it is often viewed in section, and the section is formed from a cut made in relation to one of the planes.

Imagine a vertical cut made along the midline from the front of the body to the back dividing it into right and left halves. The flat surfaces formed in each cut half illustrate the **median** or **midsagittal plane**. Figure 117 shows the direction of the cut that forms the midsagittal plane. Figure 118 shows a midsagittal section through the brain when cut in this plane and viewed from the side.

Any plane parallel to the midsagittal or median plane is called a **parasagittal** or **paramedian plane** (*para* meaning besides) (Fig. 119).

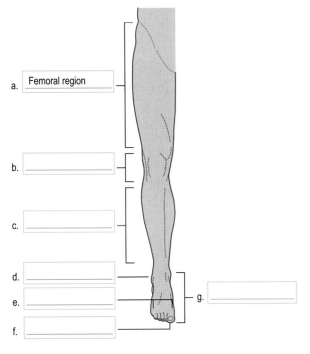

a. Femoral region

b.

c.

d.

e.

f.

g.

Figure 115   Leg regions.

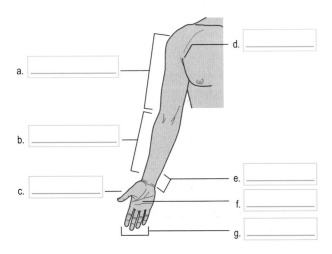

a.

b.

c.

d.

e.

f.

g.

Figure 116   Arm regions.

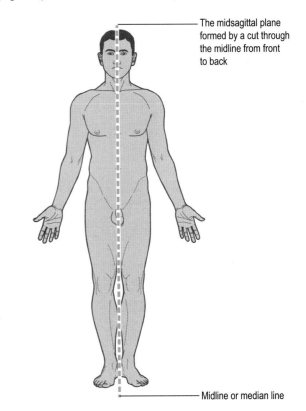

The midsagittal plane formed by a cut through the midline from front to back

Midline or median line

Figure 117   The midsagittal or median plane.

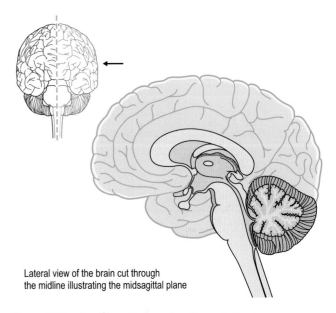

Lateral view of the brain cut through the midline illustrating the midsagittal plane

Figure 118   A midsagittal section through the brain.

Two other planes are shown in Figures 120 and 121. A horizontal cut illustrates the **horizontal** or **transverse plane** (Fig. 120). This is the equivalent of a cross-section through the body dividing it into superior and inferior portions.

A vertical side cut divides the body into anterior and posterior portions at right angles to the sagittal plane and illustrates the **frontal** or **coronal plane** (Fig. 121).

Figure 122 summarizes the three main planes of the body.

 Word Exercise 7

Match each description in Column A to a plane in Column C by inserting a number in Column B.

Column A	Column B	Column C
(a) divides the body into superior and inferior portions		1. midsagittal plane
(b) a plane parallel to the median plane		2. transverse plane
(c) divides the body into right and left halves		3. frontal plane
(d) divides the body into anterior and posterior portions		4. parasagittal plane

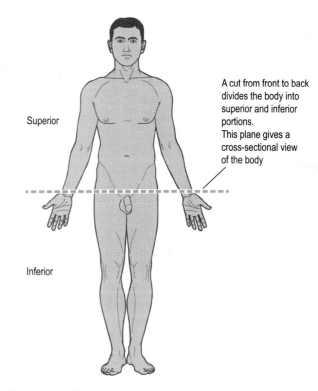

A cut from front to back divides the body into superior and inferior portions.
This plane gives a cross-sectional view of the body

Superior

Inferior

Figure 120   The horizontal or transverse plane.

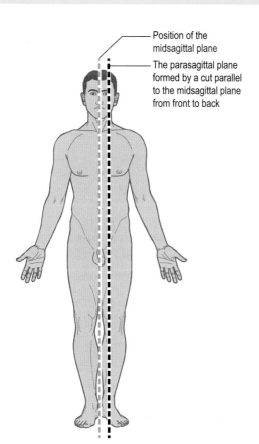

Position of the midsagittal plane

The parasagittal plane formed by a cut parallel to the midsagittal plane from front to back

Figure 119   The parsagittal or paramedian plane.

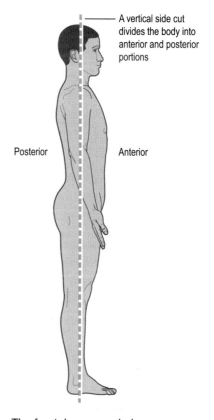

A vertical side cut divides the body into anterior and posterior portions

Posterior   Anterior

Figure 121   The frontal or coronal plane.

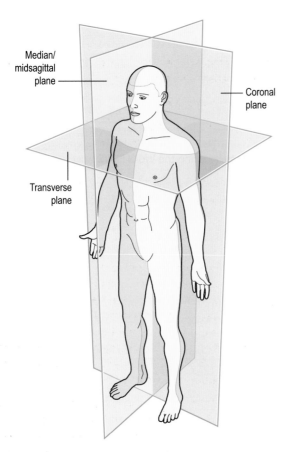

Figure 122   The planes of the body.

Locating parts of the body

There are a large number of locative prefixes that act as prepositions when placed in front of word roots. These tell us about the position of structures within the body. Use the list of locative prefixes below to complete the next two exercises.

Locative prefixes	
Above	epi-, hyper-, super-, supra-
Across	trans-
After	meta-, post-
Against	anti, contra-
Around	circum-, peri-
Away	ab-, apo-, ef-
Back	dorsi-, dorso-, post-, re-, retro-
Backward	opistho-, retro (also means back/behind)
Before/front	ante-, pre-, pro-, ventr-
Below	hypo-, infra-, sub-
Behind/after	dorsi-, dorso-, post-
Beside	para-
Between	inter-

Down	de-
Front / in front	pro-, ventr-
In/inside	em-, en-, endo-, in-, intra-
Left	laevo- (Am. levo-)
Middle	medi-, meso-
Out/outside	ec-, ect-, ef-, exo-, extra-
Right	dextro-
Side	later-
Through	dia-, per-
To/towards/near	ad-, af-
Under	infra-, sub-
Upon	epi-
Within	intra-

Word Exercise 8

Use the locative prefix list to fill in each blank with an appropriate prefix:

(a) The region beside the nose _____ nasal region

(b) Disc between vertebrae _____ vertebral disc

(c) Region upon the stomach _____ gastric region

(d) Pertaining to after a ganglion _____ ganglionic

(e) Condition of right displacement of heart _____ cardia

(f) Nerve below orbit of eye _____ orbital nerve

Word Exercise 9

Use your Exercise Guide and the locative prefix list to find the meaning of:

(a) peri/cardi/al _____

(b) intra/ven/ous _____

(c) inter/cost/al _____

(d) retro/verted uterus _____

(e) supra/hepat/ic _____

(f) infra/stern/al _____

(g) pre/ganglion/ic

(h) extra/placent/al

(i) sub/epiderm/al

Some of the locative prefixes we have listed are incorporated into words that indicate the direction of movement of parts of the body. Before noting some examples, we need to describe the main actions of muscles.

Muscles that bend limbs by decreasing the angles between articulating bones are called **flexors**, and those that increase the angles after they have flexed are called **extensors**. The action of flexors is known as **flexion** and that of extensors, **extension**. Examples of prefixes that indicate direction of movements at joints are shown in bold:

Abduction — the movement of a part away from the midline (*ad-* meaning away from).

Adduction — the movement of a part towards the midline (*ad-* meaning to)

Circumduction — the movement in which the distal ends of a bone move in a circle (*circum-* meaning around); not a separate plane of movement

Protraction — the movement of a part forward/in front, eg, the jaw (*pro-* meaning in front/before)

Retraction — the movement of a protracted part back (*re-* meaning back/contrary)

Elevation — the upward movement of a body part, eg, the jaw (from Latin *elevare* meaning to raise)

Depression — the downward movement of a body part (*de-* meaning down/from)

Dorsiflexion — the movement that bends the foot back (upwards) from the anatomical position (*dorsi-* meaning back)

Plantar flexion — the movement that bends the foot downwards from the anatomical position (*plantar* meaning pertaining to the sole of the foot)

Inversion — the movement of the sole inward so the soles face each other (*in-* meaning in/inward)

Eversion — the movement of the sole outwards, so the soles face away from each other (*e-* meaning out from)

Pronation — the movement of the forearm that turns the palm of the hand posteriorly or inferiorly when the forearm is flexed (from Latin *pronare* meaning bend forward)

Supination — the movement of the forearm that turns the palm of the hand anteriorly or superiorly when the forearm is flexed (from Latin *supinare* meaning bend backward)

CASE HISTORY 20

The object of this exercise is to understand words associated with a patient's medical history.

To complete the exercise:

- Read through the passage on an unusual fracture of the tibia; unfamiliar words are underlined, and you can find their meaning using the Word Help.

- Write the meaning of the medical terms shown in bold print on the lines that follow the Word Help.

An unusual fracture of the tibia

A 13-year-old male was referred to the Orthopaedic Department after sustaining a hyperextension injury to his right knee during a school football match. He had immediate onset of pain and swelling during the first few hours following the injury. On admission, he could not bear weight on the knee, and flexion and extension exacerbated the pain. His medical record indicated no previous injury to his right lower extremity, and he appeared to be in good health.

Examination of the right lower extremity revealed a knee effusion with soft tissue swelling and diffuse tenderness over the **proximal** tibial growth plate. There were **superficial** skin lacerations on the **anterior** and **medial** surface of his right thigh. He could not **dorsiflex** or evert his foot, and sensation in the **lateral** calf and foot was reduced. Vascular insufficiency in the injured extremity was assessed; the popliteal, dorsalis pedis and posterior tibial pulses were palpable with good **distal** refilling.

Lateral and **anteroposterior** radiographs demonstrated a proximal tibial fracture classified as a Salter-Harris type III. The intraarticular fracture extended along the articular surface into the medial and lateral plateaus. The epiphyseal plate was anteriorly displaced on the metaphysis.

He underwent open reduction and internal fixation with a 3-mm Steinmann pin; recovery was uneventful, and his articular surface was preserved.

Word Help

calf the fleshy back part of the leg below the knee

dorsalis pedis pulse the pulse on the dorsal foot (the upper part of the foot)

effusion a fluid discharge into a part/escape of fluid into an enclosed space

epiphyseal pertaining to the epiphysis, the end of a long bone separated from the main shaft by a cartilage plate

evert turn the sole of the foot outward at the ankle joint; lift up the lateral edge of the foot

extension increasing the angle between two bones (here straightening the leg)

exacerbated increased severity of symptoms

flexion decreasing the angle between two bones (here bending the leg)

hyperextension forcible overextending of a limb (here extending the knee joint so far that the lower leg bends forwards)

intraarticular within a joint or inside the cavity of a joint

laceration a tear in a tissue

lower extremity a leg (hip, thigh, leg, ankle and foot taken as one structure)

metaphysis the wider part at the end of the main shaft of a long bone adjacent to the epiphysis

open reduction an operation that exposes bones for restoration of displaced tissue

orthopaedic pertaining to orthopaedics (study of the locomotor/movement system)

palpable able to be felt using light pressure with the fingers

plateau a flat region (here the expanded end of the tibia that articulates with the femur)

popliteal pulse pertaining to the pulse behind the knee

posterior tibial pulse the pulse in the foot posterior to the lower end of the tibia

radiograph here meaning an X-ray picture/recording

Salter-Harris type III a classification system for growth plate injuries

tibial pertaining to the tibia

vascular pertaining to blood vessels

Now, write the meaning of the following words from the Case History without using your dictionary lists:

(a) proximal

(b) superficial

(c) anterior

(d) medial

(e) dorsiflex

(f) lateral

(g) distal

(h) anteroposterior

(Answers to the Case History exercise are given in the Answers to Word Exercises on page 383.)

Quick Reference

Combining forms relating to anatomical parts and positions of the body:

Anter/o	front/anterior
Axill/o	armpit
Brachi/o	arm
Bucc/o	cheek
Carp/o	carpal / wrist bones
Cephal/o	head
Crani/o	cranium
Crur/o	leg
Digit/o	finger/toe
Faci/o	face
Femor/o	femur/thigh
Hallux	great toe
Ili/o	ilium/flank
Infer/o	towards the feet / inferior
Later/o	side
Mamm/o	breast / mammary gland
Nas/o	nose
Or/o	mouth
Ot/o	ear
Palm/o	palm
Patell/o	patella / knee cap
Ped/o	foot
Phalang/o	phalange/finger/toe
Pollex	thumb
Poster/o	back/posterior
Super/o	towards the head / superior
Tars/o	tarsus / ankle bones
Vol/o	palm

Abbreviations

Some common abbreviations related to anatomical position are listed next. Note that some are not standard, and their meaning may vary from one healthcare setting to another. There is a more extensive list for reference on page 369.

Ant.	anterior
DIST, Dist	distal
Inf.	inferior
Lat.	lateral
LLQ	left lower quadrant
LUQ	left upper quadrant
Med.	medial
Post.	posterior
Prox.	proximal
RLQ	right lower quadant
RUQ	right upper quadrant
Sup.	superior

Associated words

Adam's apple the laryngeal prominence, a protrusion in front of the neck formed by the thyroid cartilage

Anatomy meaning to cut apart, now the branch of science concerned with the bodily structure of humans and other animals especially revealed by dissection

Appendage a thing that is added or attached to something larger or more important; an outgrowth such as a tail

Aspect that part of a surface facing in any designated direction

Axis an imaginary line through the centre (Am. center) of a body or about which a structure revolves; a line around which body parts are arranged

Body the trunk or animal frame with its organs; the largest or main part of an organ; any mass or collection of material

Calf the fleshy back part of the leg beneath the knee

Capitate state of having a head; of the head

Caudate state of having a tail; of the tail

Circumflex bending around something; curved

Corpus body

Ectopic pertaining to being out of place

Eminence a projection from a surface

Girdle an encircling structure or part; a ring of bones that may be incomplete

Groin the junction of the upper thigh with the abdomen

Hamstring one of the tendons of the group of muscles (the 'ham') situated at the back of the thigh, the muscles flex the knee

Hiatus a gap, a pause or break in continuity

Instep the arched middle part of the foot between the toes and ankle

Loin the part of the back between the thorax and pelvis

Morphology the study of the form and structure of an organism, organ or part

Nape the back of the neck

Pars a division or part

Prominence a protrusion or projection

Shin the prominent anterior edge of the tibia

Soma the body as distinguished from the mind; the body tissue as distinguished from reproductive (germ) cells

Stratum a layer

Trunk the main part of the body to which the head and limbs are attached; a truncus

NOW TRY THE WORD CHECK

WORD CHECK

This self-check exercise lists all the word components used in this unit. First, write down the meaning of as many word components as you can. Then, check your answers using the Exercise Guide and Quick Reference box or the Glossary of Word Components (pp. 383–410).

Prefixes

ab-	
ad-	
af-	
ante	
anti-	
apo-	
circum-	
contra-	
dextro-	
dia-	
dorso-	
ec-	
ect-	
ef-	
em-	
en-	
endo-	
exo-	
extra-	
in-	
infra-	
inter-	
intra-	
laevo- (Am. levo-)	
edi-	
meso-	
para-	
per-	
peri-	
pre-	
pro-	
retro-	
super-	
supra-	
trans-	
ventro-	

Combining forms of word roots

anter/o

axill/o

brachi/o

bucc/o

cardi/o

carp/o

cephal/o

chondr/o

cost/o

crani/o

crur/o

derm/o

digit/o

faci/o

femor/o

-ganglion

gastr/o

hallux

hepat/o

ili/o

infer/o

later/o

mamm/o

nas/o

or/o

ot/o

palm/o

patell/o

ped/o

phalang/o

placent/o

pollex

poster/o

stern/o

super/o

tars/o

ven/o

verteb/o

vol/o

Suffixes

-ac

-al

-ary

-ia

-iac

-ic

-ous

-ver(ted)

NOW TRY THE SELF-ASSESSMENT

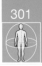

SELF-ASSESSMENT

Test 20A

Combining forms relating to parts of body

Match each meaning in Column C with a combining form of a word root in Column A by inserting the appropriate number in Column B.

Column A	Column B	Column C
(a) abdomin/o		1. head
(b) axill/o		2. leg
(c) brachi/o		3. great toe
(d) carp/o		4. ankle bones / tarsus
(e) cephal/o		5. palm (i)
(f) crani/o		6. palm (ii)
(g) crur/o		7. knee
(h) digit/o		8. finger/toe (i)
(i) femor/o		9. finger/toe (ii)
(j) hallux		10. pelvis
(k) ili/o		11. thumb
(l) palm/o		12. thigh/femur
(m) patell/o		13. abdomen
(n) ped/o		14. skull/cranium
(o) pelv/i		15. thorax
(p) phalang/o		16. foot
(q) pollex		17. arm
(r) tars/o		18. armpit
(s) thorac/o		19. ilium/flank
(t) vol/o		20. wrist bones

Score

20

Test 20B

Locative prefixes

Match each meaning in Column C with a locative prefix in Column A by inserting the appropriate number in Column B.

Column A	Column B	Column C
(a) ab-		1. through (i)
(b) ad-		2. through (ii)
(c) circum-		3. backward/behind
(d) dextro-		4. across
(e) dia-		5. between
(f) ec-		6. side
(g) en-		7. around (i)
(h) epi-		8. around (ii)
(i) infra-		9. away
(j) inter-		10. before / in front of
(k) laevo- (Am. levo-)		11. beside
(l) later-		12. towards
(m) para-		13. after/behind
(n) per-		14. right
(o) peri-		15. upon
(p) post-		16. in
(q) pre-		17. above
(r) retro-		18. left
(s) supra-		19. below
(t) trans-		20. out

Score

20

Test 20C

Write the meaning of:

(a) interphalangeal

(b) dextroversion

(c) retrobuccal

(d) supracostal

(e) intranasal

Score

5

Test 20D

Build words that mean:

(a) pertaining to the side

(b) a turning towards the left

(c) pertaining to after a ganglion

(d) pertaining to below the liver

(e) pertaining to across the skin

Score

5

Check answers to Self-Assessment Tests on page 366.

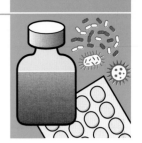

UNIT 21
PHARMACOLOGY AND MICROBIOLOGY

OBJECTIVES

Once you have completed Unit 21, you should be able to do the following:

- understand the meaning of medical words relating to pharmacology and microbiology

- deduce the use or action of drugs from their classification

- understand common medical abbreviations associated with pharmacology and microbiology

EXERCISE GUIDE

Use this list of word components and their meanings to complete the word exercises in this unit.

Prefixes

a-	without
an-	without
anti-	against
dia-	through
neo-	new
oxy-	quick
retro-	back/backward

Roots / Combining forms

acid/o	acid
aem-	blood (Am. -em)
aesthet/o	sensation/sensitivity (Am. esthet/o)
anxi/o	anxiety
alges/i/o	sense of pain
bacill/o	bacillus/bacilli
bacteri/o	bacterium/bacteria
bio-	life/living
bronch/i/o	bronchus / bronchial tubes
cocc/o	coccus/cocci
cycl/o	ciliary body
cyt/o	cell
dynam/o	force/power (of movement)
em- (Am.)	blood
epilept/o	epilepsy

esthet/o (Am.)	sensation/sensitivity
estr/o (Am.)	estrogen/estrus
fibrin/o	fibrin (a protein that forms the fibres of blood clots)
fung/i/o	fungus
gonad/o	gonads / reproductive organs
haem/o	blood (Am. hem/o)
hem/o (Am.)	blood
helmint/h/o	worms
hypn/o	sleep
immun/o	immune/immunity
kerat/o	epidermis/cornea
kinet/o	motion/movement
lact/i/o	milk
muc/o	mucus
oestr/o	oestrogen/oestrus (Am. estr/o)
pharmac/o	drug
plas/m/o	growth
prurit/o	itching
psych/o	mind
(r)rhythm/o	rhythm
septic/o	sepsis/infection
staphylococc/o	staphylococcus/staphylococci
spasm/o/d	spasm
spirill/o	spirillum/spirilla
streptococc/o	streptococcus/streptococci

thyroid/o	thyroid	**-in**	nonspecific suffix indicating a chemical
toc/o	labour/birth (Am. labor)	**-ine**	substance thought to be derived from
tox/ic/o	poison / poisonous to		ammonia
troph/o	nourish/stimulate	**-ist**	specialist
tuss/i	cough	**-ite**	end product
ur/o	urine	**-ity**	state/condition
vir/o	virus/virion	**-ive**	pertaining to / type of drug
		-logist	specialist who studies
		-logy	study of
Suffixes		**-lytic**	drug that breaks down… / pertaining to
			breakdown
-aemia	condition of blood (Am. -emia)	**-oid**	resembling
-al	pertaining to / type of drug	**-ose**	carbohydrate/sugar/starch
-ase	an enzyme	**-osis**	abnormal condition/disease of
-cidal	pertaining to killing or destroying	**-plegic**	drug that paralyses / condition of paralysis
-cide	agent that kills or destroys / killing	**-rrhea (Am.)**	excessive discharge/flow
-emia (Am.)	condition of blood	**-rrhoea**	excessive discharge/flow (Am. -rrhea)
-form	having the form/structure of	**-static**	pertaining to stopping / agent that stops
-gen	precursor / agent that produces	**-tic**	pertaining to/type of drug, equivalent to -ic
-gnosy	process of judgment/knowledge	**-uria**	condition of urine
-ia	condition of	**-y**	process/condition
-ic	type of drug / pertaining to		

Pharmacology

Pharmacology is the science that deals with the study of drugs. By drugs we mean medicinal substances that can be used to treat, prevent or diagnose disease and illness. Research into the properties and potential use of substances showing physiological activity has enabled the pharmaceutical industry to market new and more effective drugs.

 Root

Pharmac

(*From a Greek word* **pharmakon**, *meaning drug.*)

Combining form   Pharmac/o

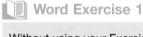 **Word Exercise 1**

Without using your Exercise Guide write the meaning of:

(a) **pharmac/o**/logy

(b) **pharmac/o**/log/ist

(c) **pharmac/o**/psych/osis

There are several specialisms related to pharmacology including:

Chemotherapy

the treatment of disease using chemical agents (a main type of treatment for cancer).

Pharmacoepidemiology

The study of the uses and effects of drugs on well-defined populations.

Pharmacodynamics

the study of the action of drugs, ie, what the drug does to the body.

Pharmacoeconomics

The study of the cost and effectiveness of drug treatments.

Pharmacognosy

the study of (*gnos-* knowledge of) crude drugs of vegetable and animal origin.

Pharmacokinetics

the study of the way drugs are absorbed, metabolized and excreted, ie, what the body does to the drug and how it moves through the body.

Pharmacy

the study of the process of preparing and dispensing medicinal drugs or a place where drugs are compounded or dispensed by a pharmacist.

Therapeutics

the branch of medicine that deals with the treatment of disease. Treatment can be **palliative**, ie, alleviates symptoms, or **curative**. In common usage, therapeutics refers mainly to the use of drugs to treat disease.

Toxicology
the study of poisons and other toxic substances and their effect on the body.

Naming drugs

Drugs are known by several different names.

1. The brand, trade or proprietary name
Following extensive research and development, pharmaceutical companies assign brand names to their products for marketing purposes. Each drug and its name are the exclusive property of the company with patent rights to its manufacture. The patent will expire after a fixed time (usually 20 years) allowing time for development costs to be recouped. When the patent expires, other companies may manufacture the drug under different brand names or under the drug's generic name.

2. The generic name
Each drug has an official generic name or nonproprietary name. This name is assigned to it in its early stage of development and is often a description of its chemical composition or class. Once the patent expires, any number of companies may manufacture a generic drug under different brand names.

3. International Nonproprietary Name (INN)
International Nonproprietary Names identify pharmaceutical substances or active pharmaceutical ingredients. The existence of this international nomenclature for pharmaceutical substances is important for the clear identification, safe prescription and dispensing of medicines to patients, and for communication and exchange of information among health professionals and scientists worldwide. An European Economic Community directive requires the use INNs and many British Approved Names (BANs) have been changed or modified to comply with the directive.

4. The chemical name
This is the scientific name based on the molecular structure of the drug, and it describes the chemical nature of each compound. A new drug is given a chemical name by the IUPAC (International Union of Pure and Applied Chemists); this can be long and complicated and is almost never used to identify the drug in a clinical or marketing situation.

Here is an example of how a commonly used analgesic drug is named:

Brand name or proprietary name	Panadol
Generic name	Paracetamol (Am. Acetaminophen)
International Nonproprietary Name	Paracetamol
Chemical name (IUPAC name)	N- (4-hydroxyphenyl)acetamide

Authoritative information about the use, structure, manufacture and the dosage of medicinal drugs is documented in large reference texts known as *pharmacopoeias*.

Product information on drugs is available to prescribers and pharmacists in a book known as a National Formulary, for example, the BNF, *British National Formulary*.

In pharmacology, certain suffixes are used to denote types of substance, eg:

Suffix	Meaning	Examples
-ase	indicates an enzyme	amy**lase**/sucr**ase**
-gen	a precursor or agent that produces or affects something	trypsino**gen**
-ic	denotes a type of medicinal drug	mucoly**tic**
-in	a nonspecific suffix denoting a chemical agent	trister**in**
-ine	a substance derived from ammonia	am**ine**/alan**ine**
-ite	a substance produced through a chemical process	metabo**lite**
-one	a hormone	cortis**one**
-ose	a type of sugar	gluc**ose**/malt**ose**

Word Exercise 2

Match each description from Column C with a biochemical name in Column A by inserting the appropriate number in Column B.

Column A	Column B	Column C
(a) lip/ase		1. a sugar
(b) rib/ose		2. a chemical agent
(c) ser/ine		3. a hormone
(d) progesto/gen		4. a medicinal drug
(e) analges/ic		5. a chemical related to ammonia
(f) aldoster/one		6. an enzyme
(g) niac/in		7. a precursor

Drug classification

Drugs can be classified by their therapeutic use or action. Exercises 3 to 14 list the classifications of drugs used to treat disorders associated with the body systems we have studied in this book.

Note. The suffixes -al, -ant, -ent, -ic and -ive are used to mean *pertaining to*, but they are also used in pharmacology to indicate a type of drug.

The action of a drug can often be deduced from its classification. To do this, we split the word classification into its components, find their meaning and then try to deduce an action or use. The technique can be practised in Word Exercises 3 to 14.

 Word Exercise 3

Many classifications have the prefix **anti-** meaning against. Using your Exercise Guide write the meaning of:

(a) **anti**/bacter/i/al _____

(b) **anti**/bio/tic _____

(c) **anti**/fung/al _____

(d) **anti**/vir/al _____

In the following examples the *i* of the prefix **anti-** is dropped for roots beginning with a vowel or the letter *h*.

(e) **ant**/acid _____

(f) **ant**/helmint/ic _____

 Word Exercise 4

Several drug classifications have the prefix **an-** meaning without. Using your Exercise Guide write the meaning of:

(a) **an**/alges/ic _____

(b) **an**/aesthet/ic
(Am. an/esthet/ic) _____

Word Exercises 5 to 14 list common types of drug associated with the systems studied in this book.

Drug classifications associated with the digestive system

 Word Exercise 5

Without using your Exercise Guide write the meaning of:

(a) anti/diarrhoe/al
(Am. antidiarrheal) _____

(b) anti/spasmod/ic
(acts on intestines) _____

Others include:

Aperient

a type of drug that promotes evacuation of the bowels, a laxative.

H₂–receptor antagonist

a type of drug that prevents the secretion of acid by the gastric mucosa (lining of the stomach) and promotes the healing of ulcers.

Laxative

promotes evacuation of the bowels.

Drug classifications associated with the respiratory system

 Word Exercise 6

Using your Exercise Guide write the meaning of:

(a) muc/o/lyt/ic _____

(b) anti/tuss/ive _____

(c) bronch/o/dilat/or
(dilate means to widen, not listed in the Exercise Guide) _____

Others include:

Antihistamine

a type of drug that counteracts the effects of histamine, a chemical that is released during allergic reactions such as asthma.

Corticosteroid

a type of drug that reduces inflammation. Corticosteroids are used for prophylaxis in the treatment of asthma by reducing inflammation in the bronchial mucosa (lining).

Decongestant

a type of drug that reduces the feeling of congestion in the nose.

Expectorant

an agent that promotes the coughing up of mucus from the lungs and bronchi.

Drug classifications associated with the cardiovascular system and blood

 Word Exercise 7

Using your Exercise Guide write the meaning of:

(a) fibrin/o/lyt/ic

(b) anti/fibrin/o/lyt/ic

(c) anti-/a/rrhythm/ic

(d) haem/o/stat/ic
(Am. hem/o/stat/ic)

Others include:

Anticoagulant

a type of drug that prevents clotting/coagulation of blood.

Antihypertensive

a type of drug that reduces high blood pressure. Antihypertensives are used to treat hypertension (high blood pressure).

Antiplatelet drug

a type of drug that decreases platelet aggregation in arteries, thereby inhibiting clot formation.

Beta-blocker

A type of drug that decreases heart activity by blocking the actions of hormones such as adrenalin; beta-blockers are used to treat angina, heart failure and high blood pressure.

Diuretic

a type of drug that promotes the excretion of urine, thereby relieving the oedema (Am. edema) of heart failure.

Inotropic

a type of drug used to increase or decrease the force of contraction of heart muscle (myocardium).

Sympathomimetic

a type of drug that mimics the action of the sympathetic nervous system; sympathomimetics are used to raise blood pressure.

Drug classifications associated with the urinary system

Antidiuretic hormone

a hormone that acts on the kidney stimulating reabsorption of water, thereby reducing the formation of urine.

Diuretic

a type of drug that promotes the excretion of urine.

Uricosuric

a type of drug that increases the excretion of uric acid in urine, thereby relieving the symptoms of gout.

Xanthine-oxidase inhibitor

a type of drug used for the palliative treatment of gout.

Drug classifications associated with the nervous system

 Word Exercise 8

Using your Exercise Guide write the meaning of:

(a) hypn/o/tic

(b) anxi/o/lyt/ic

(c) anti/epilep/tic

(d) anti/psych/o/tic

Others include:

Antidepressant

a type of drug that prevents or relieves depression.

Antiemetic

a type of drug that prevents vomiting (emesis).

CNS stimulant

a type of drug that has limited use for treating narcolepsy (a recurrent, uncontrollable desire to sleep).

Opioid analgesic

a type of drug that relieves moderate to severe pain particularly of visceral origin (opioid refers to a synthetic narcotic resembling but not derived from opium).

Drug classifications associated with the eye

Word Exercise 9

Using your Exercise Guide write the meaning of:

(a) cycl/o/pleg/ic

Others include:

Eye lotion

a solution used for irrigating the eye.

Local anaesthetic (Am. anesthetic)

a type of drug that reduces sensation in the eye.

Miotic

a type of drug used to treat glaucoma that narrows the pupil.

Mydriatic

a type of drug that dilates the pupil for eye examination.

Topical antiinfective preparation

an antibacterial, antifungal or antiviral agent that is applied directly to the eye.

Topical corticosteroid

an antiinflammatory steroid that is applied directly to the eye.

Drug classifications associated with the ear

Topical antiinfective preparation

an antibacterial or antifungal applied directly to the external ear for treatment of otitis externa.

Topical astringent

a type of drug used to treat inflammation that dries tissue.

Drug classifications associated with the mouth and nose

Oral antihistamine

a type of drug that reduces the symptoms of histamine; it is used for treatment of nasal allergy.

Systemic nasal decongestant

a type of drug used for symptomatic relief in chronic nasal congestion.

Topical decongestant

a type of drug applied directly to the nose as drops or spray to relieve congestion.

Drug classifications associated with the skin

Word Exercise 10

Using your Exercise Guide write the meaning of:

(a) anti/prurit/ic

(b) kerat/o/lyt/ic

Others include:

Antiseptic

an agent that prevents sepsis; it inhibits the growth of micro-organisms but does not necessarily kill them.

Desloughing agent

an agent that removes dead tissue from a wound.

Emollient

an agent that softens or soothes the skin.

Vehicle

an inert substance added to a drug that gives it a suitable consistency for transfer into the body; vehicles do not possess therapeutic properties.

Drug classifications associated with the musculoskeletal system

Nonsteroidal antiinflammatory drug (NSAID)

a type of drug that in full dose has analgesic and antiinflammatory effects. NSAIDs are used to treat painful inflammatory conditions such as rheumatic disease; aspirin is a familiar example.

Relaxant

a type of drug that blocks the neuromuscular junction and produces relaxation of muscles; they are widely used in anaesthesia.

Uricosuric

a type of drug that promotes the excretion of uric acid in the urine, thereby relieving the symptoms of gout.

Drug classifications associated with the reproductive system

 Word Exercise 11

Using your Exercise Guide write the meaning of:

(a) oxy/toc/ic

(b) gonad/o/trop/in

Without using your Exercise Guide write the meaning of:

(c) anti-/oestr/o/gen
    (Am. anti-/estr/o/gen)

Others include:

Oral contraceptive

a type of drug that prevents conception, ie, the fertilization of an egg by a sperm. Family planning pills contain sex hormones that inhibit the release of eggs from the ovary, thereby preventing a pregnancy.

Prostaglandin

a type of drug used to induce abortion, augment labour and minimize blood loss from the placental site.

Sex hormone

a type of hormone used for hormone replacement therapy (HRT). In women, small doses of the female sex hormone oestrogen are used to relieve menopausal symptoms. In castrated males, sex hormones called androgens are used for replacement therapy.

Drug classifications associated with the endocrine system

(This section deals with examples of drug classifications other than those that act on the reproductive system.)

 Word Exercise 12

Without using your Exercise Guide write the meaning of:

(a) anti/thyroid

Others include:

Antidiabetic

a drug that is used to treat non-insulin-dependent diabetes; it acts against diabetes by increasing insulin secretion.

Corticosteroid

a steroid produced by the adrenal cortex or its synthetic equivalent used for replacement therapy. Corticosteroids are used when secretion by the adrenal glands is insufficient.

Human growth hormone

a growth hormone of human origin (somatotrophin) used to stimulate growth in patients of short stature. This has been replaced by somatotropin, a biosynthetic human growth hormone that has a similar effect.

Insulin

insulin is a hormone that lowers blood glucose in patients with diabetes mellitus. Many different forms of insulin, eg, short-, intermediate- and long-acting are available for injection.

Drug classifications associated with oncology

Drugs used in oncology aim to prevent the replication of cancer cells and destroy them by interfering with their metabolism. The process of using drugs in this way to destroy tumours is called **chemotherapy**.

 Word Exercise 13

Using your Exercise Guide write the meaning of:

(a) cyt/o/tox/ic

(b) anti/neo/plas/t/ic

Others include:

Alkylating drugs

drugs that damage DNA (genes) and interfere with the replication of cancer cells.

Antimetabolite

a drug that combines with and inhibits vital cell enzymes.

Vinca alkaloids

drugs originally derived from the plant species *Vinca* that have the ability to directly interrupt the process of cell division.

Drug classifications associated with the immune system

Drugs can be used to stimulate or suppress the activity of the immune system. The system needs to be suppressed to prevent rejection of transplanted organs in their recipients. These drugs are also used to treat autoimmune disease (*auto-* meaning self; **autoimmunity** is an abnormal response of the immune system to the body's own tissues).

 Word Exercise 14

Without using your Exercise Guide write the meaning of:

(a) immun/o/suppress/ant
(suppress means
prevent/stop)

(b) immun/o/stimul/ant
(stimul- means speed
up or increase)

(c) cyt/o/toxic immun/o/
suppress/ant

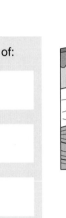

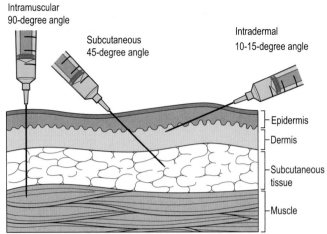

Routes of drug administration

Drugs are administered to the body via many different routes. The choice of route usually depends on pharmacokinetics, which is the way a drug is absorbed, metabolized and excreted as well as its effect. The table below shows the main routes through which a substance is administered into the body. Figure 123 shows examples of the parenteral route of drug administration.

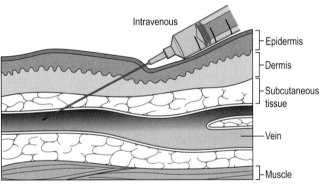

Figure 123 Examples of the parenteral route of drug administration. (Adapted from Weller BF, Bailliere's Nurses Dictionary, 26th edition, 2014, Ballière Tindall.)

Topical Route	Here a drug is applied directly to where its action is required. Examples include:	
Route	*Application*	*Example of the Form of Dosage*
Cutaneous	On to the skin	Local anaesthetic (Am. anesthetic) as an ointment, spray, or liquid
Inhalation	Into the lungs	Asthma medication as an aerosol from a metered-dose inhaler
Ophthalmic	On to the conjunctiva	Antibiotic eye drops
Otic	Into the external ear	Antibiotic ear drops or corticosteroids
Vaginal	Into the vagina	Suppository, a solid medicinal preparation that dissolves in the vagina

Enteral route	Enteral means pertaining to the intestine, but in practice it involves administration into any part of the gastrointestinal tract; the drugs have a systemic effect. Examples include:	
Route	*Application*	*Example of the Form of Dosage*
Oral	By mouth	Tablets, capsules, liquids or drops

Buccal	Between gums and cheek	Orally disintegrating tablet, thin-film drug delivery, lozenges, oral spray
Rectal	Via the anus and rectum	Suppository or enema
Sublingual	Under the tongue	Orally disintegrating tablet, thin-film drug delivery, lozenges, oral spray

Parenteral route	Here a drug is administered in a way other than through the gastrointestinal system, usually by injection. Examples include:	
Route	*Application*	*Example of the Form of Dosage*
Intraarterial	Into an artery	Liquid containing a drug
Intraarticular	Into a joint	Liquid antibiotics and corticosteroids
Intradermal	Into the skin	Liquid such as a vaccine
Intramuscular	Into a muscle	Liquid containing a drug

Intrathecal	Into the space around the spinal cord	Antibiotic in liquid form or analgesic liquid from a spinal 'pain' pump
Intravenous	Into a vein	Liquid containing a drug or nutrients
Subcutaneous	Under the skin	Liquid containing a drug

Abbreviations

Some common abbreviations related to drug administration are listed next. Note that some are not standard, and their meaning may vary from one healthcare setting to another. There is a more extensive list for reference on page 369.

a.c.	before food (ante cibum)
b.d.s.	twice a day (bis die sumendum)
cap., caps, capsul.	capsule
disp.	dispense
IM, i/m	intramuscular
IV, i/v	intravenous
o.m.	every morning (omni mane)
OTC	over the counter (nonprescription drugs)
PCA	patient-controlled analgesia
p.c.	after meals (post cibum)
p.r.n.	when required (pro re nata)
PV	per vagina
q.d.s.	four times a day (quater die sumendum)
Rx	prescription, recipe
tab	tablet
t.d.s.	three times a day (ter die sumendum)
ung.	ointment, unguentum

Microbiology

Microbiology is the study of small organisms (*micro-* small, *bio-* life, *logy-* study of). In the field of health, pathogenic microorganisms such as bacteria, protozoa, fungi and viruses are responsible for infectious disease. Swabs, fluids and tissues taken from patients suspected of having an infection are sent to the microbiology laboratories for analysis. The microbiology laboratory is often part of the pathology department in a large hospital. This section examines words associated with microorganisms.

Microbiology is divided into the following specialties:

Bacteriology	study of bacteria
Mycology	study of fungi
Virology	study of viruses
Protozoology	the study of protozoa (single-celled animals)

Naming microorganisms

Species of microorganisms are given Latin names according to the binomial (two name) system. The first name denotes the group or **genus** to which the organism belongs and always begins with a capital letter. The second name is the **species** or specific name, and this begins with a lower case letter, eg:

> *Salmonella typhi*: *Salmonella* is the genus, *typhi* the species.
> *Clostridium tetani*: *Clostridium* is the genus, *tetani* the species.

Often the name of the genus is abbreviated if it is widely used, as in *E. coli* for *Escherichia coli* and *Staph. aureus* for *Staphylococcus aureus*.

The species name of microorganisms is sometimes formed from words that indicate:

their colour	eg, *Staphylococcus aureus* (from aurum, meaning gold)
the place where they are found	eg, *Staphylococcus epidermidis* (in the epidermis of the skin)
the disease they cause	eg, *Bacillus anthracis* (causes anthrax)
the scientist who studied or named them	eg, *Escherichia coli* (after Dr Theodor Escherich, German physician, 1857–1911)

Bacteriology

Bacteria are small single-celled organisms that can only be seen with an optical microscope. There are thousands of different types classified according to their shape, group arrangement, colony characteristics, structure and chemical characteristics. The combining form **bacteri/o** is used to mean bacteria in general (from Greek *bakte-rion* meaning staff).

Classification of bacteria using the Gram staining reaction

For more than a century, bacteria have been classified using the **Gram** staining reaction, named after Christian Gram who devised it in 1884. His method is based upon the ability of bacteria to retain the purple crystal violet–iodine complex when stained and treated with organic solvents:

> **Gram-positive bacteria** (Gram +ve) retain the stain and appear purple.
> **Gram-negative bacteria** (Gram −ve) cannot retain the purple dye complex and need to be stained with a red dye before they can be seen with an optical microscope.

Classification by shape and grouping

Individual bacteria have one of three basic shapes: they are either spherical, cylindrical or spiral. Spherical cells are called **cocci** (singular **coccus**), cylindrical cells **bacilli** (singular **bacillus**) and helical or spiral cells **spirilla** (singular **spirillum**).

The coccus (plural cocci). The word coccus comes from a Greek word *kokkos* meaning berry. They are usually round but can be ovoid or flattened on one side when adhering to another cell. Cocci can grow in several different arrangements or groups depending on the plane of cell division and whether the new cells remain together. Each arrangement is typical of a species and contributes to an organism's classification. When a coccus divides in one plane and the two new cells remain together, the arrangement is called a **diplococcus**.

When cocci divide repeatedly in one plane and remain together to form a twisted row of cells, they are called **streptococci** (*strepto-* from a Greek word meaning twisted, singular strep-tococcus). Others divide in three planes and remain together in irregular, grape-like patterns; these are called **staphylococci** (*staphylo-* from a Greek word meaning grapes, singular staphy-lococcus). See Figure 124(a) to (d) for examples:

Some cocci are of great medical importance, eg:

Gram +ve

Streptococcus pneumoniae causes pneumonia and meningitis.
Staphylococcus aureus causes serious infection in hospitals (MRSA, methicillin-resistant *Staphylococcus aureus*).

Gram −ve

Neisseria gonorrhoeae causes gonorrhoea.
Neisseria meningitidis causes meningitis.
(*Neisseria* are sometimes seen in pairs and are grouped as diplococci.)

The bacillus (plural bacilli). These are rod-shaped bacteria (*bacillus* is a Latin word meaning a stick or rod); they are also classified using the Gram staining procedure (see Fig. 124(e)). There are large differences in the length and width of bacilli, and their ends can be square, rounded or tapered.

Some bacilli are of medical importance, eg:

Gram +ve

Bacillus anthracis causes anthrax. It produces highly resistant spores that are difficult to destroy except at high temperatures.
Clostridium tetani, found in soil, causes tetanus.

Gram −ve

Escherichia coli is found in the human gut; certain strains are pathogenic.
Salmonella typhi causes typhoid.

Gram-negative bacilli that appear curved in shape (like a comma) are called vibrios (see Fig. 124(f)), eg:

Vibrio cholerae causes cholera, a water-borne infection.

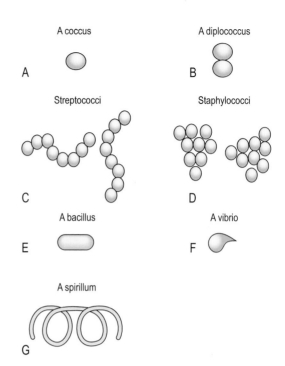

Figure 124   Shapes and group arrangements of bacteria. (a) a coccus (b) a diplococcus (c) streptococci (d) staphylococci (e) a bacillus (f) a vibrio (g) a spirillum.

The spirillum (plural spirilla). The spirilla are spiral or helical-shaped bacteria that look like tiny corkscrews (see Fig. 124(g)). Those that belong to the genus *Spirillum* consist of Gram −ve, non-flexuous (nonflexible), spiral-shaped filaments. Another group distinguished by their flexibility belongs to the genus *Spirochaeta.* (Note: the use of this group is becoming obsolete, and most of the bacteria assigned to this group have been transferred to other genera.) Examples are:

Spirillum minus causes rat-bite fever in man.
Treponema pallidum is a spirochaete (Am. spirochete) that belongs to the order *Spirochaetales* and causes syphilis.

It should be noted that the cells of a given species are rarely arranged in exactly the same pattern. It is the predominant arrangement that is important when studying bacteria.

Some terms denoting shape, for example bacillus, may be used as generic names as in *Bacillus anthracis.*

Culture and sensitivity testing

Infected swabs, fluids and tissues are sent to microbiology laboratories for **culture and sensitivity testing**. To culture an organism, it is placed at an optimum temperature in a special culture medium (broth or agar jelly) that contains all the nutrients required for growth. In ideal conditions the microorganism multiplies rapidly, producing a huge clone of identical cells. Samples from the culture are then exposed to a range of different antibiotics. If an organism is sensitive to a particular antibiotic, it will be destroyed or its growth inhibited. Antibiotics that are found to destroy the cultured organisms are administered to the patient to try and rid them of the infection.

Word Exercise 15

Match a bacterium in Column C with a description in Column A by inserting a number in Column B.

Column A	Column B	Column C
(a) A bacterium that appears rod-shaped and purple following staining with the Gram staining procedure		1. diplococci
(b) A rod that appears comma-shaped and pink following staining with the Gram staining procedure		2. Staphylococcus aureus
(c) Cocci arranged into a twisted chain that infects the lungs		3. Gram –ve Vibrio cholerae
(d) Gold-coloured cocci arranged into irregular grape-like groups that cause serious suppurative infections, sometimes resistant to common antibiotics		4. Gram –ve E. coli
(e) Cocci belonging to the genus Neisseria that arrange themselves into pairs		5. Gram +ve Bacillus anthracis
(f) A helical bacterium that causes syphilis		6. Streptococcus pneumoniae
(g) A bacterium that appears rod-shaped and pink following staining with the Gram procedure		7. Treponema pallidum (a spirochaete)

Word Exercise 16

Using your Exercise Guide write the meaning of:

(a) **bacteri/o**/log/ist

(b) **streptococc**/al

(c) **bacteri**/ur/ia

(d) **bacteri**/cid/al

(e) **bacteri/o**/stat/ic

(f) **bacteri/o**/lyt/ic

(g) **bacill**/aem/ia (Am. **bacill**/em/ia)

(h) **strept/o**/septic/aem/ia (Am. **strept/o**/septic/em/ia)

(i) **spirill**/osis

Mycology

Fungi are non-green plants that act as decomposers in the environment, breaking down the dead bodies of plants and animals. The group includes the familiar mushrooms and toadstools and microscopic moulds and yeasts.

Certain types of moulds and yeasts are pathogenic and infect the body, causing disease. When they infect the skin, they are called **dermatophytes** (dermat/o meaning skin, -phyte meaning plant). A common condition is Athlete's foot caused by several species of fungi (eg, Tri-chophyton rubrum) that infect skin between the toes. In warm, moist conditions the fungi grow and digest the skin causing it to itch and split. The fungal spores that generate the infection are usually picked up on changing room floors, so the condition is common among sports enthusiasts. Athlete's foot is easily treated and harmless, unlike some fungal infections found in tropical climates.

When round, red patches of skin infected with fungi begin to heal in the centre first, they often take on a ring-like appearance, and because of this the infection became inaccurately known as 'ringworm'. The medical name for Athlete's foot is **Tinea pedis** or ringworm of the foot (Tinea is a Latin word meaning gnawing worm, and -pedis means the foot). Other superficial fungal infections of the skin are named in a similar way: **Tinea capitis** (ringworm of the head), **Tinea corporis** (ringworm of the body).

Fungal infections are life-threatening in patients whose immune system is compromised; for example, Candida albicans can cause serious infections of the mouth, digestive system and reproductive systems in AIDS patients. This type of infection is known as **candidiasis** (from Latin *candidus* meaning white and *-iasis* meaning abnormal condition).

Fungi are named according to the binomial system with a generic and specific name, as in *Candida albicans*.

Root

Myc

(*From a Greek word* **mykes**, *meaning fungus.*)

Combining forms   Myc/o

 Word Exercise 17

Without using your Exercise Guide, write the meaning of:

(a) **myc**/osis

(b) **mycot**/ic

(c) **myc**/o/**tox**/in

(d) **myc**/o/**toxic**/osis

Root

Fung

(*From a Greek word* **fungus**, *meaning mushroom. Here fung/i/o means fungus or fungal infection.*)

Combining forms   Fung/i/o, fungos-

 Word Exercise 18

Without using your Exercise Guide, write the meaning of:

(a) **fung**/i/form

(b) **fung**/i/tox/ic

(c) **fung**/i/cide

(d) **fung**/i/stat/ic

Using your Exercise Guide, find the meaning of:

(e) **fung**/oid

(f) **fungos**/ity

Virology

A virus (virion) is an extremely small infectious particle that does not show the usual characteristics of life; for example, it does not move, respire, feed or respond to stimuli.

Viruses do reproduce but only within a specific host cell. (Note: a host is an organism that harbours a parasite.) When a virus comes into contact with a host cell, it inserts its genes into the cell. Once inside the viral genes alter the metabolism of the host cell and instruct it to make new viruses. The host cell fills with copies of the original virus and may burst, releasing the new infectious particles into the surrounding environment.

Viruses have characteristic shapes, different chemical structures and different methods of replication. They can only be seen in an electron microscope that produces a large magnification and has the ability to resolve their fine detail. Characteristics of viruses and the conditions they cause are incorporated into their common names. In the examples given next, the words have been split to show their meaning.

Onco/rna/virus

type of virus that causes cancer (onc/o) and contains ribonucleic acid (-rna-).

Pico/rna/virus

type of virus that is very small (pico-) and contains ribonucleic acid (-rna-).

Retro/virus

type of virus that carries the enzyme reverse transcriptase (retro means back, the enzyme converts viral RNA back to DNA).

Rhino/virus

type of virus that infects the nose (rhin/o means nose).

Entero/virus

type of virus that infects the intestines.

Bacterio/phage

type of virus that uses a bacterium as a host.

Viruses are responsible for many serious infectious diseases including smallpox, measles, influenza, poliomyelitis, ebola and AIDS.

Note there are several complex scientific systems of virus classification in use, but they are not relevant to our study of common medical terms and have been omitted.

Root

Vir

(*From a Greek word* **virus**, *meaning poison. Here vir/o means virus, a minute infectious particle that replicates only within a living host cell.*)

Combining forms   Vir/o/u

Word Exercise 19

Without using your Exercise Guide, write the meaning of:

(a) **vir/u**/cide

(b) **vir/o**/log/ist

(c) anti/retr/o/**vir**/al

(d) **vir**/ur/ia

Using your Exercise Guide, find the meaning of:

(e) **vir**/aem/ia
(Am. **vir**/em/ia)

(f) **vir/o**/lact/ia

Protozoology

This is a branch of medicine concerned with single-celled animals called protozoa. Some of these organisms are pathogenic parasites responsible for serious disease. Infection with protozoa is generally referred to as a **protozo**iasis (-*iasis* meaning abnormal condition of and in this case infection with protozoa). Examples are given next:

Plasmodium falciparum
(a type of sporozoan) that causes malaria.
Trypanosoma gambiense
(a type of flagellate) that causes African sleeping sickness.
Entamoeba histolytica
(a type of amoeba) that causes amoebic (Am. amebic) dysentery.

Note:

Aetiology (Am. **etiology**) is the study or science of the cause of disease.
Epidemiology is the study of how often diseases occur in different groups of people and why.
Public health officials use epidemiological information to plan and evaluate strategies to prevent illness in particular populations and to manage patients in whom disease has already developed.

CASE HISTORY 21

The object of this exercise is to understand words associated with a patient's medical history. To complete the exercise:

* Read through the passage on HIV infection; unfamiliar words are underlined, and you can find their meaning using the Word Help.

* Write the meaning of the medical terms shown in bold print on the lines that follow the Word Help.

HIV infection

Mr U, a 38-year-old homosexual man, presented to the Accident and Emergency Department with a fever, nonproductive cough and dyspnoea (Am. dyspnea). During the previous 7 days, he had become increasingly short of breath and complained of an inability to sleep because he was hot and sweating profusely. He was a nonsmoker and had no haemoptysis (Am. hemoptysis). Mr U informed the medical staff that he had been diagnosed HIV positive 3 years earlier but had declined **antiretroviral** therapy.

On examination, he appeared pale and thin, and he indicated that he had lost a considerable amount of weight over the past 2 months. He was pyrexial (Temp. 39.1°C), tachycardic (121 beats/min) and tachypnoeic (Am. tachypneic) (28 breaths/min).

Examination of his mouth revealed white patches with surrounding inflammation indicative of a severe **candidiasis**; swabs were taken and sent for analysis. He was short of breath with poor lung expansion, and a chest X-ray showed diffuse bilateral shading. His serum biochemistry and liver function were normal.

Mr U was admitted to the ward with a clinical diagnosis of PCP or other atypical pneumonia and started on the **antibacterial** co-trimoxazole (trimethoprim-sulfamethoxazole, TMP-SMX) in two daily doses and the **antibiotic** azithromycin given as an infusion over 1 hour. He was also given an intravenous steroid methylprednisolone to reduce inflammation in his alveoli and improve gaseous exchange.

The next day a bronchoscopy was performed, and the washings were sent to the **microbiology** laboratory for culture and sensitivity testing. The results confirmed the diagnosis of *Pneumocystis carinii* infection, and haematology reported a CD4 count of less than 50 cells mm^{-3}, indicating Mr U had developed AIDS. His mouth infection was confirmed as *Candida albicans*, and he was prescribed the **antifungal** itraconazole.

Following administration of his high dose of co-trimoxazole, Mr U developed severe nausea and was given the **antiemetic** metoclopramide parenterally before his infusions.

Two weeks later, he was clinically much improved, and a **pharmaceutical plan** was devised prior to his discharge. He was advised that he required antiretroviral therapy and counselled on the possibility of side effects. He was given a discharge medication of sufficient oral co-trimoxazole to complete his initial course of treatment and instructed on a prophylactic dose regimen.

Word Help

AIDS acquired immune deficiency syndrome

atypical not conforming to the usual type, in microbiology applied to strains of unusual type

bilateral pertaining to both sides

bronchoscopy technique of viewing/examining the bronchial tree

Candida albicans a yeast-like fungus belonging to the genus *Candida* that infects the digestive and reproductive systems

CD4 cluster designation/cluster of differentiation. Refers to clusters of chemicals (cell surface markers) found on the surface of leucocytes (Am. leukocytes). CD4 molecules found on lymphocytes called Helper T-cells act as the receptor molecules for HIV. The depletion of CD4 lympho-cytes by HIV leads to the development of AIDS

culture and sensitivity testing growing microorganisms in the laboratory and testing them for sensitivity to antibiotics

dyspnoea difficult/laboured breathing (Am. dyspnea)

haemoptysis spitting/coughing up of blood (Am. hemoptysis)

HIV human immunodeficiency virus

HIV positive presence of antibodies to the human immu-nodeficiency virus in the blood; it indicates the virus has infected the body

infusion slow introduction of a therapeutic agent into a vein

nonproductive not producing (sputum)

parenterally the word means pertaining to beyond the intestine, but in practice it refers to administering a drug in a way other than through the gastrointestinal system, eg, by injection

PCP *Pneumocystis carinii* pneumonia

Pneumocystis carinii a protozoa-like organism that causes pneumonia, an opportunistic infection commonly seen in AIDS patients

prophylactic pertaining to preventative treatment

pyrexial having a fever/elevation of body temperature above normal

regimen a regulated scheme (eg, of taking drugs/ medication)

tachycardic pertaining to a fast heart beat

tachypnoeic pertaining to fast breathing (Am. tachypneic)

washing a solution that has contacted a surface and is to be used for analysis

---

Now write the meaning of the following words from the case study without using your dictionary lists:

(a) antiretroviral

(b) candidiasis

(c) antibacterial

(d) antibiotic

(e) microbiology

(f) antifungal

(g) antiemetic

(h) pharmaceutical plan

(Answers to the Case History exercise are given in the Answers to Word Exercises beginning on page 358.)

Quick Reference

Combining forms relating to the pharmacology and microbiology:

cocc/o	coccus (a berry-shaped bacterium)
bacill/o	bacillus (a rod-like bacterium)
bacteri/o	bacterium/bacteria
fung/i	fungus
helmint/h/o	worm
myc/o	fungus
pharmac/o	drug
spirill/o	a spiral-shaped bacterium of genus *Spirillum*
staphylococc/o	staphylococcus / a bunch of cocci
streptococc/o	streptococcus / a chain of cocci
toxic/o	poison
vibri/o	a comma-shaped bacterium of genus Vibrio
vir/o/u	virus/virion

Abbreviations

Some common abbreviations related to microbiology and infectious disease are listed next. Note that some are not standard, and their meaning may vary from one healthcare setting to another. There is a more extensive list for refer-ence on page 369.

ABX	antibiotics
AFB	acid-fast bacilli
AMR	antimicrobial resistance
BCG	bacille (bacillus) Calmette-Guérin (causes tuberculosis)
BET	bacterial endotoxin test
C + S	culture and sensitivity test
EBV	Epstein-Barr virus
GNC	Gram-negative coccus

GPC	Gram-positive coccus
HBV	hepatitis B virus
Hib	*Haemophilus influenzae* type b
HIV	human immunodeficiency virus
HSV	Herpes simplex virus
MRSA	methicillin-resistant S. aureus
NGU	non-gonococcal urethritis
PCN	penicillin

Associated words

Aerobe an organism that lives and grows in the presence of oxygen

Anaerobe an organism that lives and grows in the absence of oxygen

Aseptic pertaining to free from microorganisms

Colony a visible cluster of microorganisms growing on a solid growth medium such as agar

Communicable of infectious disease, able to be transmitted to someone else

Contagion the transmission of infection by direct or indirect contact; an infectious disease

Culture the propagation of microorganisms in a nutrient medium in the laboratory

Disinfectant a chemical that destroys infectious microorganisms

Disposition a tendency to develop a disease or condition

Flora the microorganisms that normally inhabit a body organ or part

Focus a localized area of disease or infection

Host the organism that harbours and nourishes a parasite (Am. harbor)

Innocuous producing no injury; not harmful

Inoculum the cells or material that is added to a growth medium to start a new culture

Instillation the act of inserting a liquid into a cavity drop by drop

Inunction the act of rubbing an oily substance into the skin; an ointment

Local affecting only a small area of the body

Morbid relating to or caused by disease

Nosocomial pertaining to hospital-acquired disease or infection

Nosology a branch of medicine that deals with the study of disease classification

Notifiable relating to a disease or incident that must by law be reported to the health authorities

Nutrient agar a jelly-like substance used in Petri dishes as a medium for growth of microorganisms

Opportunistic refers to infection that attacks patients who are ill or immunocompromised

Placebo substance with no therapeutic value used as a control in testing new drugs or prescribed for psychological benefit

Regimen a strictly regulated scheme, system or programme

Sequela a morbid condition occurring after a disease and resulting from it

Sporadic pertaining to isolated cases of disease with no clear connection between them

Strain a genetic variant or subtype of a microorganism

Vector an organism that carries organisms or parasites from one host to another

Virulence the power of a microorganism to overcome host resistance; the relative ability to cause disease

Virulent dangerously infectious or poisonous

Zoonosis a disease of animals that is transmissible to humans

NOW TRY THE WORD CHECK

WORD CHECK

This self-check exercise lists all the word components used in this unit. First, write down the meaning of as many word components as you can. Then, check your answers using the Exercise Guide and Quick Reference box or the Glossary of Word Components (pp. 383–410).

Prefixes

a-	
an-	
anti-	
auto-	
dia-	
neo-	
oxy-	
retro-	

Roots / Combining forms

acid/o	
aesthet/o	
anxi/o	
alges/i/o	
bacill/o	
bacteri/o	
bio-	
bronch/i/o	
cocc/o	
cycl/o	
cyt/o	

dynam/o	
epilept/o	
esthet/o (Am.)	
estr/o (Am.)	
fibrin/o	
fung/i	
gonad/o	
haem/o	
helmint/h/o	
hem/o (Am.)	
hypn/o	
immun/o	
kerat/o	
kinet/o	
lact/i/o	
muc/o	
oestr/o	
pharmac/o	
plas/m/o	
prurit/o	
psych/o	
(r)rhythm/o	
septic/o	
spasm/o/d	
spirill/o	
staphylococc/o	
streptococc/o	
thyroid/o	
tox/ic/o	
troph/o	

tuss/i	
ur/o	
vir/o	

Suffixes

-aemia	
-al	
-ase	
-cid(e)	
-emia (Am.)	
-form	
-gen	
-gnosy	
-ia	
-ic	
-ite	
-ive	
-logist	
-logy	
-lytic	
-oid	
-ose	
-osis	
-plegia	
-rrhea (Am.)	
-rrhoea	
-uria	
-y	

NOW TRY THE SELF-ASSESSMENT

SELF-ASSESSMENT

Test 21A

Prefixes and suffixes

Match each meaning in Column C with a prefix or suffix in Column A by inserting the appropriate number in Column B.

Column A	Column B	Column C
(a) an-		1. quick
(b) anti-		2. knowledge/process of judgment
(c) -ase		3. chemical derived from ammonia
(d) -cide		4. abnormal condition/disease
(e) -gen		5. condition of rhythm
(f) -gnosy		6. process/condition
(g) -ose		7. study of
(h) -ic		8. drug that breaks down…/pertaining to breakdown
(i) -in		9. without
(j) -ine		10. end product of a process
(k) -ite		11. excessive discharge/flow
(l) -ive		12. enzyme
(m) -logy		13. against
(n) -logist		14. nonspecific suffix indicating a chemical
(o) -lytic		15. type of drug / pertaining to (i)
(p) -osis		16. type of drug / pertaining to (ii)
(q) oxy-		17. agent that kills
(r) -rrhoea (Am. rrhea)		18. specialist who studies
(s) -rrhythmia		19. precursor/agent that produces
(t) -y		20. sugar

Score

20

Test 21B

Combining forms of word roots

Match each meaning in Column C with a combining form of a word root in Column A by inserting the appropriate number in Column B.

Column A	Column B	Column C
(a) acid/o		1. poison
(b) aesthet/o (Am. esthet/o)		2. worms
(c) alges/i/o		3. itching
(d) anxi/o		4. fungus (i)
(e) bacteri/o		5. fungus (ii)
(f) bio-		6. bacteria
(g) dynam/o		7. drug
(h) fung/i		8. life
(i) helmint/h/o		9. sensation
(j) hypn/o		10. mind
(k) kinet/o		11. nourish/stimulate
(l) muc/o		12. cough
(m) myc/o		13. anxiety
(n) pharmac/o		14. force/power of movement
(o) prurit/o		15. virus/virion
(p) psych/o		16. pain
(q) toxic/o		17. acid
(r) troph/o		18. motion/ movement
(s) tuss/i		19. sleep
(t) vir/o		20. mucus

Score

20

Test 21C

Write the meaning of:

(a) toxicology

(b) mycotoxicosis

(c) pharmacist

(d) chemotherapeutic agent

(e) microbiologist

Score

5

Test 21D

Build words that mean:

(a) specialist who studies bacteria

(b) drug that acts against living things

(c) the study of protozoa

(d) agent that stops the growth of bacteria

(e) pertaining to killing viruses

Score

5

Test 21E

Match each drug action from Column A with a drug classification from Column C by inserting the appropriate number in Column B.

Column A	Column B	Column C
(a) acts against worms		1. anaesthetic (Am. anesthetic)
(b) acts to kill cancer cells		2. analgesic
(c) reduces sensation		3. antacid
(d) acts to reduce coughing		4. anthelmintic
(e) neutralises stomach acid		5. antibiotic
(f) acts to break up mucus		6. anticoagulant
(g) acts to promote the excretion of urine		7. antidiabetic

Column A	Column B	Column C
(h) acts to dilate bronchi		8. antihistamine
(i) used to treat schizophrenia		9. antihypertensive
(j) used to induce labour		10. antipruritic
(k) acts to lower blood sugar of non-insulin-dependent diabetics		11. antipsychotic
(l) acts to reduce pain		12. antitussive
(m) reduces the immune response		13. anxiolytic
(n) used to treat glaucoma		14. bronchodilator
(o) dilates the pupil for examination		15. contraceptive
(p) promotes evacuation of the bowels		16. cytotoxic
(q) prevents the effects of histamine		17. diuretic
(r) used to induce sleep		18. gonadotrophin
(s) used to reduce high blood pressure		19. hypnotic
(t) used to reduce anxiety		20. immunosup-pressant
(u) used to prevent itching		21. laxative
(v) used to prevent conception/pregnancy		22. miotic
(w) stimulates/nourishes the reproductive organs		23. mucolytic
(x) prevents blood clotting		24. mydriatic
(y) destroys bacteria and fungi		25. oxytocic

Score

25

Test 21F

Match each description from Column A with the name of an organism from Column C by inserting the appropriate number in Column B.

Test your recall of the meanings of word components in Units 16 to 21 by completing the appropriate self-assessment tests in Unit 22 on pages 331–332.

Column A	**Column B**	**Column C**
(a) a round, berry-like bacterium		1. bacillus
(b) a rod-like bacterium		2. bacteriophage
(c) a comma-shaped bacterium		3. coccus
(d) a spiral-shaped bacterium		4. dermatophyte
(e) a cancer-forming virus that contains RNA		5. diplococci
(f) a plant (fungus) that infects the skin		6. oncornavirus
(g) round berry-like bacteria that occur in chains		7. Plasmodium, a protozoan
(h) round berry-like bacteria that occur in bunches		8. rhinovirus
(i) a virus that infects the nose		9. spirillum
(j) berry-like bacteria that group in pairs		10. staphylococci
(k) a single-celled animal that causes malaria		11. streptococci
(l) a virus that infects bacteria		12. vibrio

Score

12

Check answers to Self-Assessment Tests on page 366.

UNIT 22
FINAL SELF-ASSESSMENT TESTS

In this section, you can assess your recall of the meaning of medical word components. The tests that follow each contain a selection of words relating to the topics studied in Units 1 to 21. Answers can be found on pages 366–368.

FINAL SELF-ASSESSMENT TESTS FOR UNITS 1 TO 5

Final Test 1: Prefixes

Match each meaning in Column C with a prefix in Column A by inserting the appropriate number in Column B.

Column A	Column B	Column C
(a) a-		1. around
(b) bi-		2. inside/within
(c) brady-		3. beside/near
(d) dextro-		4. below normal / reduced
(e) dys-		5. slow
(f) endo-		6. right
(g) epi-		7. large (i)
(h) hyper-		8. large (ii)
(i) hypo-		9. all
(j) inter-		10. fast
(k) macro-		11. small
(l) mega-		12. upon / above in position
(m) micro-		13. many
(n) normo-		14. varied/irregular
(o) pan-		15. between
(p) para-		16. normal
(q) peri-		17. painful/difficult
(r) poikilo-		18. without
(s) poly-		19. above normal / excessive
(t) tachy-		20. two

Score

20

Final Test 2: Combining forms of medical word roots

Match each meaning in Column C with a combining form of a word root in Column A by inserting the appropriate number in Column B.

Column A	Column B	Column C
(a) angi/o		1. abdomen/abdominal wall
(b) ather/o		2. nose
(c) cardi/o		3. stomach
(d) cholecyst/o		4. platelet
(e) cost/o		5. tissue
(f) cyt/o		6. anus/rectum
(g) erythrocyt/o		7. liver
(h) gastr/o		8. atheroma (fatty plaque)
(i) haem/o (Am. hem/o)		9. organ
(j) hepat/o		10. diaphragm
(k) hist/o		11. vessel
(l) lapar/o		12. vein
(m) laryng/o		13. cell
(n) leucocyt/o (Am. leuk/o)		14. lung
(o) myel/o		15. disease
(p) organ/o		16. pulse
(q) path/o		17. gallbladder
(r) phleb/o		18. rib
(s) phren/o		19. larynx
(t) pneumon/o		20. heart
(u) proct/o		21. myelocyte/marrow
(v) reticul/o		22. red blood cell
(w) sphygm/o		23. blood
(x) rhin/o		24. white blood cell
(y) thrombocyt/o		25. immature erythrocyte

Score

25

Final Test 3: Suffixes

Match each meaning in Column C with a suffix in Column A by inserting the appropriate number in Column B.

Column A	Column B	Column C
(a) -algia		1. condition of the urine
(b) -clysis		2. opening into/an opening
(c) -genesis		3. enlargement
(d) -gram		4. breakdown
(e) -graphy		5. disease of
(f) -ia		6. study of
(g) -ic		7. specialist
(h) -ist		8. condition of pain
(i) -itis		9. a recording/X-ray
(j) -logy		10. pertaining to
(k) -lysis		11. technique of viewing/examining
(l) -megaly		12. infusion/injection into
(m) -pathy		13. incision into
(n) -scope		14. formation of
(o) -scopy		15. instrument to view/examine
(p) -stomy		16. pertaining to being poisonous
(q) -tomy		17. condition of
(r) -toxic		18. pertaining to stimulating/inducing
(s) -tropic		19. technique of making a recording/X-ray
(t) -uria		20. inflammation of

Score: 20

Final Test 4: Suffixes

Match each meaning in Column C with a suffix in Column A by inserting the appropriate number in Column B.

Column A	Column B	Column C
(a) -aemia (Am. -emia)		1. formation of
(b) -ary		2. a cutting instrument
(c) -centesis		3. condition of paralysis
(d) -chromia		4. condition of narrowing
(e) -cytosis		5. tumour (Am. tumor)/swelling
(f) -desis		6. surgical repair/reconstruction
(g) -dynia		7. pertaining to
(h) -ectasis		8. excessive discharge/excessive flow
(i) -meter		9. surgical fixation (i)
(j) -metry		10. surgical fixation (ii)
(k) -oma		11. involuntary contraction
(l) -osis		12. stopping/cessation of movement
(m) -penia		13. puncture to remove fluid
(n) -pexy		14. condition of pain
(o) -plasty		15. dilation/stretching
(p) -plegia		16. structure/anatomical part
(q) -poiesis		17. condition of/disease of
(r) -ptysis		18. technique of measuring
(s) -rrhage		19. a measuring instrument
(t) -rrhoea (Am. -rrhea)		20. condition of cells (too many)
(u) -spasm		21. condition of blood
(v) -stasis		22. bursting forth of blood
(w) -stenosis		23. condition of deficiency
(x) -tome		24. spitting up
(y) -um		25. condition of haemoglobin (Am. hemoglobin)/colour

Score: 25

FINAL SELF-ASSESSMENT TESTS FOR UNITS 6 TO 10

Final Test 5: Prefixes

Match each meaning in Column C with a prefix in Column A by inserting the appropriate number in Column B.

Column A	Column B	Column C
(a) agora-		1. deficiency/ few
(b) ambly-		2. grey (grey matter of the CNS)
(c) auto-		3. through
(d) bin-		4. open place
(e) di-		5. out / away from
(f) dia-		6. same/equal
(g) diplo-		7. four (i)
(h) en-		8. four (ii)
(i) ex-		9. under
(j) hemi-		10. beside/near
(k) intra-		11. dry
(l) iso-		12. after/behind
(m) meso-		13. old man/old age
(n) mono-		14. in/within (i)
(o) oligo-		15. in/within (ii)
(p) para-		16. one (i)
(q) polio-		17. one (ii)
(r) post-		18. self
(s) pre-		19. middle
(t) presby-		20. before / in front of
(u) quadri-		21. dull/dim
(v) sub-		22. half
(w) tetra-		23. two/double (i)
(x) uni-		24. two/double (ii)
(y) xero-		25. two/double (iii)

Score ___
25

Final Test 6: Combining forms of medical word roots

Match each meaning in Column C with a combining form of a word root in Column A by inserting the appropriate number in Column B.

Column A	Column B	Column C
(a) adenoid-		1. kidney (i)
(b) aesthesi/o (Am. esthesi/o)		2. kidney (ii)
(c) alges/i		3. dura mater
(d) azot/o		4. thymus gland
(e) cyst/o		5. pain
(f) dur/o		6. bladder (i)
(g) encephal/o		7. bladder (ii)
(h) immun/o		8. lymph vessel
(i) lith/o		9. nerve
(j) lymphaden/o		10. sensation
(k) lymphangi/o		11. serum
(l) nephr/o		12. ureter
(m) neur/o		13. urinary tract / urine
(n) phag/o		14. spleen
(o) psych/o		15. stone
(p) pyel/o		16. brain
(q) py/o		17. mind
(r) ren/o		18. adenoids
(s) ser/o		19. renal pelvis
(t) splen/o		20. urethra
(u) thym/o		21. lymph node
(v) ureter/o		22. pus
(w) urethr/o		23. eating/ consuming
(x) ur/o		24. immunity
(y) vesic/o		25. urea/nitrogen

Score ___
25

Final Test 7: Combining forms of medical word roots

Match each meaning in Column C with a combining form of a word root in Column A by inserting the appropriate number in Column B.

Column A	Column B	Column C
(a) audi/o		1. eustachian tube / auditory tube
(b) aur/i		2. angle of anterior chamber of the eye
(c) auricul/o		3. pupil
(d) blephar/o		4. sclera
(e) chromat/o		5. auricle/pinna
(f) cochle/o		6. lens
(g) cor/e/o		7. malleus (an ear ossicle)
(h) cycl/o		8. ear drum / ear membrane
(i) dacry/o		9. stapes (an ear ossicle)
(j) goni/o		10. uvea
(k) incud/o		11. iris
(l) irid/o		12. ear (i)
(m) lacrim/o		13. ear (ii)
(n) malle/o		14. eye (i)
(o) myring/o		15. eye (ii)
(p) ocul/o		16. middle ear (the tympanum)
(q) ophthalm/o		17. hearing
(r) opt/o		18. cochlea
(s) ot/o		19. incus (an ear ossicle)
(t) phac/o		20. ciliary body
(u) scler/o		21. sight
(v) salping/o		22. tear (i)
(w) stapedi/o		23. tear (ii)
(x) tympan/o		24. colour/haemoglobin (Am. hemoglobin)
(y) uve/o		25. eyelid

Score: 25

Final Test 8: Suffixes

Match each meaning in Column C with a suffix in Column A by inserting the appropriate number in Column B.

Column A	Column B	Column C
(a) -al		1. abnormal condition / disease of
(b) -cele		2. stitching/suturing
(c) -eal		3. act of crushing
(d) -ectomy		4. tumour (Am. tumor)/boil
(e) -ferous		5. condition of softening
(f) -genic		6. condition of urine (excretion of)
(g) -iasis		7. presence of stones / abnormal condition of stones
(h) -ity		8. swelling/protrusion
(i) -lapaxy		9. pertaining to carrying
(j) -lithiasis		10. instrument that fragments, eg, using shock waves
(k) -malacia		11. instrument that crushes
(l) -phyma		12. condition of bursting forth of blood/bleeding
(m) -ptosis		13. pertaining to (i)
(n) -rrhagia		14. pertaining to (ii)
(o) -rrhaphy		15. pertaining to (iii)
(p) -tic		16. removal of
(q) -tripsy		17. falling/displacement
(r) -triptor		18. pertaining to forming
(s) -trite		19. to wash out/evacuate
(t) -uresis		20. state/condition of

Score: 20

Final Test 9: Suffixes

Match each meaning in Column C with a suffix in Column A by inserting the appropriate number in Column B.

Column A	Column B	Column C
(a) -agogic		1. thing / a structure
(b) -ar		2. to carve
(c) -chalasis		3. pertaining to circular motion
(d) -conus		4. heat
(e) -graph		5. instrument that records
(f) -emphraxis		6. pertaining to (i)
(g) -erysis		7. pertaining to (ii)
(h) -gyric		8. cone-like protrusion
(i) -iatry		9. prick/puncture
(j) -kinesis		10. splitting/parting
(k) -metrist		11. drag / draw / suck out
(l) -mileusis		12. wasting away
(m) -nyxis		13. nourishment/ development
(n) -ous		14. blocking/stopping up
(o) -phthisis		15. medical treatment
(p) -plasia		16. slackening/ loosening
(q) -schisis		17. pertaining to inducing/an agent that stimulates
(r) -thermy		18. specialist who measures
(s) -trophy		19. condition of movement
(t) -us		20. condition of growth (of cells)

Score ☐ 20

Final Test 10: Prefixes

Match each meaning in Column C with a prefix in Column A by inserting the appropriate number in Column B.

Column A	Column B	Column C
(a) a-		1. large
(b) an-		2. under/below
(c) crypto-		3. above normal / excessive
(d) dys-		4. inside/within
(e) endo-		5. below normal / reduced
(f) epi-		6. beside/near
(g) hyper-		7. yellow
(h) hypo-		8. little/small amount
(i) macro-		9. hidden
(j) oligo-		10. difficult/painful
(k) ortho-		11. many
(l) pachy-		12. straight/correct
(m) para-		13. after
(n) peri-		14. dry
(o) poly-		15. across/through
(p) post-		16. without/not (i)
(q) sub-		17. without/not (ii)
(r) trans-		18. around
(s) xantho-		19. upon/above in position
(t) xero-		20. thick

Score ☐ 20

FINAL SELF-ASSESSMENT TESTS FOR UNITS 11 TO 15

Final Test 11: Combining forms of medical word roots

Match each meaning in Column C with a combining form of a word root in Column A by inserting the appropriate number in Column B.

Column A	Column B	Column C
(a) arthr/o		1. sweat
(b) balan/o		2. movement
(c) cheil/o		3. jaw
(d) chondr/o		4. epidermis
(e) dermat/o		5. bone
(f) gingiv/o		6. foreskin/prepuce
(g) gnath/o		7. cartilage
(h) hidr/o		8. muscle
(i) kerat/o		9. lip
(j) kinesi/o		10. joint
(k) kyph/o		11. glans penis
(l) lei/o		12. vas deferens
(m) my/o		13. vertebra
(n) onych/o		14. smooth
(o) orchi/o		15. striated muscle
(p) oste/o		16. penis
(q) phall/o		17. testis/testicle
(r) posth/o		18. skin
(s) rhabd/o		19. crooked/hunched
(t) rhin/o		20. tendon
(u) spondyl/o		21. scaly
(v) squam/o		22. hair
(w) tendin/o		23. nail
(x) trich/o		24. gum
(y) vas/o		25. nose

Score [25]

Final Test 12: Suffixes

Match each meaning in Column C with a suffix in Column A by inserting the appropriate number in Column B.

Column A	Column B	Column C
(a) -agogue		1. condition of softening
(b) -auxis		2. condition of muscle tone
(c) -blast		3. increase
(d) -cide		4. condition of eating
(e) -clasis		5. slipping
(f) -clast		6. a plant-like growth / a plant, eg, a fungus
(g) -dynia		7. slight paralysis
(h) -globin		8. condition of having voice
(i) -ism		9. immature germ cell / cell that forms
(j) -kymia		10. condition of pain
(k) -malacia		11. formation
(l) -oid		12. breakdown / surgical breakdown
(m) -olisthesis		13. agent that kills / killing
(n) -paresis		14. pertaining to inducing / an agent that stimulates
(o) -phagia		15. protein
(p) -phonia		16. condition of involuntary muscle twitching
(q) -phyte		17. resembling
(r) -poiesis		18. a cell that breaks something
(s) -rrhexis		19. rupturing
(t) -tonia		20. process of / state or condition of

Score [20]

FINAL SELF-ASSESSMENT TESTS FOR UNITS 16 TO 21

Final Test 13: Prefixes

Match each meaning in Column C with a prefix in Column A by inserting the appropriate number in Column B.

Column A	Column B	Column C
(a) acro-		1. before (i)
(b) an-		2. before (ii)
(c) ana-		3. before (iii)
(d) ante-		4. against
(e) anti-		5. without/not
(f) auto-		6. through/across
(g) dia-		7. first
(h) eu-		8. many
(i) hypo-		9. extremity/point
(j) meta-		10. beyond
(k) multi-		11. none
(l) neo-		12. self
(m) nulli-		13. second
(n) oxy-		14. below normal/ reduced
(o) pre-		15. new
(p) primi-		16. good
(q) pro-		17. quick
(r) retro-		18. backward (i)
(s) secundi-		19. backward (ii)
(t) ultra-		20. changed in form or position

Score

20

Final Test 14: Combining forms of medical word roots

Match each meaning in Column C with a combining form of a word root in Column A by inserting the appropriate number in Column B.

Column A	Column B	Column C
(a) aden/o		1. vagina
(b) andr/o		2. breast (i)
(c) cine/o		3. breast (ii)
(d) colp/o		4. birth
(e) echo-		5. slice/section
(f) endometr/i		6. pregnancy
(g) -gravida		7. labour (Am. labor)
(h) helmint/h/o		8. fungus
(i) hyster/o		9. gland
(j) kal/i		10. midwifery/ obstetrics
(k) lact/o		11. fallopian tube / uterine tube
(l) mamm/o		12. to bear / bring forth (as in pregnancy)
(m) mast/o		13. drug
(n) myc/o		14. potassium (K^+)
(o) nat/o		15. uterus
(p) obstetr-		16. ovary
(q) oophor/o		17. milk
(r) -para		18. worm
(s) pharmac/o		19. echo / ultrasound echo
(t) radi/o		20. movement / motion picture
(u) salping/o		21. thyroid gland
(v) toc/o		22. endometrium
(w) tom/o		23. virus/virion
(x) thyr/o		24. X-ray/radiation
(y) vir/o		25. male

Score

25

Final Test 15: Suffixes

Match each meaning in Column C with a suffix in Column A by inserting the appropriate number in Column B.

Column A	Column B	Column C
(a) -arche		1. agent that suppresses or removes
(b) -ase		2. pertaining to stopping / agent that stops or controls
(c) -cidal		3. condition of small size
(d) -er		4. beginning
(e) -form		5. treatment
(f) -fuge		6. condition of holding back/reducing
(g) -gnosy		7. stopping
(h) -ischia		8. pertaining to a tube or a uterine tube
(i) -ite		9. enzyme
(j) -ive		10. having the form/ structure of
(k) -micria		11. carbohydrate/ sugar/starch
(l) -ose		12. condition of the urine (excretion of)
(m) -pathia		13. process of/state or condition of
(n) -pause		14. dripping
(o) -static		15. type of drug
(p) -staxis		16. end product
(q) -therapy		17. condition of disease
(r) -tubal		18. process of judging/ having knowledge of
(s) -uresis		19. one who
(t) -y		20. pertaining to killing

Score [ ] / 20

Final Test 16: Locative prefixes

Match each meaning in Column C with a locative prefix in Column A by inserting the appropriate number in Column B.

Column A	Column B	Column C
(a) ab-		1. around
(b) ad-		2. between
(c) circum-		3. against
(d) contra-		4. inside
(e) de-		5. middle
(f) dextro-		6. through/across (i)
(g) dorso-		7. through/across (ii)
(h) epi-		8. away from, eg, the midline
(i) extra-		9. back/dorsal surface
(j) in-		10. right
(k) infra-		11. left
(l) inter-		12. outside
(m) laevo- (Am. levo-)		13. side
(n) later-		14. down/loss of
(o) medi-		15. backward
(p) per-		16. upon
(q) retro-		17. to/towards, eg, the midline
(r) supra-		18. below
(s) trans-		19. front/ventral surface
(t) ventr-		20. above

Score [ ] / 20

FINAL SELF-ASSESSMENT TESTS OF MEDICAL SPECIALTIES REFERRED TO IN UNITS 1 TO 21

Final Test 17: Medical specialties

Match each medical specialty in Column A with a meaning in Column C by inserting the appropriate number in Column B.

Column A	Column B	Column C
(a) andrology		1. study of tumours (Am. tumors)
(b) cardiology		2. study of the stomach and intestines
(c) endocrinology		3. study of the urinary system
(d) gastroenterology		4. study of tissues
(e) histology		5. study of the kidney
(f) microbiology		6. specialty dealing with the musculoskeletal system
(g) nephrology		7. study and treatment of mental disease
(h) neonatology		8. study of single-celled animals that cause disease
(i) neuropathology		9. study of the heart
(j) oncology		10. study of disease
(k) orthopaedics (Am. orthopedics)		11 study of the male (urogenital system)
(l) otorhinolaryngology		12. study of the newborn child
(m) pathology		13. study of the ear, nose and larynx
(n) protozoology		14. study of the ductless glands
(o) psychiatry		15. study of diseases of the nervous system
(p) urology		16. study of microorganisms

Score | 16

Final Test 18: Medical specialties

Match each medical specialty in Column A with a meaning in Column C by inserting the appropriate number in Column B.

Column A	Column B	Column C
(a) anaesthesiology		1. study of the nervous system
(b) dermatology		2. study of the female (reproductive system)
(c) gynaecology (Am. gynecology)		3. study of the eye
(d) haematology (Am. hematology)		4. study of virions (viruses)
(e) immunopathology		5. study of the nose
(f) neurology		6. specialty dealing with pregnancy and childbirth
(g) obstetrics		7. study of drugs
(h) ophthalmology		8. study of the skin
(i) otology		9. study of the lungs
(j) paediatrics (Am. pediatrics)		10. study of blood
(k) pharmacology		11. study of rheumatism
(l) pulmonology		12. study of behaviour (the mind)
(m) rheumatology		13. the study and practice of anaesthesia (Am. anesthesia)
(n) rhinology		14. specialty dealing with childhood diseases and injuries
(o) psychology		15. study of diseases of the immune system
(p) virology		16. study of the ear

Score | 16

ANSWERS TO WORD EXERCISES

Introduction

Word Exercise 1

(a) Gastropathy
(b) Gastroscopy
(c) Hepatitis
(d) Hepatomegaly
(e) Hepatoma

Word Exercise 2

(a) Duodenojejunostomy
(b) Tracheobronchitis
(c) Gastroenterostomy
(d) Laryngopharyngectomy
(e) Osteoarthropathy

Word Exercise 3

(a) Endodontic
(b) Prosthodontist
(c) Pararectal
(d) Monocular
(e) Perisplenitis

Unit 1 Levels of Organization

Word Exercise 1

(a) Cyt, word root meaning cell; o, combining vowel; pathy, suffix meaning disease
(b) Disease of cells
(c) Study of disease
(d) Study of cell disease
(e) Breakdown/disintegration of cells
(f) Pertaining to poisonous to cells
(g) Specialist who studies cells

Word Exercise 2

(a) Erythr/o, combining form meaning red; cyte, suffix meaning cell (note. this is a compound suffix containing the root, -cyt- meaning cell + (e) used to end a name)
(b) Red cell

Word Exercise 3

(a) Melanocyte
(b) Fibrocyte
(c) Lympho/lymphocyte (lymph cell)
  Spermato/spermatocyte (sperm cell)
  Oo/oocyte (egg cell)
  Granulo/granulocyte (granular cell)
  Chondro/chondrocyte (cartilage cell)

Word Exercise 4

(a) Bone forming cell/immature bone cell
(b) Fibre forming cell/immature fibre cell
(c) A cell that forms blood cells/an immature blood cell

Word Exercise 5

(a) The chemistry of tissues (refers to the study of)
(b) Study of tissue disease
(c) Person who specializes in study of tissues
(d) Breakdown/disintegration of tissues

Word Exercise 6

(a) Small
(b) Instrument to view small objects
(c) Technique of viewing very small objects with a microscope
(d) Specialist who views small things (a specialist in microscopy)
(e) Study of small life (microorganisms: bacteria, fungi, protozoa, etc.)

Word Exercise 7

(a) Pertaining to an organ or originating in an organ
(b) The formation of organs
(c) Pertaining to formation of organs
(d) Pertaining to nourishing/stimulating organs

Case History 1

(a) The study of tissues / a department that studies tissues
(b) Specialist who studies disease/diseased organs
(c) Pertaining to the study of cells or pertaining to cytology
(d) Technique of viewing small things (here cells)
(e) White (blood) cell
(f) Lymph cell
(g) Study of small forms of life, ie, bacteria, fungi, protozoa, etc.
(h) Pertaining to causing disease

Unit 2 The Digestive System

Word Exercise 1

(a) Instrument to view the oesophagus (Am. esophagus)
(b) Removal of oesophagus (Am. esophagus)
(c) Incision into the oesophagus (Am. esophagus)
(d) Inflammation of the oesophagus (Am. esophagus)

Word Exercise 2

(a) Instrument to view the stomach
(b) Removal of part or all of the stomach
(c) Incision into the stomach
(d) Inflammation of the stomach, especially the lining
(e) Gastropathy
(f) Gastrology
(g) Epigastric
(h) Gastrologist
(i) Gastroscopy

Word Exercise 3

(a) Inflammation of the intestines
(b) Disease of the intestines
(c) Incision into the intestine
(d) Opening into the intestine (often to connect to stomach, ileum, jejunum or abdominal wall)
(e) Intestinal stone (compacted material in intestine)
(f) Enterology
(g) Enterologist
(h) Study of the stomach and intestines (plus associated structures, eg, liver and pancreas)
(i) Disease of the stomach and intestines
(j) Inflammation of the stomach and intestines (often due to infection)
(k) Technique of viewing or examining the stomach and intestines

Word Exercise 4

(a) Removal of the pylorus and stomach
(b) Technique of viewing the pylorus (with an endoscope)

Word Exercise 5

(a) Formation of an opening (anastomosis) between the duodenum and another part of the small intestine
(b) Formation of an opening (anastomosis) between one part of the jejunum and another part of the jejunum
(c) Pertaining to the duodenum and jejunum
(d) Ileostomy
(e) Ileitis

Word Exercise 6

(a) Large colon
(b) Inflammation of the appendix
(c) Removal of the colon
(d) Opening into the colon (usually a connection between the colon and the abdominal wall; it acts as an artificial anus)
(e) Caecostomy (Am. cecostomy)
(f) Appendicectomy (Am. appendectomy)
(g) Gastrocolostomy
(h) Colonoscope

Word Exercise 7

(a) Pertaining to beside the rectum
(b) Pertaining to the anus and rectum
(c) Inflammation around the anus/rectum
(d) Administration of fluid into the anus/rectum (enema)
(e) Condition of pain in the anus/rectum
(f) Proctoscope
(g) Proctocaecostomy (Am. proctocecostomy)
(h) Caecosigmoidostomy (Am. cecosigmoidostomy)
(i) Sigmoidoscope
(j) Sigmoidoscopy

Word Exercise 8

(a) Inflammation of the peritoneum
(b) Technique of viewing or examining the peritoneum

Word Exercise 9

(a) Breaking down of the pancreas
(b) Enlargement of the liver
(c) Liver tumour (Am. tumor)
(d) Pertaining to poisonous to the liver
(e) Formation of an opening between the hepatic duct and stomach
(f) Pertaining to the pancreatic duct and duodenum

Word Exercise 10

(a) Condition of absence of bile
(b) Bile stone
(c) Abnormal condition of stones in the bile duct (or gallbladder)
(d) Condition of bile in the blood
(e) Condition of bile in the urine
(f) Incision into the gallbladder
(g) Removal of the gallbladder
(h) Abnormal condition of gallbladder stones (stones in the gallbladder)
(i) X-ray film demonstrating bile ducts (vessels)
(j) Technique or process of making a cholangiogram

(k) Abnormal condition of common bile duct stones (stones in the common bile duct)
(l) Incision into the common bile duct to remove stones

Word Exercise 11

(a) Visual examination of the abdomen (ie, abdominal cavity) with a laparoscope
(b) Incision through the abdominal wall

Word Exercise 12

(a) Capsule endoscopy (2)
(b) Enteroscope (4)
(c) Endoscope (6)
(d) Enteroscopy (7)
(e) Endoscopy (9)
(f) Endoscopist (8)
(g) Colonoscopy (3)
(h) Proctoscope (1)
(i) Sigmoidoscopy (10)
(j) Panendoscopy (5)

Case History 2

(a) Abnormal condition of stones in the bile (in the gallbladder or bile duct)
(b) Pertaining to the region upon/above the stomach (epigastrium)
(c) Pertaining/relating to bile
(d) Study of the stomach and intestines
(e) Pertaining to using a laparoscope (instrument to view the abdomen)
(f) Removal of the gallbladder
(g) Inflammation of the gallbladder
(h) Pertaining to the nose and stomach (here a tube passed through the nose into the stomach)

Unit 3 The Respiratory System

Word Exercise 1

(a) Instrument used to view or examine the nose
(b) Disease of the nose
(c) Condition of pain in the nose
(d) Inflammation of the nose
(e) Excessive flow/discharge from the nose
(f) Surgical repair of the nose
(g) Technique of viewing the nose

Word Exercise 2

(a) A tube that passes from nose to stomach (for suction or feeding)
(b) A tube that passes from nose to oesophagus (Am. esophagus) (for suction or feeding)

Word Exercise 3

(a) Condition of pain in the pharynx
(b) Excessive flow/discharge from the pharynx
(c) Pharyngoplasty
(d) Pharyngorhinitis
(e) Pharyngoscope

Word Exercise 4

(a) Study of the larynx
(b) Removal of the larynx and pharynx
(c) Laryngoscope
(d) Laryngoscopy
(e) Laryngorhinology

Word Exercise 5

(a) Incision into the trachea
(b) Pertaining to within the trachea
(c) Formation of an opening into the trachea (to establish a safe airway) or the opening itself

Word Exercise 6

(a) Bronchoplegia
(b) Bronchogram
(c) Bronchography
(d) Bronchiectasis
(e) A structure, the bronchus
(f) Stitching/suturing of the bronchi
(g) Abnormal condition of bronchial fungi (fungi in the bronchi)
(h) Originating in the bronchi/pertaining to formation of the bronchi
(i) Involuntary contraction of the bronchi (smooth muscle)
(j) Pertaining to the trachea and bronchi
(k) Instrument used to view or examine the bronchi
(l) Discharge or excessive flow of mucus from the bronchi
(m) Inflammation of the larynx, trachea and bronchi
(n) Formation of an opening between a bronchus and the oesophagus (Am. esophagus)

Word Exercise 7

(a) Incision into the lung
(b) Suturing of the lung
(c) Disease/abnormal condition of the lungs
(d) Pneumonectomy
(e) Pneumonopathy
(f) Puncture of the lung (by surgery)
(g) Fixation of a lung by surgery (to thoracic wall)

Word Exercise 8

(a) A thorax containing air and blood (in the pleural cavity)
(b) Technique of making an X-ray after injection of air

(c) Without breathing (temporary, due to low levels of carbon dioxide in blood)
(d) Difficult/painful breathing
(e) Above normal breathing (higher rate and depth)
(f) Below normal breathing (low rate and depth)
(g) Fast breathing
(h) Slow breathing

Word Exercise 9

(a) Lobotomy
(b) Lobectomy

Word Exercise 10

(a) Pertaining to the lungs
(b) Pertaining to the lungs

Word Exercise 11

(a) Inflammation of the pleura
(b) Puncture of the pleura
(c) Pleurography
(d) Condition of pain in the pleura
(e) Adhesion/fixation of pleura

Word Exercise 12

(a) Pertaining to the diaphragm and stomach
(b) Pertaining to the diaphragm and liver
(c) Condition of paralysis of the diaphragm

Word Exercise 13

(a) Thoracopathy
(b) Thoracotomy
(c) Puncture of the thorax (by surgery)
(d) Instrument used to view the thorax
(e) Abnormal condition of narrowing of the thorax

Word Exercise 14

(a) Pertaining to between the ribs
(b) Pertaining to originating in the ribs / pertaining to forming ribs
(c) Inflammation of rib cartilage

Word Exercise 15

(a) Bronchoscope (3)
(b) Laryngoscopy (4)
(c) Rhinoscope (8)
(d) Pharyngoscope (6)
(e) Bronchoscopy (7)
(f) Rhinologist (1)
(g) Tracheostomy tube (5)
(h) Laryngoscope (2)

Word Exercise 16

(a) Thoracoscope (5)
(b) Stethoscope (7)
(c) Spirometer (6)
(d) Spirography (3)
(e) Nasal speculum (1)
(f) Nasogastric tube (8)
(g) Pleurography (2)
(h) Spirometry (4)

Case History 3

(a) Pertaining to the lungs
(b) Removal of a lobe (here of the lung)
(c) Difficult/painful breathing
(d) Abnormal condition of blue (appearance of skin and mucous membranes)
(e) Spasmodic (involuntary) contractions of the bronchi / bronchial tubes
(f) Condition of below normal supply of oxygen (to tissues)
(g) Condition of above normal carbon dioxide (in the blood)
(h) Condition of the lung (in which there is inflammation of the spongy tissue of the lung due to infection)

Unit 4 The Cardiovascular System

Word Exercise 1

(a) Pertaining to the heart
(b) Condition of pain in the heart
(c) Instrument used to view the heart
(d) Instrument that records the heart (beat, force and form of)
(e) Tracing/recording made by a cardiograph
(f) Condition of fast heart rate
(g) Cardiomegaly
(h) Cardioplasty
(i) Cardiopathy
(j) Cardiology
(k) A structure, the heart muscle
(l) Disease of heart muscle
(m) Stitching/suturing of the heart
(n) Instrument that records electrical activity of the heart
(o) Inflammation inside the heart (its lining)
(p) Inflammation of all of the heart
(q) Condition of slow heart beat
(r) Condition of right heart (heart displaced to right)
(s) Technique of recording sounds of the heart
(t) Technique of recording (ultrasound) echoes of the heart
(u) A tracing of the electrical activity of the heart

Word Exercise 2

(a) Pericarditis
(b) Fixation of the heart pericardium (pericardium to the heart)

(c)   Puncture of the pericardium (by surgery)
(d)   Removal of the pericardium (part of)

Word Exercise 3

(a)   Valvoplasty
(b)   Valvectomy
(c)   Instrument for cutting a heart valve
(d)   Pertaining to a valve
(e)   Incision into a valve

Word Exercise 4

(a)   Sudden contraction of a blood vessel
(b)   Pertaining to without blood vessels
(c)   Vasculitis
(d)   Vasculopathy

Word Exercise 5

(a)   X-ray picture of blood vessels (usually arteries)
(b)   X-ray picture of the (major) vessels and heart
(c)   Technique of making an angiocardiogram
(d)   Angiology
(e)   Angioplasty
(f)   Tumour (Am. tumor) formed from blood vessels (non-malignant)
(g)   Dilatation of blood vessels
(h)   Formation of blood vessels
(i)   Abnormal condition of hardening of blood vessels

Word Exercise 6

(a)   Aortopathy
(b)   Aortography

Word Exercise 7

(a)   Arteriorrhaphy
(b)   Arteriosclerosis
(c)   Removal of the inside (lining) of an artery
(d)   Abnormal condition of arterial death (breakdown of arteries)
(e)   Abnormal condition of narrowing of arteries

Word Exercise 8

(a)   X-ray picture of a vena cava
(b)   Technique of making an X-ray / tracing of the venae cavae

Word Exercise 9

(a)   Dilatation of a vein (a varicosity or varicose vein)
(b)   Injection or infusion into a vein (of nutrients or medicines)

(c)   Pertaining to veins / of the nature of veins
(d)   Venogram
(e)   Venography

Word Exercise 10

(a)   Dilatation of veins and arteries
(b)   Injection/infusion into a vein
(c)   Incision into vein
(d)   Cessation of movement of blood in a vein
(e)   Instrument used to measure vein pressure (pressure within a vein)
(f)   Concretion or stone within a vein

Word Exercise 11

(a)   Formation of a clot
(b)   Inflammation of a vein associated with a thrombus
(c)   Removal of a thrombus and the lining of an artery
(d)   Thrombosis
(e)   Thrombectomy
(f)   Formation of clots
(g)   Disintegration/breakdown of clots

Word Exercise 12

(a)   Formation of atheroma
(b)   Blockage caused by an embolus composed of atheroma or fragments of atheromatous plaques

Word Exercise 13

(a)   Surgical repair of an aneurysm
(b)   Suturing/stitching of an aneurysm

Word Exercise 14

(a)   Instrument that measures the pulse force (pressure and volume)
(b)   Instrument that measures pulse pressure (arterial blood pressure)
(c)   Technique of measuring the pulse
(d)   Instrument that records the pulse
(e)   Tracing/picture/recording of the pulse
(f)   Instrument that records the pulse and heart beat

Word Exercise 15

(a)   Cardioscope (6)
(b)   Cardiograph (4)
(c)   Electrocardiograph (5)
(d)   Cardiovalvotome (2)
(e)   Angiocardiography (3)
(f)   Sphygmomanometer (1)

Word Exercise 16

(a) Echocardiography (6)
(b) Sphygmocardiograph (5)
(c) Stethoscope (7)
(d) Phonocardiogram (1)
(e) Electrocardiogram (3)
(f) Phlebomanometer (4)
(g) Sphygmodynamic (2)

Case History 4

(a) Study of the heart
(b) Pertaining to veins / of the nature of veins
(c) Condition of fast heart beat
(d) Instrument that records the electrical activity of the heart
(e) Enlargement of the heart
(f) Pertaining to two ventricles (right and left)
(g) Pertaining to the heart
(h) Drug that induces dilatation of blood vessels

Unit 5 The Blood

Word Exercise 1

(a) The study of blood
(b) Study of blood diseases
(c) Pertaining to the force and movement of the blood (study of)
(d) Formation of the blood
(e) Cessation of blood flow/stopping of bleeding by clotting
(f) A structure containing blood in the pericardium (blood in the pericardial sac)
(g) Spitting up of blood
(h) Haematoma (Am. hematoma)
(i) Haemolysis (Am. hemolysis)
(j) Haematuria (Am. hematuria)
(k) Haemorrhage (Am. hemorrhage)
(l) Condition of too many cells in blood (it refers to conditions in which there is an increase in the number of circulating red blood cells)
(m) Condition of without blood (it refers to condition of reduced number of red cells and/or quantity of haemoglobin (Am. hemoglobin))
(n) Condition of decay of blood (due to infection)
(o) Instrument that measures haemoglobin (Am. hemoglobin)
(p) Blood protein
(q) Condition of haemoglobin (Am. hemoglobin) in the urine
(r) Condition of abnormal decrease of haemoglobin (colour) (Am. hemoglobin)
(s) Condition of abnormal increase of haemoglobin (colour) (Am. hemoglobin)
(t) Pertaining to normal concentration of haemoglobin (colour) (Am. hemoglobin)

Word Exercise 2

(a) Condition of reduction in number of red blood cells
(b) Formation of red blood cells
(c) Immature germ cell that gives rise to red blood cells
(d) Formation of red blood cells
(e) Breakdown of red blood cells
(f) Condition of too many red cells in the blood, ie, too many erythrocytes
(g) Abnormal condition of too many small cells (small erythrocytes)
(h) Abnormal condition of too many large cells (large erythrocytes)
(i) Abnormal condition of too many elliptical cells (elliptical erythrocytes)
(j) Abnormal condition of too many unequal cells (unequal sized erythrocytes)
(k) Abnormal condition of too many irregular/varied cells (variable shaped erythrocytes)
(l) Pertaining to normal cells (red blood cells of normal size)

Word Exercise 3

(a) Reticuloblast
(b) Reticulocytosis
(c) Reticulopenia

Word Exercise 4

(a) Leucopenia (Am. leukopenia)
(b) Leucopoiesis (Am. leukopoiesis)
(c) Formation of white blood cells
(d) Condition of white blood (synonymous with leukocythaemia, a malignant cancer of white blood cells)
(e) Abnormal condition of white cells (an increase in white blood cells, usually transient in response to infection)
(f) Tumour (Am. tumor) of leucocytes (Am. leukocytes)
(g) Immature germ cell that gives rise to leucocytes (Am. leukocytes)
(h) Abnormal condition of too many white germ cells (results in proliferation of leucocytes (Am. leukocytes))
(i) Pertaining to poisonous to white cells (leucocytes, Am. leukocytes)

Word Exercise 5

(a) Marrow cell (a cell that forms white blood cells called polymorphonuclear granulocytes)
(b) Condition of marrow fibres (replacement of bone marrow with fibrous tissue) (Am. fiber)
(c) Myeloblast
(d) Myeloma

Word Exercise 6

(a) Condition of reduction in the number of platelets (thrombocytes)
(b) Formation of platelets (thrombocytes)
(c) Breakdown of platelets (thrombocytes)
(d) Disease of platelets (thrombocytes)

Word Exercise 7

(a) Withdrawal of blood, removal of red cells and re-transfusion of the remainder
(b) Withdrawal of blood, removal of thrombocytes and re-transfusion of the remainder
(c) Withdrawal of blood, removal of leucocytes and re-transfusion of the remainder

Word Exercise 8

(a) Plasmapheresis (4)
(b) Differential count (3)
(c) Haematocrit (2)
(d) Haemoglobinometer (5)
(e) Blood count (1)

Case History 5

(a) Spitting/coughing up of blood
(b) Condition of reduction of all cells (ie, all types of cells in the blood)
(c) Pertaining to leukaemia/white blood (a cancer of the white blood cells)
(d) Pertaining to normal colour (here meaning normal haemoglobin)
(e) Pertaining to normal cells (here normocyte refers to an erythrocyte of a typical shape and size)
(f) Condition of a reduction in granulocytes (types of white blood cells)
(g) Condition of reduction in thrombocytes/platelets
(h) Condition of without blood (actually a reduction in erythrocytes and haemoglobin (Am. hemoglobin))

Unit 6 The Lymphatic System and Immunology

Word Exercise 1

(a) Abnormal condition of lymph cells (too many cells)
(b) Condition of bursting forth of lymph (from lymph vessels)
(c) Technique of making an X-ray/tracing of lymphatic vessels
(d) X-ray picture/tracing of a lymph vessel
(e) Dilatation of lymph vessels
(f) Tumour (Am. tumor) of lymphoid tissue
(g) Removal of a lymph node

(h) Disease of a lymph node
(i) Inflammation of a lymph node

Word Exercise 2

(a) Enlargement of the spleen
(b) Enlargement of the spleen and liver
(c) Surgical fixation of the spleen
(d) Hernia/protrusion of the spleen
(e) Condition of softening of the spleen
(f) Breakdown/disintegration of the spleen
(g) Technique of making an X-ray picture of the spleen or a description of the spleen
(h) X-ray picture of the splenic and portal veins

Word Exercise 3

(a) Tonsillitis
(b) Tonsillectomy
(c) Pertaining to the tonsils and pharynx
(d) Instrument used to cut the tonsils

Word Exercise 4

(a) Thymocyte
(b) Thymopathy
(c) Thymocele
(d) Abnormal condition of ulceration of the thymus gland
(e) Pertaining to the thymus gland and lymphatics

Word Exercise 5

(a) Immunology
(b) Immunopathology
(c) Formation of immunity
(d) Self-immunity (the immune system acts against itself, producing an autoimmune disease)
(e) A protein of the immune system (an antibody)

Word Exercise 6

(a) Serology

Word Exercise 7

(a) Condition of pus in the blood (infection in blood)
(b) Pertaining to generating pus
(c) Flow of pus (usually referring to pus flowing from the teeth sockets)
(d) Formation of pus

Word Exercise 8

(a) Tonsillotome (3)
(b) Lymphangiography (4)
(c) Lymphadenography (6)

(d) Lymphogram (2)
(e) Splenoportogram (1)
(f) Lymphography (5)

Case History 6

(a) Inflammation of the tonsils
(b) Enlargement of the spleen
(c) Disease of lymph nodes
(d) Pertaining to a lymph node
(e) Study of tissue disease (here refers to a section of the pathology laboratory)
(f) Tumour (Am. tumor) of the lymph (tissue)
(g) Lymph cell
(h) Type of lymphocyte that secretes antibodies (named after the bursa of Fabricus in birds)

Unit 7 The Urinary System

Word Exercise 1

(a) Pertaining to the kidney and stomach
(b) X-ray / tracing of the kidney
(c) Technique of making an X-ray / tracing of the kidney

Word Exercise 2

(a) Falling kidney (downward displacement)
(b) Abnormal condition of water in a kidney (a swelling)
(c) A swelling/hernia of a kidney
(d) Condition of pain in a kidney
(e) Nephropexy
(f) Nephroplasty
(g) Nephrotomy
(h) Nephrolithiasis
(i) Nephrectomy
(j) Inflammation of glomeruli (producing pus)
(k) Disease of glomeruli
(l) Abnormal condition of hardening of glomeruli

Word Exercise 3

(a) Inflammation of the renal pelvis and kidney
(b) Incision to remove a pelvic stone (a stone from the renal pelvis)
(c) Disease/abnormal condition of a renal pelvis and kidney
(d) Pyeloplasty
(e) Pyelogram

Word Exercise 4

(a) Hernia/protrusion of the ureter
(b) Removal of a ureterocele
(c) Water in the ureter (a ureter swollen with urine)
(d) Condition of excessive flow of blood from the ureter
(e) Stitching/suturing of the ureter

(f) Dilatation of a ureter
(g) Visual examination of the ureters and kidneys
(h) Formation of an opening into the ureter
(i) Ureteroenterostomy
(j) Ureterocolostomy

Word Exercise 5

(a) Inflammation of the bladder
(b) Removal of a bladder stone
(c) Inflammation of the bladder and renal pelvis
(d) Falling/displacement of the bladder
(e) Instrument used to view the bladder
(f) Formation of an opening between the bladder and rectum/anus
(g) Cystometer (measures contractile force and changes in pressure)
(h) Cystometry
(i) Cystometrogram

Word Exercise 6

(a) Vesicostomy
(b) Vesicotomy
(c) Infusion/injection into the bladder
(d) Pertaining to the bladder
(e) Opening between the bladder and sigmoid colon (to drain urine)
(f) Pertaining to the bladder and ureters

Word Exercise 7

(a) Process of measuring the urethra
(b) Inflammation of the urethra and trigone (of the bladder)
(c) Fixation (by surgery) of the urethra
(d) Urethralgia
(e) Urethrorrhagia
(f) Urethroscopy
(g) Tumour (Am. tumor)/boil in the urethra
(h) Instrument for cutting the urethra
(i) Abnormal condition of narrowing of the urethra
(j) Condition of pain in the urethra

Word Exercise 8

(a) Of the nature of / pertaining to carrying urine
(b) Urine splitting/separating for analysis
(c) Instrument used to measure urine

Word Exercise 9

(a) Technique of recording the urinary tract (X-ray)
(b) Person specializing in the study of the urinary tract
(c) Formation of urine
(d) Condition of little urine (diminished secretion of)
(e) Condition of albumin in the urine

(f)   Condition of urea (too much) in the urine
(g)   Condition of much urine
(h)   Condition of painful difficult (flow) of urine
(i)   Condition of blood in the urine
(j)   Condition of pus in the urine
(k)   Condition of too much calcium in the urine

Word Exercise 10

(a)   Inflammation of kidney due to stones
(b)   Condition of calculi or stones in the urine
(c)   Formation of stones
(d)   Incision to remove a kidney stone (eg, by a small incision through the skin percutaneous nephrolithotomy)
(e)   Instrument used to crush stones
(f)   Washing of stones from bladder following crushing
(g)   Instrument that uses shock waves to destroy stones
(h)   The procedure of breaking stones using shock waves from a lithotriptor
(i)   Excretion of stones in the urine

Word Exercise 11

(a)   Diathermy (8)
(b)   Cystoscope (10)
(c)   Lithotriptor (7)
(d)   Urinometer (9)
(e)   Hemodialyzer (2)
(f)   Ureteroscopy (4)
(g)   Urethrotome (3)
(h)   Cystometer (5)
(i)   Urethroscope (6)
(j)   Lithotrite (1)

Word Exercise 12

(a)   Retrograde pyelography (6)
(b)   Haemodialysis (4)
(c)   Lithotripsy (8)
(d)   Catheterization (7)
(e)   Urography (3)
(f)   Urodynamics (1)
(g)   Litholapaxy (2)
(h)   Ureterorenoscopy (5)

Case History 7

(a)   Abnormal condition of stones in the urinary tract
(b)   Pertaining to the urethra
(c)   Condition of painful/difficult urine (urination)
(d)   Condition of blood in the urine
(e)   Disease of the urinary tract
(f)   Technique of making a tracing/X-ray of the renal pelvis
(g)   Technique of breaking up stones using a lithotriptor
(h)   Condition of above normal calcium levels in the urine

Unit 8 The Nervous System

Word Exercise 1

(a)   Study of the nerves/nervous system
(b)   Disease of the nervous system
(c)   Condition of pain in nerves
(d)   A nerve fibre tumour (Am. tumor) (arises from connective tissue around nerves)
(e)   Inflammation of many nerves
(f)   Pertaining to formation of nerves / originating in nerves
(g)   Neurosclerosis
(h)   Neuromalacia
(i)   Neurologist
(j)   Wasting/decay of nerves or nervous tissue
(k)   Pertaining to affinity for/stimulating nervous tissue
(l)   Injury to nerves
(m)   Nerve glue cell/neuroglial cell
(n)   A tumour (Am. tumor) of gliocytes/gliacytes/neuroglial cells (nerve glue cells)

Word Exercise 2

(a)   Disease of a plexus
(b)   Pertaining to the formation of a plexus/originating in a plexus

Word Exercise 3

(a)   Hernia/protrusion of the cranial contents from the head (syn. encephalocele)
(b)   Pertaining to without a head
(c)   Pertaining to a tumour (Am. tumor) of blood within the head (actually a collection of blood in subperiosteal tissue, the result of an injury)
(d)   Meaning a thing (baby) with water in the head; it is an abnormal expansion of the ventricles within the brain caused by an accumulation of cerebrospinal fluid
(e)   Microcephalic
(f)   Cephalogram
(g)   Cephalometry
(h)   Pertaining to having a large head
(i)   Pertaining to a turning motion of the head

Word Exercise 4

(a)   Tumour of the brain (Am. tumor)
(b)   Abnormal condition of pus (infection) of the brain
(c)   Pertaining to without a brain
(d)   Instrument that records electrical activity of the brain
(e)   Encephalography
(f)   Electroencephalography
(g)   Encephalopathy
(h)   Encephalocele
(i)   Tracing/picture of the brain made using (echoes) reflected ultrasound

(j)   The middle brain
(k)   Inflammation of the grey matter of the brain (Am. gray)

Word Exercise 5

(a)   Cerebrosclerosis (syn. encephalosclerosis)
(b)   Cerebromalacia (syn. encephalomalacia)
(c)   Cerebral

Word Exercise 6

(a)   Ventriculoscopy
(b)   Ventriculotomy
(c)   Opening between the ventricles and cistern
        (subarachnoid space)

Word Exercise 7

(a)   Craniotomy
(b)   Craniometry
(c)   Intracranial

Word Exercise 8

(a)   Pertaining to before a ganglion
(b)   Pertaining to after a ganglion
(c)   Having the form of a ganglion

Word Exercise 9

(a)   Meningitis
(b)   Meningocele
(c)   Meningorrhagia
(d)   Hernia / protrusion of the meninges and brain (through a
        defect in the cranium)
(e)   Inflammation of the meninges and brain
(f)   Disease of the meninges and brain
(g)   Tumour (Am. tumor) of the meninges
(h)   Pertaining to above/upon the dura
(i)   Swelling/tumour (Am. tumor) of blood beneath the dura

Word Exercise 10

(a)   Inflammation of spinal nerve roots and their associated
        ganglia
(b)   Inflammation spinal nerve roots and their associated
        peripheral nerves
(c)   Incision into a spinal nerve root (syn. rhizotomy)

Word Exercise 11

(a)   Inflammation of the spinal cord and meninges
        (syn. meningomyelitis)
(b)   Hernia/protrusion of the meninges and spinal cord
        through a defect in the spinal column
(c)   Inflammation of the spinal cord and spinal nerve roots

(d)   Inflammation of the spinal cord and brain
(e)   Wasting of the spinal cord
(f)   Inflammation of the grey matter of the spinal cord
(g)   Myelosclerosis
(h)   Myelomalacia
(i)   Myelography
(j)   Condition of abnormal/difficult development/growth (of
        cells) of the spinal cord (a neural tube defect)
(k)   Without nourishment of the spinal cord (wasting away /
        poor growth)
(l)   Abnormal condition of tubes (cavities) in the spinal cord

Word Exercise 12

(a)   Instrument used to measure the spine (curvature)
(b)   Puncture of the spine to remove fluid (syn. lumbar
        puncture)
(c)   Splitting of the spine (a congenital fissure of one or
        more vertebrae)

Word Exercise 13

(a)   Condition of paralysis of all four limbs
(b)   Condition of paralysis of half the body, right or left side
(c)   Condition of near/beside/beyond paralysis (lower limbs)
(d)   Condition of two parts paralyzed (similar parts on either
        side of the body)
(e)   Condition of paralysis of four limbs (synonymous with
        quadriplegia)

Word Exercise 14

(a)   A specialist who studies anaesthesia (Am. anesthesia)
        and anaesthetics (Am. anesthetics)
(b)   A specialist who administers anaesthetics (Am. anes-
        thetics)
(c)   Condition of without sensation of half the body (one side)
(d)   To cause to become without sensation
(e)   Condition of decreased sensation
(f)   Condition of increased sensation
(g)   Post-anaesthetic/post-anaesthesia (Am. post-
        anesthetic/post-anesthesia)
(h)   Pre-anaesthetic/pre-anaesthesia (Am. pre-anesthetic/
        pre-anesthesia)

Word Exercise 15

(a)   Abnormal condition of stupor/deep sleep (drug induced)
(b)   Treatment with narcotics (a type of psychotherapy)

Word Exercise 16

(a)   Condition of sensing pain
(b)   Condition of without sensation of pain
(c)   Condition of excessive / above normal sensation of pain
(d)   Pertaining to a loss of pain/a drug that reduces pain

Word Exercise 17

(a) Study of the mind (behaviour)
(b) Pertaining to the mind; pertaining to the psyche; influenced by the mind; mental as opposed to physical
(c) Disease of the mind
(d) Abnormal condition/disease of the mind (a severe mental disease such as schizophrenia)
(e) Drug that acts on/has an affinity for the mind (affects behaviour, emotion or perception)
(f) Pertaining to mind and body (actually body symptoms of mental origin)
(g) Specialized medical study and treatment of the mind by a doctor

Word Exercise 18

(a) Condition of fear of heights (peaks, extremities)
(b) Condition of fear of open spaces
(c) Condition of fear of water
(d) Condition of fear of cancer
(e) Condition of fear of death/dead bodies

Word Exercise 19

(a) Pertaining to forming/causing epileptic fits
(b) Pertaining to following/after an epileptic fit
(c) Having the form of epilepsy

Word Exercise 20

(a) Encephalography (5)
(b) Positron emission tomography (4)
(c) Ventriculoscopy (6)
(d) Tendon hammer (1)
(e) Tomograph (2)
(f) Craniometry (3)

Word Exercise 21

(a) MRI (3)
(b) Lumbar puncture (6)
(c) Myelography (5)
(d) Computed tomography (1)
(e) Electroencephalography (2)
(f) Echoencephalography (4)

Case History 8

(a) Pertaining to the (blood) vessels of the cerebrum/brain
(b) Condition of half paralysis (it refers to one side of the body)
(c) Condition of beyond sensation (numbness) of half (one side) of the body / it refers to abnormal sensations
(d) Loss of sensation of half (one side) of the body
(e) Pertaining to the cerebrum/cerebral hemispheres

(f) Pertaining to within the cranium/skull
(g) Study of nerves or the nervous system; here it refers to a department that studies and treats disorders of the nervous system
(h) Pertaining to above normal / exaggerated reflexes

Unit 9 The Eye

Word Exercise 1

(a) Ophthalmoscope
(b) Ophthalmologist
(c) Ophthalmoplegia
(d) Ophthalmitis
(e) Ophthalmomycosis
(f) Condition of pain in the eye
(g) Pertaining to circular movement of the eye
(h) Inflammation of the optic nerve
(i) Inflammation of all of the eye
(j) Instrument used to measure eye tension (the pressure within the eye)
(k) Condition of mucus discharge of the eye
(l) Condition of dryness of the eye
(m) In eye (displacement of the eyes into their sockets)
(n) Out eye (bulging eyes)

Word Exercise 2

(a) Pertaining to one eye
(b) Pertaining to one eye
(c) Pertaining to two eyes
(d) A nerve that stimulates eye movement/action
(e) Pertaining to the eye and nose
(f) Picture/tracing of the electrical activity of the eye
(g) Pertaining to a circular movement of the eye

Word Exercise 3

(a) Instrument that measures sight
(b) Technique of measuring sight
(c) Person who measures sight (specializes in optometry)
(d) Instrument for measuring the muscles of sight (the power of the ocular muscles)

Word Exercise 4

(a) Condition of double vision
(b) Condition of old man's vision
(c) Condition of dim vision
(d) Condition of half colour vision (faulty colour vision in half the field of view)
(e) Condition of painful/difficult/bad vision
(f) Condition of without half vision (blindness in one half of the visual field in one or both eyes)

Word Exercise 5

(a) Blepharoplegia
(b) Blepharospasm
(c) Blepharoptosis
(d) Blepharorrhaphy
(e) Flow of pus from the eyelid
(f) Inflammation of the eyelid glands (meibomian glands)
(g) Condition of sticking together of the eyelids
(h) Slack, loose eyelids (causes drooping)

Word Exercise 6

(a) Incision into the sclera
(b) Dilatation of the sclera
(c) Instrument to cut the sclera

Word Exercise 7

(a) Inflammation of the sclera and cornea
(b) Measurement of the cornea (actually the curvature of the cornea)
(c) Instrument to cut the cornea
(d) Surgical repair of the cornea (a corneal graft)
(e) Puncture of the cornea
(f) Abnormal condition of corneal ulcers (ulceration of the cornea)
(g) Puncture of the cornea (to remove a cataract)
(h) Carving or reshaping of the cornea
(i) A cone-like protrusion of the cornea

Word Exercise 8

(a) Iridoptosis
(b) Iridokeratitis
(c) Motion/movement of the iris (contraction and expansion)
(d) Separation of the iris
(e) Hernia/protrusion of the iris (through the cornea)
(f) Inflammation of the sclera and iris
(g) Condition of paralysis of the iris
(h) Inflammation of the cornea and iris

Word Exercise 9

(a) Inflammation of the iris and ciliary body
(b) Condition of paralysis of the ciliary body
(c) Heating through the ciliary body (to destroy tissue)

Word Exercise 10

(a) Goniometer
(b) Gonioscope
(c) Goniotomy

Word Exercise 11

(a) Condition of paralysis of the pupil
(b) Measurement of pupils (diameter)

Word Exercise 12

(a) Condition of equal pupils
(b) Condition of unequal pupils
(c) Surgical fixation of the pupil into a new position
(d) Surgical repair of the pupil

Word Exercise 13

(a) Inflammation of the choroid and ciliary body
(b) Inflammation of the sclera and choroid

Word Exercise 14

(a) Tumour (Am. tumor) of germ cells of the retina
(b) Condition of softening of the retina
(c) Splitting (separation of the retina)
(d) Disease of the retina
(e) Technique of viewing the retina
(f) Electroretinogram
(g) Retinochoroiditis (syn. with choroidoretinitis)
(h) Choroidoretinitis (syn. with retinochoroiditis)

Word Exercise 15

(a) Swelling of the optic disc
(b) Retinopapillitis

Word Exercise 16

(a) Phacomalacia
(b) Phacoscope
(c) Phacosclerosis
(d) Aphakia
(e) Removal of the lens bladder (capsule)
(f) Sucking out of the lens

Word Exercise 17

(a) Instrument to measure scotomas
(b) Technique of measuring scotomas
(c) Instrument used to record scotomas

Word Exercise 18

(a) Lacrimotomy
(b) Nasolacrimal

Word Exercise 19

(a) Technique of making an X-ray of the lacrimal sac (tear bladder or tear cyst)

(b)   Formation of an opening between the lacrimal sac and nose
(c)   A tear stone
(d)   Abnormal condition of narrowing of the lacrimal duct (or lacrimal apparatus)
(e)   Flow of mucus from the lacrimal sac
(f)   Condition of pus in the lacrimal sac

Word Exercise 20

(a)   Ophthalmoscope (4)
(b)   Dacryocystogram (1)
(c)   Keratome (5)
(d)   Pupillometry (8)
(e)   Optometry (7)
(f)   Scotometry (2)
(g)   Ophthalmotonometer (3)
(h)   Optomyometer (6)

Word Exercise 21

(a)   Sclerotome (5)
(b)   Optometer (4)
(c)   Keratometry (6)
(d)   Pupillometer (8)
(e)   Phacoscope (7)
(f)   Retinoscopy (1)
(g)   Tonography (2)
(h)   Dacryocystography (3)

Case History 9

(a)   Specialist who measures sight
(b)   Condition of double vision
(c)   Condition of pain in the eye
(d)   Inflammation of the optic nerve
(e)   Inflammation of the optic disc
(f)   A dark area/region of reduced vision within a visual field
(g)   Pertaining to the eye
(h)   Condition of paralysis of the eye

Unit 10 The Ear

Word Exercise 1

(a)   Otology
(b)   Otoscope
(c)   Otosclerosis
(d)   Otopyosis
(e)   Technique of viewing the ear (with an otoscope)
(f)   Study of the ear, nose and larynx
(g)   Abnormal condition of fungi in the ear
(h)   Excessive flow of pus from the ear
(i)   Condition of small ears
(j)   Condition of large ears

Word Exercise 2

(a)   Auriscope
(b)   Pertaining to two ears
(c)   Pertaining to within the ear
(d)   Pertaining to or having two ear auricles or pinnae

Word Exercise 3

(a)   Myringotomy
(b)   Myringotome
(c)   Myringomycosis

Word Exercise 4

(a)   Tympanoplasty
(b)   Tympanocentesis
(c)   Tympanostomy
(d)   Inflammation of the middle ear and/or ear drum
(e)   Incision into the middle ear and/or ear drum

Word Exercise 5

(a)   Blocking up of the eustachian tube / pharyngotympanic tube
(b)   Pertaining to the eustachian tube (or pharyngotympanic tube) and pharynx

Word Exercise 6

(a)   Stapedectomy
(b)   Incision into the stapes tendon

Word Exercise 7

(a)   Incision into the malleus

Word Exercise 8

(a)   Pertaining to the incus and malleus
(b)   Pertaining to the incus and stapes
(c)   Pertaining to the malleus and incus

Word Exercise 9

(a)   Cochleostomy
(b)   Electrocochleography

Word Exercise 10

(a)   Labyrinthitis
(b)   Labyrinthectomy

Word Exercise 11

(a)   Incision into the vestibule
(b)   Pertaining to originating in the vestibule

Word Exercise 12

(a) Mastoidalgia
(b) Mastoidotomy
(c) Mastoidectomy
(d) Tympanomastoiditis

Word Exercise 13

(a) Audiology
(b) Instrument that measures hearing
(c) A tracing/recording of hearing made by an audiometer
(d) Technique of measuring hearing/using an audiometer

Word Exercise 14

(a) Audiometer (6)
(b) Audiometry (1)
(c) Aural speculum (7)
(d) Auriscope (2)
(e) Otoscopy (3)
(f) Aural syringe (4)
(g) Grommet (5)

Case History 10

(a) Condition of pain in the ear
(b) Technique of viewing/examining the ear
(c) Specialist who measures hearing
(d) A tracing/recording of hearing (ability)
(e) Study of the ear and its disorders
(f) Technique of measuring the tympanic membrane (actually the measurement of the mobility and impedance of the membrane)
(g) Incision into the tympanic membrane/ear drum
(h) Opening into the tympanum/tympanic membrane

Unit 11 The Skin

Word Exercise 1

(a) Abnormal condition of the skin
(b) Above/upon the skin, the outer layer of the skin
(c) A skin plant (fungus that infects skin)
(d) Thick skin
(e) Yellow skin
(f) Self-surgical repair of skin (using one's own skin for a graft)
(g) Condition of dry skin
(h) Specialist who studies skin and diseases of the skin
(i) Dermatomycosis
(j) Dermatome
(k) Hypodermic/subdermal
(l) Intradermal

Word Exercise 2

(a) Abnormal condition of the epidermis caused by excessive exposure to the sun
(b) Abnormal condition of the epidermis (above normal thickening)
(c) Tumour (Am. tumor) of the epidermis
(d) Breakdown/disintegration of the epidermis

Word Exercise 3

(a) A nerve that produces a hair action (it erects the hair in cold conditions)

Word Exercise 4

(a) Abnormal condition of hair plants (fungal infection with *Trichophyton*)
(b) Abnormal condition of hair
(c) Condition of sensitive hairs
(d) Condition of split hairs
(e) Broken or ruptured hairs

Word Exercise 5

(a) Excessive flow of sebum
(b) A sebaceous stone (actually hardened sebum)
(c) Pertaining to stimulating the sebaceous glands

Word Exercise 6

(a) Abnormal condition of sweating (excess)
(b) Condition of increased/above normal sweating
(c) Formation of sweat
(d) Abnormal condition of without sweating
(e) Inflammation of sweat glands

Word Exercise 7

(a) Abnormal condition of a hidden nail (ingrowing)
(b) Condition of increased growth of nails
(c) Difficult/poor growth of nails (malformation)
(d) Without nourishment/wasting away of nails
(e) Condition beside a nail (inflammation)
(f) Splitting/parting of nails
(g) Condition of nail eating (actually biting)
(h) Onycholysis
(i) Onychomycosis
(j) Onychitis
(k) Rupture/breaking of nails
(l) Condition of without nails
(m) Condition of thickened nails

Word Exercise 8

(a) Melanocyte
(b) Melanosis

(c) Tumour (Am. tumor) of melanin (melanocytes), highly malignant

Word Exercise 9

(a) Excision biopsy (4)
(b) Dermatome (5)
(c) Medical laser (2)
(d) PUVA (6)
(e) Epilation (1)
(f) Electrolysis (3)

Case History 11

(a) Study of the skin
(b) Specialist who studies the skin and its disorders
(c) Pertaining to above normal epidermis, ie, a thickening of the epidermis
(d) Pertaining to the skin/of the nature of skin
(e) Disintegration/breakdown of the nails
(f) Pertaining to the epidermis or keratin
(g) Tumour (Am. tumor) formed from an epithelium/ epithelial cell
(h) Tumour (Am. tumor) of melanin/melanocytes

Unit 12 The Nose and Mouth

Word Exercise 1

(a) Study of the mouth
(b) Condition of excessive flow (of blood) from mouth
(c) Disease of the mouth
(d) Stomatodynia/stomatalgia
(e) Stomatomycosis

Word Exercise 2

(a) Pertaining to the mouth
(b) Pertaining to inside the mouth
(c) Pertaining to the mouth and pharynx
(d) Pertaining to the mouth and nose

Word Exercise 3

(a) Glossology
(b) Glossodynia
(c) Glossopharyngeal (eg, glossopharyngeal nerve IX)
(d) Condition of paralysis of the tongue
(e) Condition of hairy tongue
(f) Protrusion/swelling of the tongue
(g) Condition of a large tongue
(h) Surgical repair of the tongue

Word Exercise 4

(a) Removal of a salivary gland
(b) Technique of making X-ray/tracing of salivary vessels/ducts

(c) Condition of much saliva (excess secretion) (syn. ptyalism)
(d) X-ray of the salivary glands and ducts
(e) Sialolith
(f) A drug that stimulates saliva (production)
(g) Condition of eating saliva and air (excessive swallowing)

Word Exercise 5

(a) Pertaining to formation of saliva/originating in saliva/by the action of saliva
(b) Excessive flow of saliva (syn. ptyalism)

Word Exercise 6

(a) Gnathalgia/gnathodynia
(b) Gnathoplasty
(c) Gnathology
(d) Stomatognathic
(e) Instrument that measures jaw force (the force of the jaw closing)
(f) Split or cleft jaw
(g) Inflammation of the jaw

Word Exercise 7

(a) Surgical repair of the lips and mouth
(b) Split/cleft lip
(c) Suturing of lips
(d) Cheilitis

Word Exercise 8

(a) Pertaining to the lips, tongue and larynx
(b) Labioglossopharyngeal

Word Exercise 9

(a) Gingivitis
(b) Gingivectomy
(c) Pertaining to the lips and gums

Word Exercise 10

(a) Palatoplegia
(b) Palatoschisis
(c) Pertaining to after the palate

Word Exercise 11

(a) Uvulectomy
(b) Uvulopalatopharyngoplasty

Word Exercise 12

(a) Condition of without speech/loss of voice
(b) Condition of difficult speech (difficulty speaking)

Word Exercise 13

(a) Odontology
(b) Odontopathy
(c) Odontalgia
(d) The science or study of tissues that support the teeth
(e) The study of the inside of teeth (pulp, dentine, etc.)
(f) A specialty of dentistry dealing with the straightening of teeth and associated facial abnormalities)
(g) Person who specializes in orthodontics
(h) A specialty of dentistry dealing with the construction of artificial teeth and other oral components

Word Exercise 14

(a) Condition of having a nasal voice (speech through the nose)
(b) Instrument that measures nose pressure (air flow in the nose)
(c) Tumour (Am. tumor)/swelling/boil of the nose
(d) Technique of viewing the nose (internally)
(e) Study of the ear, nose and larynx
(f) Condition of excessive flow of blood (from nose)

Word Exercise 15

(a) Hollow/cavity in bone / an anatomical part
(b) Inflammation of the sinuses and bronchi
(c) Inflammation of a sinus
(d) An X-ray/tracing of a sinus

Word Exercise 16

(a) Antroscope
(b) Antrotympanic
(c) Incision into the antrum
(d) Pertaining to the antrum and nose
(e) Swelling/protrusion of the antrum
(f) Pertaining to the antrum and cheek
(g) Formation of an opening into the antrum

Word Exercise 17

(a) Pertaining to the face
(b) Condition of paralysis of the face
(c) Surgical repair of the face

Word Exercise 18

(a) Antroscope (3)
(b) Sialoangiography (5)
(c) Gnathodynamometer (1)
(d) Rhinomanometer (6)
(e) Prosthesis (4)
(f) Glossography (2)

Case History 12

(a) Inflammation of the nose
(b) Technique of viewing/examining the nose
(c) Inflammation of a sinus
(d) Study of the ears, nose and larynx (here referring to the department that studies disorders of these areas)
(e) Pertaining to towards the back of the nose
(f) Pertaining to the antrum (here referring to the maxillary sinus or antrum of Highmore)
(g) Pertaining to within the nose
(h) Formation of an opening into the antrum (here into the maxillary sinus or antrum of Highmore)

Unit 13 The Muscular System

Word Exercise 1

(a) Pertaining to muscle and nerve
(b) Disease of heart muscle
(c) Poor nourishment (growth) of muscle (muscular dystrophy)
(d) Inflammation of a muscle
(e) Abnormal condition of muscle fibres (the muscle is replaced by fibrous tissue) (Am. fiber)
(f) Myosclerosis
(g) Myoma
(h) Myoglobin
(i) Myospasm
(j) Condition of involuntary twitching of muscle
(k) Condition of muscle tone (abnormal increased tone and delayed relaxation)
(l) Slight paralysis of muscle
(m) Rupture of a muscle
(n) Condition of softening of a muscle
(o) Myography
(p) Electromyography
(q) Myogram

Word Exercise 2

(a) Tumour (benign) of striated muscle (Am. tumor)
(b) Breakdown of striated muscle

Word Exercise 3

(a) Pertaining to affinity for/stimulating muscle
(b) Pertaining to the muscles of the diaphragm
(c) Poor nourishment (growth) of muscle, an inherited disease

Word Exercise 4

(a) Condition of sensation of movement
(b) Instrument that measures movement of muscle
(c) Pertaining to forming movements
(d) Condition of above normal movement
(e) Dyskinesia

Word Exercise 5

(a) Condition of pain in a tendon
(b) Instrument used to cut tendons
(c) Inflammation of tendons
(d) Study of tendons
(e) Tenomyoplasty
(f) Tenomyotomy
(g) Suturing of an aponeurosis
(h) Inflammation of an aponeurosis

Word Exercise 6

(a) Pertaining to a straight child; now a branch of surgery that deals with the restoration of function in the musculoskeletal system

Word Exercise 7

(a) Myography (5)
(b) Electromyography (4)
(c) Myogram (2)
(d) Kinesimeter (6)
(e) Orthosis (1)
(f) Electromyogram (3)

Case History 13

(a) Difficult/poor nourishment (of a tissue)
(b) False, above normal nourishment (here the muscles look large and over-nourished, but the enlargement is due to disease processes within the muscle)
(c) Pertaining to dystrophy
(d) Technique of recording the electrical activity of muscle
(e) Pertaining to disease of muscle
(f) A recording/tracing of the electrical activity of muscle
(g) Without nourishment (wasting away)
(h) Pertaining to heart muscle

Unit 14 The Skeletal System

Word Exercise 1

(a) A bone plant (a pathological growth of bone)
(b) Abnormal condition of passages (pores) in bone
(c) Condition of softening of the bones
(d) Abnormal condition of stone-like or brittle bones
(e) Breaking of bone (by surgery)
(f) A cell that breaks down bone
(g) Bad nourishment of bone (poor growth)
(h) Osteoblast
(i) Osteolytic
(j) Osteotome
(k) Osteologist

Word Exercise 2

(a) Instrument used to view within a joint
(b) Abnormal condition of pus in a joint
(c) Technique of making an X-ray of joints
(d) Inflammation of many joints
(e) Fixation of a joint by surgery (it induces ossification between two bones to reduce movement and pain)
(f) Breaking of a joint (actually breaking adhesions within a joint to improve mobility)
(g) Arthroscopy
(h) Arthrocentesis
(i) Arthrogram
(j) Arthropathy
(k) Artholith
(l) Arthroplasty

Word Exercise 3

(a) Inflammation of joint synovia (inflammation of a synovial membrane)
(b) Removal of the synovial membranes / synovia
(c) Tumour (Am. tumor) / swelling of a synovial membrane

Word Exercise 4

(a) A plant-like growth of cartilage (a pathological growth of cartilage)
(b) Pertaining to/of the nature of cartilage and bone
(c) Abnormal condition of passages (pores) in cartilage
(d) Bad nourishment of cartilage (poor growth)
(e) Condition of softening of cartilage
(f) Pertaining to cartilage of a rib
(g) Pertaining to within cartilage
(h) Chondralgia
(i) Chondrogenesis
(j) Chondrolysis
(k) Abnormal condition of cartilage that has calcified (an abnormal increase in calcium in cartilage)

Word Exercise 5

(a) Condition of pain in the vertebrae
(b) Abnormal condition of pus in vertebrae
(c) Spondylolysis
(d) Spondylopathy
(e) Spondylitis, eg, ankylosing spondylitis in which vertebrae fuse
(f) Slipping/forward displacement of vertebrae

Word Exercise 6

(a) Resembling a disc
(b) Pertaining to forming a disc / originating in a disc
(c) Discography
(d) Discectomy

Word Exercise 7

(a) Inflammation of bone marrow
(b) Abnormal condition of fibrous bone marrow (fibres present in bone marrow)

Word Exercise 8

(a) Osteotome (4)
(b) Arthrodesis (3)
(c) Replacement arthroplasty (5)
(d) Arthrocentesis (1)
(e) Arthrography (2)

Word Exercise 9

(a) Claviculoplasty
(b) Craniomalacia
(c) Intercostal
(d) Phalangectomy
(e) Pelvic
(f) Olecranarthritis
(g) Tibiofemoral
(h) Scapulodesis
(i) Metatarsalgia
(j) Acetabuloplasty
(k) Mandibuloplasty
(l) Maxillitis
(m) Sternocostal
(n) Ischiococcygeal

Word Exercise 10

(a) Pertaining to between the phalanges (finger or toe bones)
(b) Condition of pain in a metatarsus or metatarsal bone
(c) Pertaining to a tarsus and metatarsus or tarsal and metatarsal bones
(d) Pertaining to a metacarpus or metacarpal bone
(e) Pertaining to the humerus and radius
(f) Pertaining to the ulna and carpus (wrist)
(g) Condition of pain in the coccyx
(h) Pertaining to the kneecap and femur
(i) Pertaining to the ilium and sacrum
(j) Pertaining to the tibia and fibula

Case History 14

(a) Specialist who studies rheumatism
(b) Condition of pain in the joints
(c) Inflammation of a bursa
(d) Inflammation of many joints
(e) Pertaining to the metacarpals and phalanges
(f) Pertaining to between the phalanges
(g) Pertaining to the metatarsal bones and phalanges
(h) Disease of joints

Unit 15 The Male Reproductive System

Word Exercise 1

(a) Disease of the testes
(b) Hernia/protrusion/swelling of testes (through scrotum)
(c) Condition of having hidden testes, ie, undescended
(d) Surgical fixation of the testes, ie, into their normal position
(e) Orchiotomy, orchidotomy less used
(f) Orchioplasty, orchidoplasty less used
(g) Orchiectomy or orchidectomy
(h) Orchialgia or orchidalgia
(i) Surgical fixation of hidden testes, ie, into their normal position

Word Exercise 2

(a) Scrotectomy
(b) Scrotoplasty
(c) Scrotocele
(d) Pertaining to through/across the scrotum

Word Exercise 3

(a) Phallocampsis
(b) Phallic
(c) Phallectomy

Word Exercise 4

(a) Balanitis
(b) Condition of bursting forth (of pus) from the glans penis
(c) Inflammation of the glans penis and prepuce

Word Exercise 5

(a) Epididymitis
(b) Epididymectomy
(c) Inflammation of the epididymis and testis

Word Exercise 6

(a) Removal of the vas deferens (a section of it to prevent transfer of sperm)
(b) Formation of an opening between the vas deferens and epididymis
(c) Technique of making an X-ray of the vas deferens and epididymis
(d) Cutting/excision of the vas deferens
(e) Stitching/suturing of the vas deferens
(f) Formation of an opening between the vas deferens and testes
(g) Formation of an opening between the vas deferens and another part of the vas deferens
(h) Incision into the vas deferens

Word Exercise 7

(a) Vesiculography
(b) Vesiculotomy
(c) Removal of the vas deferens and seminal vesicles

Word Exercise 8

(a) Incision into the prostate gland and bladder
(b) Enlargement of the prostate gland
(c) Removal of the prostate gland
(d) Removal of the prostate gland and seminal vesicles

Word Exercise 9

(a) Pertaining to carrying semen
(b) Condition of semen in the urine
(c) Tumour (Am. tumor) of semen (actually the germ cells of the testis)

Word Exercise 10

(a) Condition of being without sperm, also used to mean without semen
(b) Condition of few sperm (low sperm count)
(c) Killing of sperms (actually an agent used as a contraceptive for killing sperm)
(d) Spermatopathia
(e) Spermatogenesis
(f) Spermatolysis
(g) Spermatorrhoea (Am. spermatorrhea)

Word Exercise 11

(a) Sperm count (5)
(b) Transurethral resection (4)
(c) Vasectomy (6)
(d) Orchidometer (3)
(e) In vitro fertilization (1)
(f) Vasoligature (2)

Case History 15

(a) Process/condition of hidden testicles (ie, undescended testicles)
(b) Fixation of testicles by surgery (an operation to fix undescended testicles in their correct position)
(c) Inflammation of the testes/testicles
(d) Pertaining to within a testicle
(e) Removal of a testicle
(f) Pertaining to sperm/semen
(g) Pertaining to through the scrotum
(h) Tumour (Am. tumor) of the semen (arising from undifferentiated germ cells in the testis)

Unit 16 The Female Reproductive System

Word Exercise 1

(a) Germ cell that produces eggs
(b) Egg cell (actually an immature ovum)
(c) Formation of eggs

Word Exercise 2

(a) Oophorectomy
(b) Oophoropexy
(c) Oophorotomy
(d) Removal of an ovarian bladder (cyst) from the ovary (an ovarian cyst)
(e) Opening into an ovary/formation of an opening into an ovary

Word Exercise 3

(a) Ovariectomy
(b) Ovariotomy
(c) Rupture/breaking of an ovary
(d) Pertaining to the ovary and oviduct
(e) Puncture of an ovary to remove fluid

Word Exercise 4

(a) Removal of an oviduct and ovary
(b) Removal of an ovary and oviduct
(c) Fixation of a fallopian tube (by surgery)
(d) Hernia/protrusion/swelling of an oviduct
(e) Inflammation of an oviduct and ovary
(f) Salpingography
(g) Salpingolithiasis
(h) Salpingoplasty

Word Exercise 5

(a) Uteralgia/uterodynia
(b) Uterosclerosis
(c) Pertaining to the uterus and fallopian tubes
(d) Technique of making an X-ray of the uterus and oviducts
(e) Pertaining to the uterus and bladder
(f) Pertaining to the uterus and rectum
(g) Pertaining to the uterus and placenta

Word Exercise 6

(a) Hysteroscope
(b) Hysteroptosis
(c) Hysterogram
(d) Technique of making an X-ray of the uterus and oviducts

(e) Formation of an opening between the uterus and oviducts
(f) Removal of the uterus, oviducts and ovaries
(g) Suturing of the neck of the uterus
(h) Incision into the neck of the uterus

Word Exercise 7

(a) Excessive dripping/bleeding from the uterus
(b) Condition of disease of the uterus with excessive loss of blood
(c) Inflammation of the uterine peritoneum (a membrane around the uterus)
(d) Inflammation of the uterine veins
(e) Abnormal condition of uterine cysts (cysts in the uterus)
(f) Abnormal condition of a falling/prolapsed uterus
(g) Metrostenosis
(h) Metromalacia
(i) Inflammation within the lining of the uterus (endometrium)
(j) Tumour (Am. tumor) of the endometrium
(k) Abnormal/disease condition of the endometrium

Word Exercise 8

(a) Excessive dripping of menses / prolonged menstruation
(b) The beginning of menstruation
(c) Stopping of menstruation (occurs in women aged 45–50 years approximately)
(d) Without menstrual flow (menstruation), eg, as in pregnancy
(e) Difficult/painful/bad menstruation
(f) Reduced flow of menses/infrequent menstruation
(g) Pertaining to before menstruation

Word Exercise 9

(a) Cervicitis
(b) Cervicectomy

Word Exercise 10

(a) Technique of viewing or examining the vagina
(b) A microscope used to view the vagina in situ (its lining)
(c) Suturing of the vagina and perineum
(d) Removal of the uterus through the vagina
(e) Hernia/protrusion/swelling of the uterus into the vagina
(f) Inflammation of the cervix and vagina
(g) Colpoperineoplasty
(h) Colpopexy

Word Exercise 11

(a) Incision into the vagina and perineum
(b) Suturing of the vagina and perineum
(c) Pertaining to the vagina and bladder

(d) Vaginomycosis
(e) Vaginopathy

Word Exercise 12

(a) Inflammation of the vulva and vagina
(b) Pertaining to the vulva and vagina

Word Exercise 13

(a) Instrument to view the rectouterine pouch
(b) Technique of viewing the rectouterine pouch (actually the examination of the female pelvic viscera through the posterior vaginal fornix)
(c) Puncture of the rectouterine pouch to remove fluid

Word Exercise 14

(a) Study of the female reproductive system (particularly diseases and disorders specific to women)
(b) Pertaining to gynaecology (Am. gynecology)

Word Exercise 15

(a) A woman's first pregnancy
(b) A woman's second pregnancy
(c) A woman who is pregnant and has been pregnant at least twice before

Word Exercise 16

(a) A woman who has had one pregnancy that resulted in a viable child
(b) A woman who has had two pregnancies that resulted in viable offspring
(c) A woman who has had more than two pregnancies that resulted in viable offspring
(d) A woman who has never borne a viable child

Word Exercise 17

(a) Study of the fetus
(b) Instrument to view the fetus
(c) Pertaining to the fetus and placenta
(d) Fetotoxic
(e) Fetometry

Word Exercise 18

(a) Pertaining to the amnion
(b) Instrument to cut the amnion
(c) Amniotomy
(d) Amnioscope
(e) Puncture of the amnion to remove amniotic fluid
(f) Pertaining to the chorion and amnion (fetal membranes)
(g) Inflammation of the chorion and amnion

Word Exercise 19

(a) Placentitis
(b) Placentopathy

Word Exercise 20

(a) Condition of difficult/painful/bad birth
(b) Study of labour (Am. labor)/birth
(c) Condition of good (normal) birth

Word Exercise 21

(a) Pertaining to a new birth
(b) Pertaining to before birth
(c) Pertaining to around/near birth
(d) Pertaining to before birth
(e) Study of neonates (new births)

Word Exercise 22

(a) Technique of making a breast X-ray
(b) Surgical reconstruction/repair of the breast
(c) Pertaining to affinity for / affecting the breast

Word Exercise 23

(a) Mastalgia
(b) Mastoptosis (pendulous breasts)
(c) Mastectomy
(d) Condition of women's breasts (abnormal condition seen in males)

Word Exercise 24

(a) Agent stimulating/promoting milk production
(b) Pertaining to carrying milk
(c) Instrument used to measure milk (its specific gravity)
(d) Hormone that acts before milk, ie, on the breast to stimulate lactation
(e) Agent that stops milk (secretion)
(f) Pertaining to forming milk/originating in milk

Word Exercise 25

(a) Agent that stimulates milk production
(b) Excessive flow of milk
(c) Condition of holding back/stopping milk (secretion)
(d) Formation of milk

Word Exercise 26

(a) Vaginal speculum (9)
(b) Colposcope (5)
(c) Pap test (7)
(d) Culdoscopy (3)
(e) Fetoscope (10)
(f) Hysteroscope (2)
(g) Amniotome (4)
(h) Lactometer (6)
(i) Obstetrical forceps (8)
(j) Tocography (1)

Case History 16

(a) Woman pregnant for the first time
(b) Without menstruation / menstrual flow
(c) Technique of recording the heart rate (of the fetus) and labour (uterine contractions) during delivery (Am. labor)
(d) Pertaining to before birth
(e) Pertaining to around birth
(f) A doctor who specializes in problems associated with childbirth/midwifery
(g) Period following birth when reproductive organs return to their normal condition (approx. 6 weeks)
(h) Pertaining to the amnion

Unit 17 The Endocrine System

Word Exercise 1

(a) Process of secreting below normal level of pituitary hormones (an underactive pituitary gland)
(b) Process of secreting above normal level of pituitary hormones (an overactive pituitary gland)
(c) Condition of small extremities, ie, hands and feet (due to deficiency of growth hormone in adulthood)
(d) Large extremities, ie, hands and feet (due to excess production of growth hormone in adulthood)

Word Exercise 2

(a) Pertaining to the thyroid gland and tongue
(b) Inflammation of the thyroid gland
(c) Thyroid protein
(d) Incision into the thyroid cartilage
(e) Condition of poisoning by the thyroid (due to overstimulation of thyroid gland)
(f) Near/beside the thyroid (the parathyroid gland)
(g) Removal of the parathyroid glands
(h) Process of secreting above normal levels of parathyroid hormones
(i) Enlargement of the thyroid gland
(j) Hyperthyroidism
(k) Hypothyroidism
(l) Thyroptosis
(m) Thyrotropic
(n) Thyrogenic

Word Exercise 3

(a) Pertaining to affinity for/acting on the pancreas
(b) Formation of insulin (from the islets of Langerhans)
(c) Tumour (Am. tumor) of the islets of Langerhans
(d) Inflammation of the islets of Langerhans
(e) Process of secreting above normal levels of insulin
(f) Condition of below normal levels of sugar in blood
(g) Condition of above normal levels of sugar in blood
(h) Condition of sugar in the urine

Word Exercise 4

(a) Adrenomegaly
(b) Adrenalectomy
(c) Adrenotropic
(d) Condition of above normal levels of sodium in the blood
(e) Condition of below normal levels of potassium in the blood
(f) Secretion of excess sodium in the urine
(g) Pertaining to nourishing the adrenal cortex
(h) Condition of above normal growth of cells of adrenal cortex

Word Exercise 5

(a) Pertaining to male and female (hermaphroditic or of doubtful sex)
(b) Tumour (Am. tumor) of the germ cells of the male, ie, the testis

Word Exercise 6

(a) Adrenal function test (4)
(b) Glucose tolerance test (3)
(c) PBI test (2)
(d) Blood glucose monitor (5)
(e) Thyroid scan (1)

Case History 17

(a) Condition of too much urine
(b) Condition of sugar in the urine
(c) Condition of above normal concentration of sugar in the blood
(d) Condition of ketones in the blood
(e) Abnormal acidity caused by ketones
(f) Pertaining to the pancreas
(g) Condition of below normal levels of sugar in the blood
(h) Pertaining to sugar in the blood

Unit 18 Radiology

Word Exercise 1

(a) Specialist who studies radiology (a physician specializing in radiology); a specialist who studies radiation

(b) An X-ray picture
(c) Technique of making an X-ray
(d) One who makes an X-ray (Am. radiologic technologist)
(e) Treatment with X-rays or other forms of radiation

Word Exercise 2

(a) Technique of making an X-ray/roentgenogram
(b) A specialist who studies roentgenology/X-rays (a physician specializing in radiology)
(c) An X-ray picture

Word Exercise 3

(a) Fluoroscope
(b) Fluoroscopical
(c) Fluorography (syn. fluororadiography and photofluorography)

Word Exercise 4

(a) Technique of making a moving X-ray recording
(b) A recording of a moving X-ray picture
(c) Technique of making a moving image (X-ray) of the vessels and heart
(d) A recording (X-ray) of the movement of the oesophagus (Am. esophagus)

Word Exercise 5

(a) An X-ray picture of a slice/section through the body
(b) Technique of making an X-ray of a slice/section through the body

Word Exercise 6

(a) A picture of sparks, ie, distribution of radioactivity within the body (synonymous with a scintiscan, an image/tracing produced by a scintiscanner)
(b) Technique of making a scintigram

Word Exercise 7

(a) A picture/tracing produced using ultrasound (syn. sonogram, sonograph, echogram)
(b) Technique of making a picture/tracing using ultrasound (syn. sonography, echography)
(c) An instrument that uses ultrasound to make a picture/tracing/recording; an ultrasound image (syn. Sonograph)

Word Exercise 8

(a) A picture/tracing made using ultrasound echoes from the brain
(b) Echogenic
(c) Echogram (syn. sonogram)

(d) Echoencephalograph
(e) Echocardiogram
(f) Echography (syn. ultrasonography)

Word Exercise 9

(a) Radiography (4)
(b) Fluoroscopy (7)
(c) Radionuclide (8)
(d) Ultrasonograph (5)
(e) Computerized tomograph (6)
(f) Radiotherapy (9)
(g) Cineradiography (10)
(h) Gamma camera (1)
(i) Echocardiography (2)
(j) Contrast medium (3)

Case History 18

(a) A recording/picture produced using X-rays
(b) Technique of recording/producing an image of a slice/ cross-section through the body
(c) Treatment using radiation/X-rays, etc.
(d) An X-ray picture of a slice/section through the body
(e) Pertaining to the killing of a tumour (Am. tumor)
(f) Radiant energy, eg, X-rays used in the treatment of cancer
(g) A device that produces high energy beams of electrons/ X-rays for radiotherapy
(h) Technique of making a recording using high-frequency sound waves

Unit 19 Oncology

Word Exercise 1

(a) Abnormal condition of tumours (Am. tumor) (Note. oncosis is also used to mean ischaemic cell death, a condition in which cellular components swell; this is not relevant to our study of cancer)
(b) Formation of tumours (Am. tumor)
(c) Pertaining to affinity for a tumour (Am. tumor)
(d) Oncogenic
(e) Oncolysis
(f) Oncologist

Word Exercise 2

(a) Pertaining to the formation of a carcinoma (a malignant tumour of an epithelium)
(b) Destruction/disintegration of a carcinoma
(c) Pertaining to stopping the growth of a carcinoma

Word Exercise 3

(a) A malignant tumour (Am. tumor) of cartilage
(b) A malignant tumour of smooth muscle
(c) A malignant tumour of striated muscle
(d) A malignant tumour of meninges
(e) A malignant tumour of blood vessels
(f) Abnormal condition of sarcomas

Case History 19

(a) A new growth (of cancer cells)
(b) Parts of a tumour (Am. tumor) that have spread from one site to another
(c) Tumour of the meninges
(d) Lump of matter (here meaning a tumour)
(e) Tumour of glial cells (neurogliacytes) in the brain
(f) A specialist who studies tumours/cancers
(g) Treatment using chemicals (cytotoxic drugs that kill cancer cells)
(h) 'Wasting away' of body tissues; malnutrition and emaciation

Unit 20 Anatomical Position

Word Exercise 1

(a) Superior
(b) Inferior
(c) Lateral
(d) Medial
(e) Anterior
(f) Dorsal
(g) Distal
(h) Proximal
(i) Superficial

Word Exercise 2

(a) Inferior
(b) Superior
(c) Medial
(d) Proximal
(e) Anterior
(f) Dorsal

Word Exercise 3

(a) 6
(b) 2
(c) 5
(d) 3
(e) 7
(f) 4
(g) 1

Word Exercise 4

(a) Pertaining to the region below cartilage (of the rib cage)
(b) Pertaining to the region upon/above the stomach
(c) Pertaining to the region of the ilium/hip

Word Exercise 5

(a) 6
(b) 1
(c) 7
(d) 2
(e) 5
(f) 8
(g) 3
(h) 4

Word Exercise 6

Leg regions

(a) femoral region
(b) patellar region
(c) crural region
(d) tarsal region
(e) digital/phalangeal region
(f) hallux region
(g) pedal region

Arm regions

(a) brachial region
(b) antebrachial region
(c) pollex region
(d) axillary region
(e) carpal region
(f) palmar/volar region
(g) digital/phalangeal region

Word Exercise 7

(a) 2
(b) 4
(c) 1
(d) 3

Word Exercise 8

(a) Paranasal
(b) Intervertebral
(c) Epigastric
(d) Postganglionic
(e) Dextrocardia
(f) Infra-orbital/suborbital

Word Exercise 9

(a) Pertaining to around the heart
(b) Pertaining to within a vein
(c) Pertaining to between the ribs
(d) A uterus turned backwards
(e) Pertaining to above the liver
(f) Pertaining to below the sternum
(g) Pertaining to before/in front of a ganglion
(h) Pertaining to outside the placenta
(i) Pertaining to under the epidermis

Case History 20

(a) Pertaining to near the point of attachment/origin
(b) Pertaining to near the surface of the body or surface of a structure
(c) Towards the front
(d) Pertaining to the median line along the centre of the body
(e) Flexing/bending back
(f) Pertaining to the side
(g) Pertaining to further away from the point of attachment/ origin
(h) From the front to the back

Unit 21 Pharmacology and Microbiology

Word Exercise 1

(a) The (scientific) study of drugs
(b) A specialist who studies drugs
(c) Abnormal condition of a drug affecting the mind / a psychosis due to drugs/any mental condition caused by drugs

Word Exercise 2

(a) 6
(b) 1
(c) 5
(d) 7
(e) 4
(f) 3
(g) 2

Word Exercise 3

(a) Drug that acts against bacteria
(b) Drug that acts against life (actually against bacteria and fungi)
(c) Drug that acts against fungi
(d) Drug that acts against viruses/virions
(e) Drug that acts against acid (neutralizes acid)
(f) Drug that acts against worms, eg, thread worms/tape-worms

Word Exercise 4

(a) The word means without pain, therefore a drug that reduces pain
(b) The word means without sensation, therefore a drug that reduces sensation

Word Exercise 5

(a) Drug that acts against (reduces symptoms of) diarrhoea (Am. diarrhea)

(b) Drug that acts against (prevents) spasm; it reduces the motility of the intestines

Word Exercise 6

(a) Drug that breaks down mucus (it reduces viscosity of mucus)
(b) Drug that acts against (prevents) coughing
(c) Drug that dilates the bronchi

Word Exercise 7

(a) Drug that breaks down fibrin of blood clots (used to remove clots/thrombi)
(b) Drug that prevents the breakdown of fibrin/clots (used to promote clotting in severe haemorrhage (Am. hemorrhage))
(c) The word means against without rhythm, therefore a drug that acts against arrhythmias (an arrhythmia is an abnormal heart beat, ie, one without rhythm)
(d) Drug that stops blood flow, thereby stimulating the clotting of blood

Word Exercise 8

(a) The word means pertaining to sleep, therefore a drug that induces sleep
(b) The word means breaking down anxiety, therefore a drug that reduces anxiety
(c) Drug that acts against (prevents) epilepsy
(d) Drug that acts against (prevents) psychosis, eg, schizophrenia

Word Exercise 9

(a) Drug that paralyzes the ciliary body of the eye

Word Exercise 10

(a) Drug that acts against (prevents) itching
(b) Drug that breaks down epidermis/keratin (used to remove warts, overgrowths of epidermis caused by a viral infection)

Word Exercise 11

(a) Drug that produces quick labour (Am. labor)/birth (used to induce birth)
(b) Drug that nourishes/stimulates the gonads
(c) Drug that acts against oestrogen (Am. estrogen), used for infertility treatment in women

Word Exercise 12

(a) Drug that acts against the thyroid (especially the synthesis of thyroid hormones)

Word Exercise 13

(a) Drug that is poisonous to cells and kills them, used to destroy cancer cells
(b) Drug that acts against new growths (tumours / cancer cells) and kills them

Word Exercise 14

(a) Drug that suppresses the immune system or immune response
(b) Drug that increases the activity of the immune system
(c) Drug used to suppress the cell-mediated immune response by killing cells (used to prevent rejection of transplanted organs)

Word Exercise 15

(a) 5
(b) 3
(c) 6
(d) 2
(e) 1
(f) 7
(g) 4

Word Exercise 16

(a) A specialist who studies bacteria
(b) Pertaining to streptococci
(c) Condition of bacteria in the urine
(d) Pertaining to killing bacteria
(e) Pertaining to stopping bacteria (growing)
(f) Pertaining to breakdown/disintegration of bacteria
(g) Condition of bacilli in the blood
(h) Condition of blood poisoning (septicaemia (Am. septicemia)) caused by streptococci
(i) Abnormal condition/disease caused by spirilla

Word Exercise 17

(a) Abnormal condition/disease of fungi (fungal infection)
(b) Pertaining to fungi
(c) A toxin/poison produced by fungi
(d) Abnormal condition/disease due to a fungal toxin or fungal poison

Word Exercise 18

(a) Having the form of a fungus
(b) Pertaining to being toxic/poisonous to fungi
(c) Agent that kills fungi
(d) Pertaining to stopping fungi (growth)
(e) Resembling fungi
(f) State/condition of fungi; a fungoid growth or excrescence

Word Exercise 19

(a) Agent that destroys or deactivates viruses (note. as viruses do not show the characteristics of life, they are destroyed rather than killed)

(b) Specialist who studies viruses

(c) Agent that acts against retroviruses (eg, HIV)

(d) Condition of (excreting) viruses in urine

(e) Condition of viruses in the blood

(f) Condition of (excreting) viruses in milk

(c) Drug that acts against bacteria

(d) Drug that acts against life (antibiotics are derived or are derivatives of chemicals produced by living microorganisms and have the capacity to kill other organisms)

(e) The study of small organisms (bacteria, fungi, protozoa, etc.)

(f) Drug that acts against fungi (eg, *Candida albicans*)

(g) Drug that acts to prevent vomiting

(h) Pertaining to a treatment regimen involving drugs

Case History 21

(a) Drug that acts against retroviruses (eg, HIV)

(b) Abnormal condition resulting from Candida (a yeast-like fungal infection)

ANSWERS TO SELF-ASSESSMENT TESTS

Unit 1 Levels of Organization

Test 1A

(a)	7	(h)	4	(o)	16
(b)	14	(i)	17	(p)	20
(c)	18	(j)	12	(q)	11
(d)	19	(k)	5	(r)	15
(e)	8	(l)	10	(s)	6
(f)	3	(m)	1	(t)	13
(g)	9	(n)	2		

Test 1B

(a) Breakdown of cartilage
(b) Breakdown of white cells
(c) Pertaining to poisonous to tissues
(d) Disease of bone; also used to mean a system of complementary medicine that manipulates and massages the musculoskeletal system
(e) Immature lymph cell/cell that forms lymphocytes

Test 1C

(a) Microcyte
(b) Pathologist
(c) Cytopathologist
(d) Chondrology
(e) Cytopathic

Unit 2 The Digestive System

Test 2A

(a)	15	(f)	4	(k)	3
(b)	14	(g)	13/12	(l)	7
(c)	10/11	(h)	5	(m)	8
(d)	2	(i)	12	(n)	6
(e)	9	(j)	1	(o)	11

Test 2B

(a)	14	(h)	17	(o)	11
(b)	20	(i)	15	(p)	13
(c)	2	(j)	7	(q)	10
(d)	5	(k)	12	(r)	4
(e)	19	(l)	3	(s)	18
(f)	9	(m)	16	(t)	8
(g)	6	(n)	1		

Test 2C

(a)	6	(h)	7	(o)	18
(b)	20	(i)	5	(p)	3
(c)	17	(j)	12	(q)	10
(d)	14	(k)	19	(r)	1
(e)	16	(l)	4	(s)	9
(f)	8	(m)	15	(t)	2
(g)	11	(n)	13		

Test 2D

(a) Inflammation of the stomach, small intestine and colon
(b) Technique of making an X-ray/recording of liver
(c) Pertaining to the ileum and rectum
(d) Technique of viewing/examining the rectum and sigmoid colon
(e) Enlargement of the pancreas

Test 2E

(a) Duodenitis
(b) Gastralgia
(c) Hepatotomy
(d) Proctology
(e) Ileoproctostomy

Unit 3 The Respiratory System

Test 3A

(a)	3	(e)	4	(i)	9
(b)	10	(f)	7/6	(j)	1
(c)	5	(g)	2		
(d)	6/7	(h)	8		

Test 3B

(a)	14	(h)	18	(o)	15
(b)	16	(i)	4	(p)	20
(c)	7	(j)	1	(q)	9
(d)	12	(k)	19	(r)	3
(e)	8	(l)	5	(s)	10
(f)	2	(m)	6	(t)	17
(g)	11	(n)	13		

Test 3C

(a)	3	(h)	13	(o)	17
(b)	19	(i)	12	(p)	9
(c)	5	(j)	10/11	(q)	11/10
(d)	18	(k)	14	(r)	20
(e)	7	(l)	2	(s)	4
(f)	15	(m)	6	(t)	8
(g)	1	(n)	16		

Test 3D

(a) Originating in bronchi / pertaining to formation of bronchi
(b) Abnormal condition of narrowing of trachea
(c) Specialist who studies lungs
(d) Condition of pain in the diaphragm
(e) Condition of paralysis of the larynx (actually the laryngeal muscles)

Test 3E

(a) Bronchoplasty
(b) Bronchoscopy
(c) Tracheorrhaphy
(d) Rhinology
(e) Costophrenic

Unit 4 The Cardiovascular System

Test 4A

(a)	6	(c)	4	(e)	2
(b)	1	(d)	5	(f)	3

Test 4B

(a)	7	(h)	20	(o)	17
(b)	6	(i)	1/2	(p)	14
(c)	4	(j)	19	(q)	12
(d)	15	(k)	18	(r)	13
(e)	3	(l)	11	(s)	5
(f)	10	(m)	9	(t)	16
(g)	8	(n)	2/1		

Test 4C

(a)	12	(h)	1	(o)	18
(b)	9/10	(i)	13	(p)	20
(c)	6	(j)	14	(q)	17
(d)	2	(k)	3	(r)	5
(e)	7	(l)	15/16	(s)	10/9
(f)	8	(m)	4	(t)	16/15
(g)	11	(n)	19		

Test 4D

(a) Inflammation of heart valves
(b) Suturing of the aorta
(c) Instrument used to view vessels
(d) Abnormal condition of narrowing of veins
(e) Inflammation of the lining of an artery due to a clot

Test 4E

(a) Phlebosclerosis
(b) Cardiocentesis
(c) Arteriopathy
(d) Phlebectomy
(e) Angiocardiology

Unit 5 The Blood

Test 5A

(a)	5	(c)	1	(e)	4
(b)	3	(d)	2		

Test 5B

(a)	10	(i)	12	(q)	5
(b)	17	(j)	9	(r)	11
(c)	6	(k)	7	(s)	16
(d)	13	(l)	2	(t)	15
(e)	19	(m)	21	(u)	24
(f)	20	(n)	4	(v)	14
(g)	22	(o)	18	(w)	8
(h)	3	(p)	23	(x)	1

Test 5C

(a) Condition of white blood cells/leucocytes (Am. leukocytes) in urine
(b) Abnormal condition of marrow cells (too many)
(c) Condition of a deficiency of reticulocytes in the blood
(d) Condition of blood with thrombocytes (too many platelets)
(e) Breakdown of phagocytes

Test 5D

(a) Haemopathy (Am. hemopathy)
(b) Thrombocytosis
(c) Haematologist (Am. hematologist)
(d) Haemotoxic/haematotoxic (Am. hemotoxic/hematotoxic)
(e) Neutropenia

Unit 6 The Lymphatic System and Immunology

Test 6A

(a) 5   (c) 2   (e) 4
(b) 3   (d) 1

Test 6B

(a) 14   (h) 10   (o) 15
(b) 5   (i) 3   (p) 11
(c) 8   (j) 13   (q) 9
(d) 4   (k) 18   (r) 20
(e) 2   (l) 17   (s) 7
(f) 1   (m) 19   (t) 12
(g) 16   (n) 6

Test 6C

(a) Excessive flow of lymph
(b) Pertaining to the spleen
(c) Dilatation of a lymph node
(d) Breakdown of the thymus gland
(e) A specialist who studies sera

Test 6D

(a) Lymphoma
(b) Lymphography
(c) Splenectomy
(d) Splenorrhagia
(e) Lymphangioma

Unit 7 The Urinary System

Test 7A

(a) 4   (d) 3   (g) 5
(b) 2   (e) 7   (h) 8
(c) 1   (f) 6

Test 7B

(a) 9   (h) 17   (o) 10
(b) 7   (i) 18   (p) 6
(c) 15   (j) 2   (q) 20
(d) 16   (k) 5   (r) 1
(e) 14   (l) 13   (s) 3
(f) 11   (m) 8   (t) 4
(g) 12   (n) 19

Test 7C

(a) 17   (h) 18   (o) 16
(b) 8/9   (i) 12   (p) 7

(c) 11   (j) 5   (q) 13
(d) 15   (k) 3/2   (r) 14
(e) 1   (l) 4   (s) 10
(f) 19   (m) 20   (t) 9 or 8
(g) 2/3   (n) 6

Test 7D

(a) Incision to remove stones from the kidney and renal pelvis
(b) Abnormal condition of narrowing of the ureter
(c) Technique of recording/making an X-ray of the bladder and urethra
(d) Hernia/protrusion of the bladder
(e) Dilatation of the pelvis

Test 7E

(a) Ureterectasis
(b) Sigmoidoureterostomy
(c) Cystography
(d) Urogram
(e) Nephrosclerosis

Unit 8 The Nervous System

Test 8A

(a) 3   (e) 6   (h) 8
(b) 1   (f) 4   (i) 7
(c) 9   (g) 2   (j) 5
(d) 10

Test 8B

(a) 7/8   (h) 13   (o) 20
(b) 19   (i) 4/3   (p) 12
(c) 15   (j) 14   (q) 1
(d) 8/7   (k) 6   (r) 11
(e) 3/4   (l) 2   (s) 9/10
(f) 18   (m) 17   (t) 10/9
(g) 16   (n) 5

Test 8C

(a) 20   (h) 7   (o) 3
(b) 10   (i) 18   (p) 2
(c) 13   (j) 6   (q) 1
(d) 8   (k) 17   (r) 14
(e) 11   (l) 16   (s) 5
(f) 19   (m) 4   (t) 9
(g) 12   (n) 15

Test 8D

(a) 14	(h) 2	(o) 4
(b) 7	(i) 17	(p) 6
(c) 19	(j) 11	(q) 15
(d) 13	(k) 8	(r) 20
(e) 3	(l) 1	(s) 9
(f) 18	(m) 16	(t) 5
(g) 12	(n) 10	

Test 8E

(a) Inflammation of the nerves and the spinal cord
(b) Incision into the spine
(c) Condition of softening of the meninges
(d) Disease of the brain and spinal cord
(e) Instrument used to view the ventricles of the brain (an endoscope for intracranial use)

Test 8F

(a) Meningopathy
(b) Cephalometer
(c) Radiculomyelitis
(d) Encephalorrhagia
(e) Neurocytology

Unit 9 The Eye

Test 9A

(a) 3	(e) 1	(h) 9
(b) 4	(f) 7	(i) 6
(c) 2	(g) 8	(j) 10
(d) 5		

Test 9B

(a) 12	(h) 20	(o) 8
(b) 17	(i) 15	(p) 7
(c) 18	(j) 6	(q) 10
(d) 19	(k) 16	(r) 2
(e) 1	(l) 4/5	(s) 9
(f) 14	(m) 3	(t) 5/4
(g) 13	(n) 11	

Test 9C

(a) 17	(h) 10	(o) 3
(b) 14	(i) 4	(p) 11
(c) 9	(j) 2	(q) 5
(d) 18	(k) 20/19	(r) 8
(e) 1	(l) 16/15	(s) 13
(f) 12	(m) 15/16	(t) 7
(g) 19/20	(n) 6	

Test 9D

(a) Surgical repair/reconstruction of the eye
(b) Surgical fixation of the retina
(c) Excessive flow of pus from tear ducts
(d) Inflammation of the sclera and iris
(e) Nerve that stimulates movement/action of the eye

Test 9E

(a) Ophthalmoscopy
(b) Blepharitis
(c) Keratopathy
(d) Retinoscope
(e) Iridoschisis

Unit 10 The Ear

Test 10A

(a) 8	(e) 3	(h) 1
(b) 5	(f) 4	(i) 6
(c) 7/5	(g) 10	(j) 2
(d) 9		

Test 10B

(a) 8/9/10	(h) 3	(o) 11
(b) 9/8/10	(i) 15	(p) 13
(c) 14	(j) 17	(q) 2
(d) 16	(k) 6	(r) 5
(e) 10/9/8	(l) 18	(s) 4
(f) 19	(m) 7	(t) 1
(g) 12	(n) 20	

Test 10C

(a) 12	(h) 17	(o) 3
(b) 5/6	(i) 11	(p) 4
(c) 7	(j) 13	(q) 1
(d) 15	(k) 18	(r) 14
(e) 20	(l) 6/5	(s) 8
(f) 2	(m) 16	(t) 9
(g) 10	(n) 19	

Test 10D

(a) Study of the ear and larynx
(b) Condition of hardening within the middle ear (around the ear ossicles)
(c) Pertaining to the stapes and vestibular apparatus
(d) Pertaining to the tympanic membrane and malleus
(e) Puncture of the mastoid process

Test 10E

(a) Vestibulocochlear
(b) Myringectomy
(c) Otoplasty
(d) Otalgia
(e) Tympanogenic

Unit 11 The Skin

Test 11A

(a) 5
(b) 4
(c) 1
(d) 6
(e) 2
(f) 3

Test 11B

(a) 18
(b) 19
(c) 17
(d) 8
(e) 13
(f) 2
(g) 16
(h) 4
(i) 3
(j) 14
(k) 6
(l) 5
(m) 10
(n) 11
(o) 20
(p) 1
(q) 7
(r) 12
(s) 15
(t) 9

Test 11C

(a) 11
(b) 7
(c) 9
(d) 1
(e) 12
(f) 2
(g) 3
(h) 6
(i) 8
(j) 4/5
(k) 10
(l) 5/4

Test 11D

(a) Abnormal condition of skin plants (a fungal infection)
(b) Epidermal cell
(c) Condition of without hair sensation
(d) Tumour (Am. tumor) of a sweat gland
(e) Abnormal condition of fungi in the epidermis

Test 11E

(a) Dermatitis
(b) Onychosis
(c) Melanonychia
(d) Dermatology
(e) Pachyonychia

Unit 12 The Nose and Mouth

Test 12A

(a) 4
(b) 8
(c) 6
(d) 5
(e) 2
(f) 7
(g) 3
(h) 1

Test 12B

(a) 19
(b) 14
(c) 13
(d) 15
(e) 16
(f) 4
(g) 17
(h) 8
(i) 7
(j) 9
(k) 18
(l) 5
(m) 1
(n) 12
(o) 6
(p) 11
(q) 20
(r) 10
(s) 3
(t) 2

Test 12C

(a) 9
(b) 13
(c) 15/16
(d) 17
(e) 18
(f) 1
(g) 7
(h) 12
(i) 16/15
(j) 5
(k) 4
(l) 2
(m) 14
(n) 19/20
(o) 8
(p) 20/19
(q) 3
(r) 11
(s) 10
(t) 6

Test 12D

(a) Instrument used to measure the power/force of the tongue
(b) Measurement of saliva
(c) Inflammation of the mouth and tongue
(d) Splitting of the jaw and palate
(e) Pertaining to formation of or originating in teeth

Test 12E

(a) Sialadenotomy
(b) Palatorrhaphy
(c) Rhinomycosis
(d) Labial
(e) Palatoplasty

Unit 13 The Muscular System

Test 13A

(a) 18
(b) 15
(c) 8
(d) 13
(e) 9
(f) 2
(g) 16/17
(h) 17/16
(i) 3
(j) 19
(k) 1
(l) 5
(m) 4
(n) 6
(o) 7
(p) 10
(q) 20
(r) 11
(s) 12
(t) 14

Test 13B

(a) Instrument that measures the electrical activity of muscle
(b) Study of movement
(c) Incision into a muscle and tendon
(d) Without nourishment of muscle (muscle wasting)
(e) Pertaining to muscle and an aponeurosis

Test 13C

(a) Myomalacia
(b) Myogenic
(c) Myopathy
(d) Tenorrhaphy
(e) Tenotomy

Unit 14 The Skeletal System

Test 14A

(a)	4	(c)	2	(e)	6
(b)	3	(d)	1	(f)	5

Test 14B

(a)	14/15	(h)	13	(o)	3
(b)	4	(i)	15/14	(p)	2
(c)	18	(j)	20	(q)	6
(d)	12	(k)	11	(r)	16
(e)	7	(l)	8	(s)	5
(f)	19	(m)	9	(t)	10
(g)	17	(n)	1		

Test 14C

(a)	5	(h)	15	(o)	19
(b)	7	(i)	16	(p)	18
(c)	9	(j)	11	(q)	4
(d)	12	(k)	10	(r)	13
(e)	17	(l)	2	(s)	6
(f)	20	(m)	1	(t)	3
(g)	14	(n)	8		

Test 14D

(a) Inflammation of a joint cartilage
(b) Stone in a bursa
(c) Binding together of vertebrae
(d) A cell that breaks down cartilage
(e) Pertaining to having a humped/hunched back

Test 14E

(a) Arthralgia
(b) Osteosynovitis
(c) Spondylomalacia
(d) Osteoarthropathy
(e) Synovial

Unit 15 The Male Reproductive System

Test 15A

(a)	3	(d)	6	(g)	4
(b)	7	(e)	2	(h)	8
(c)	5	(f)	1		

Test 15B

(a)	16	(h)	13	(o)	14
(b)	18	(i)	20	(p)	19
(c)	3	(j)	12/11	(q)	2
(d)	9	(k)	1	(r)	5
(e)	15	(l)	7	(s)	6
(f)	17	(m)	10	(t)	4
(g)	11/12	(n)	8		

Test 15C

(a)	4	(f)	15	(k)	13
(b)	14	(g)	2	(l)	7
(c)	8	(h)	3	(m)	9
(d)	1	(i)	6	(n)	10
(e)	12	(j)	5	(o)	11

Test 15D

(a) Removal of the testes and epididymes
(b) Flow from the penis (abnormal)
(c) Removal of the epididymes and vas deferens
(d) Tying off of the vas deferens
(e) Condition of sperm in the urine

Test 15E

(a) Orchidorrhaphy/orchiorrhaphy
(b) Prostatalgia
(c) Epididymovasostomy
(d) Scrotitis
(e) Prostatorrhoea (Am. prostatorrhea)

Unit 16 The Female Reproductive System

Test 16A

(a)	3	(d)	6	(g)	8
(b)	4	(e)	2	(h)	7
(c)	1	(f)	5		

Test 16B

(a)	5	(h)	17	(o)	18
(b)	10/11	(i)	7	(p)	8
(c)	12	(j)	15	(q)	16
(d)	19	(k)	3	(r)	1
(e)	20	(l)	13	(s)	14
(f)	2	(m)	6	(t)	9
(g)	4	(n)	11/10		

Test 16C

(a)	22	(j)	4	(r)	9
(b)	17/18	(k)	13/12/14	(s)	7

(c) 16
(d) 8
(e) 1
(f) 12/13/14
(g) 24
(h) 2/3
(i) 3/2
(l) 5
(m) 10
(n) 19
(o) 20/21
(p) 21/20
(q) 11
(t) 23
(u) 15
(v) 14/12/13
(w) 18/17
(x) 25
(y) 6

Test 16D

(a) An instrument that measures labour (Am. labor); it measures uterine contractions
(b) Removal of the ovaries and uterus
(c) Surgical fixation of the breasts
(d) Rupture of the uterus
(e) Disease of the uterus

Test 16E

(a) Culdoplasty
(b) Salpingostomy
(c) Amniorrhexis
(d) Colpoptosis
(e) Colpocytology

Unit 17 The Endocrine System

Test 17A

(a) 4
(b) 3
(c) 7
(d) 2
(e) 5
(f) 6
(g) 1
(h) 8

Test 17B

(a) 16
(b) 11
(c) 20
(d) 1
(e) 19
(f) 8
(g) 18
(h) 10
(i) 15
(j) 2
(k) 7
(l) 3
(m) 17
(n) 5
(o) 6
(p) 9
(q) 4
(r) 12
(s) 14
(t) 13

Test 17C

(a) Removal of the thyroid gland and parathyroid gland
(b) A pituitary cell
(c) Enlargement of the adrenal
(d) Pertaining to acting on/affinity for sugar
(e) Condition of above normal level of ketones in the blood

Test 17D

(a) Hyperinsulinism
(b) Hyponatraemia (Am. hyponatremia)

(c) Thyrotrophic
(d) Adrenotropic
(e) Hypoparathyroidism

Unit 18 Radiology

Test 18A

(a) 11
(b) 8
(c) 13
(d) 15
(e) 20
(f) 17
(g) 14
(h) 12
(i) 19
(j) 9
(k) 3
(l) 1
(m) 2
(n) 18
(o) 16
(p) 10
(q) 7
(r) 4
(s) 6
(t) 5

Test 18B

(a) A device that uses X-rays to obtain images of sections through the body
(b) A specialist who makes ultrasound images
(c) The treatment of disease using radiation from an external source (external beam radiotherapy)
(d) An element that spontaneously decays emitting radiation
(e) Technique of using ultrasound to make an image of a slice or section through the body

Test 18C

(a) Brachytherapy
(b) Radiopaque
(c) Scintiangiography
(d) Echocardiography
(e) Echoencephalography

Unit 19 Oncology

Test 19A

(a) 9
(b) 20
(c) 10
(d) 14
(e) 12
(f) 3
(g) 1
(h) 16
(i) 17
(j) 18
(k) 4
(l) 2
(m) 19
(n) 13
(o) 11
(p) 6
(q) 5
(r) 15
(s) 7
(t) 8

Test 19B

(a) Malignant tumour (Am. tumor) of fibrous tissue
(b) Malignant glandular tumour of stomach
(c) Malignant tumour of liver cells
(d) Malignant, disordered tumour of the thyroid (refers to appearance of backward growth, ie, becoming disordered)
(e) Malignant tumour originating in the bronchus

Test 19C

(a) Lymphosarcoma
(b) Chondroma
(c) Osteosarcoma
(d) Neoplasia
(e) Oncotherapy

Unit 20 Anatomical Position

Test 20A

(a) 13	(h) 8/9	(o) 10
(b) 18	(i) 12	(p) 9/8
(c) 17	(j) 3	(q) 11
(d) 20	(k) 19	(r) 4
(e) 1	(l) 5/6	(s) 15
(f) 14	(m) 7	(t) 6/5
(g) 2	(n) 16	

Test 20B

(a) 9	(h) 15	(o) 8/7
(b) 12	(i) 19	(p) 13
(c) 7/8	(j) 5	(q) 10
(d) 14	(k) 18	(r) 3
(e) 1/2	(l) 6	(s) 17
(f) 20	(m) 11	(t) 4
(g) 16	(n) 2/1	

Test 20C

(a) Pertaining to between the phalanges (fingers and toes)
(b) A turning to the right
(c) Pertaining to behind/back of the cheek
(d) Pertaining to above the ribs
(e) Pertaining to within the nose

Test 20D

(a) Lateral
(b) Laevoversion (Am. levoversion)
(c) Post-ganglionic
(d) Infrahepatic or subhepatic
(e) Transdermal or percutaneous

Unit 21 Pharmacology and Microbiology

Test 21A

(a) 9	(h) 15/16	(o) 8
(b) 13	(i) 14	(p) 4
(c) 12	(j) 3	(q) 1
(d) 17	(k) 10	(r) 11
(e) 19	(l) 15/16	(s) 5
(f) 2	(m) 7	(t) 6
(g) 20	(n) 18	

Test 21B

(a) 17	(h) 4/5	(o) 3
(b) 9	(i) 2	(p) 10
(c) 16	(j) 19	(q) 1
(d) 13	(k) 18	(r) 11
(e) 6	(l) 20	(s) 12
(f) 8	(m) 5/4	(t) 15
(g) 14	(n) 7	

Test 21C

(a) Study of poisons
(b) Abnormal condition/disease caused by poisoning with fungi / fungal toxins
(c) A drug specialist (a person who dispenses drugs)
(d) Chemical/drug used for treatment of disease (used in treatment of cancer, chemotherapy)
(e) A specialist who studies microorganisms

Test 21D

(a) Bacteriologist
(b) Antibiotic
(c) Protozoology
(d) Bacteriostatic
(e) Virucidal

Test 21E

(a) 4	(h) 14	(o) 24	(v) 15
(b) 16	(i) 11	(p) 21	(w) 18
(c) 1	(j) 25	(q) 8	(x) 6
(d) 12	(k) 7	(r) 19	(y) 5
(e) 3	(l) 2	(s) 9	
(f) 23	(m) 20	(t) 13	
(g) 17	(n) 22	(u) 10	

Test 21F

(a) 3	(h) 10
(b) 1	(i) 8
(c) 12	(j) 5
(d) 9	(k) 7
(e) 6	(l) 2
(f) 4	
(g) 11	

Unit 22 Final Self-Assessment Tests

Final Test 1

(a) 18	(f) 2	(k) 7/8	(p) 3
(b) 20	(g) 12	(l) 8/7	(q) 1
(c) 5	(h) 19	(m) 11	(r) 14
(d) 6	(i) 4	(n) 16	(s) 13
(e) 17	(j) 15	(o) 9	(t) 10

Final Test 2

(a)	11	(f)	13	(k)	5	(p)	9	(u)	6
(b)	8	(g)	22	(l)	1	(q)	15	(v)	25
(c)	20	(h)	3	(m)	19	(r)	12	(w)	16
(d)	17	(i)	23	(n)	24	(s)	10	(x)	2
(e)	18	(j)	7	(o)	21	(t)	14	(y)	4

Final Test 3

(a)	8	(f)	17	(k)	4	(p)	2
(b)	12	(g)	10	(l)	3	(q)	13
(c)	14	(h)	7	(m)	5	(r)	16
(d)	9	(i)	20	(n)	15	(s)	18
(e)	19	(j)	6	(o)	11	(t)	1

Final Test 4

(a)	21	(f)	9/10	(k)	5	(p)	3	(u)	11
(b)	7	(g)	14	(l)	17	(q)	1	(v)	12
(c)	13	(h)	15	(m)	23	(r)	24	(w)	4
(d)	25	(i)	19	(n)	10/9	(s)	22	(x)	2
(e)	20	(j)	18	(o)	6	(t)	8	(y)	16

Final Test 5

(a)	4	(h)	14/15	(n)	16/17	(t)	13
(b)	21	(i)	5	(o)	1	(u)	7/8
(c)	18	(j)	22	(p)	10	(v)	9
(d)	23/24/25	(k)	15/14	(q)	2	(w)	8/7
(e)	24/25/23	(l)	6	(r)	12	(x)	17/16
(f)	3	(m)	19	(s)	20	(y)	11
(g)	25/23/24						

Final Test 6

(a)	18	(f)	3	(k)	8	(p)	19	(u)	4
(b)	10	(g)	16	(l)	1/2	(q)	22	(v)	12
(c)	5	(h)	24	(m)	9	(r)	2/1	(w)	20
(d)	25	(i)	15	(n)	23	(s)	11	(x)	13
(e)	6/7	(j)	21	(o)	17	(t)	14	(y)	7/6

Final Test 7

(a)	17	(f)	18	(k)	19	(p)	14/15	(u)	4
(b)	12/13	(g)	3	(l)	11	(q)	15/14	(v)	1
(c)	5	(h)	20	(m)	23/22	(r)	21	(w)	9
(d)	25	(i)	22/23	(n)	7	(s)	13/12	(x)	16
(e)	24	(j)	2	(o)	8	(t)	6	(y)	10

Final Test 8

(a)	13/14/15	(f)	18	(k)	5	(p)	15/13/14
(b)	8	(g)	1	(l)	4	(q)	3
(c)	14/15/13	(h)	20	(m)	17	(r)	10
(d)	16	(i)	19	(n)	12	(s)	11
(e)	9	(j)	7	(o)	2	(t)	6

Final Test 9

(a)	17	(f)	14	(k)	18	(p)	20
(b)	6/7	(g)	11	(l)	2	(q)	10
(c)	16	(h)	3	(m)	9	(r)	4
(d)	8	(i)	15	(n)	7/6	(s)	13
(e)	5	(j)	19	(o)	12	(t)	1

Final Test 10

(a)	16/17	(f)	19	(k)	12	(p)	13
(b)	17/16	(g)	3	(l)	20	(q)	2
(c)	9	(h)	5	(m)	6	(r)	15
(d)	10	(i)	1	(n)	18	(s)	7
(e)	4	(j)	8	(o)	11	(t)	14

Final Test 11

(a)	10	(f)	24	(k)	19	(p)	5	(u)	13
(b)	11	(g)	3	(l)	14	(q)	16	(v)	21
(c)	9	(h)	1	(m)	8	(r)	6	(w)	20
(d)	7	(i)	4	(n)	23	(s)	15	(x)	22
(e)	18	(j)	2	(o)	17	(t)	25	(y)	12

Final Test 12

(a)	14	(f)	18	(k)	1	(p)	8
(b)	3	(g)	10	(l)	17	(q)	6
(c)	9	(h)	15	(m)	5	(r)	11
(d)	13	(i)	20	(n)	7	(s)	19
(e)	12	(j)	16	(o)	4	(t)	2

Final Test 13

(a)	9	(f)	12	(k)	8	(p)	7
(b)	5	(g)	6	(l)	15	(q)	3/1/2
(c)	18/19	(h)	16	(m)	11	(r)	19/18
(d)	1/2/3	(i)	14	(n)	17	(s)	13
(e)	4	(j)	20	(o)	2/3/1	(t)	10

Final Test 14

(a)	9	(f)	22	(k)	17	(p)	10	(u)	11
(b)	25	(g)	6	(l)	2/3	(q)	16	(v)	7
(c)	20	(h)	18	(m)	3/2	(r)	12	(w)	5
(d)	1	(i)	15	(n)	8	(s)	13	(x)	21
(e)	19	(j)	14	(o)	4	(t)	24	(y)	23

Final Test 15

(a)	4	(f)	1	(k)	3	(p)	14
(b)	9	(g)	18	(l)	11	(q)	5
(c)	20	(h)	6	(m)	17	(r)	8
(d)	19	(i)	16	(n)	7	(s)	12
(e)	10	(j)	15	(o)	2	(t)	13

Final Test 16

(a) 8	(f) 10	(k) 18	(p) 6/7
(b) 17	(g) 9	(l) 2	(q) 15
(c) 1	(h) 16	(m) 11	(r) 20
(d) 3	(i) 12	(n) 13	(s) 7/6
(e) 14	(j) 4	(o) 5	(t) 19

Final Test 18

(a) 13	(f) 1	(k) 7	(p) 4
(b) 8	(g) 6	(l) 9	
(c) 2	(h) 3	(m) 11	
(d) 10	(i) 16	(n) 5	
(e) 15	(j) 14	(o) 12	

Final Test 17

(a) 11	(f) 16	(k) 6	(p) 3
(b) 9	(g) 5	(l) 13	
(c) 14	(h) 12	(m) 10	
(d) 2	(i) 15	(n) 8	
(e) 4	(j) 1	(o) 7	

ABBREVIATIONS

The abbreviations and acronyms listed here have been extracted from recent health care publications and the medical records of patients. Students should be aware that whilst certain abbreviations are standard, others are not, and their meaning may vary from one health care setting to another. Abbreviations with several meanings should be carefully interpreted to avoid confusion.

A	anaemia (Am. anemia)
AAA	abdominal aortic aneurysm/acute anxiety attack
AAAAA	aphasia, agnosia, agraphia, alexia and apraxia
A&E	accident and emergency
AAFB	acid alcohol fast bacilli
AB1	one abortion
AB, Ab, ab	abortion / antibody
ABC	airway, breathing, circulation
Abdo	abdomen
ABE	acute bacterial endocarditis
ABG	arterial blood gases
abor	abortion
ABR	auditory brainstem evoked responses
ABX	antibiotics
AC	air conduction
a.c.	ante cibum (before meals/food)
ACBS	aortocoronary bypass surgery
Acc, accom	accommodation of eye
ACE	angiotensin converting enzyme
ACh	acetyl choline
ACL	anterior cruciate ligament (of the knee)
ACS	acute confused state
ACTH	adrenocorticotrophic hormone
ACU	acute care unit
AD, ad	Alzheimer disease/auris dextra (right ear)
ADA	adenosine deaminase
ADC	AIDS dementia complex
ADD	attention deficit disorder
ADH	antidiuretic hormone
ADHD	attention deficit hyperactivity disorder
ADL	aids to daily living
ad lib	as desired
ADR	adverse drug reaction
ADT	admission, discharge and transfer
ADU	acute duodenal ulcer
AED	antiepileptic drug
AEM	ambulatory electrocardiogram monitoring
AF	amniotic fluid/atrial fibrillation
AFB	acid-fast bacilli
AFP	Alpha-fetoprotein
A/G	albumin/globulin ratio
Ag	antigen
AGA	appropriate for gestational age
AGL	acute granulocytic leukaemia (Am. leukemia)
AGN	acute glomerulonephritis
AI	aortic incompetence / aortic insufficiency / artificial insemination
AID	artificial insemination by donor
AIDS	acquired immunodeficiency syndrome
AIED	autoimmune inner ear disease
AIH	artificial insemination by husband
A/K	above knee (amputation)
alb	albumin (protein)
ALD	alcoholic liver disease
ALG	antilymphocyte immunoglobulin
ALL	acute lymphocytic leukaemia (Am. leukemia)
ALS	amyotrophic lateral sclerosis (Lou Gehrig disease)
ALs	activities of living
ALT	alanine aminotransferase / alanine transaminase
amb	ambulant/ambulatory (walking)
AMD	age-related macular degeneration
AMI	acute myocardial infarction
AML	acute myeloid leukaemia (Am. leukemia)
AMR	antimicrobial resistance
ANC	absolute neutrophil count
ANF	antinuclear factor
ANS	autonomic nervous system
ANT, ant.	anterior
antib	antibiotic
A&O	alert and orientated
AOB	alcohol on breath
AP	antepartum/anteroposterior/appendicectomy/auscultation and percussion
APB	atrial premature beat
APH	antepartum haemorrhage (Am. hemorrhage)
APPY	appendicectomy
APSAC	acylated plasminogen streptokinase activator complex (anistreplase)
APTT	activated partial thromboplastin time
aq	aqueous/water
A–R	apical–radial (pulse)
ARC	aids-related complex
ARD	acute respiratory disease
ARDS	acute respiratory distress syndrome
ARF	acute renal failure
ARM	artificial rupture of membranes/age-related maculopathy
ARMD	age-related macular degeneration

AS	alimentary system / aortic stenosis / auris sinistra (left ear)
A–S	Adams–Stokes attack
5-ASA	5-aminosalicylic acid (aspirin)
ASC	altered state of consciousness
ASCVD	arteriosclerotic cardiovascular disease
ASD	atrial septal defect
ASHD	arteriosclerotic heart disease
ASO	antistreptolysin O
ASOM	acute suppurative otitis media
AST	aspartate transaminase
Astigm	astigmatism of eye
ASX	asymptomatic
ATG	antithymocyte immunoglobulin
ATN	acute tubular necrosis
ATP	adenosine triphosphate
ATS	anti-tetanus serum
AU	auris utraque (both ears)
Au	gold
AuD, aud	audiology/auditory
auris dextra	the right ear
AV	arteriovenous / atrioventricular bundle/ atrioventricular node / aortic valve
AVM	arteriovenous malformation
AVP	arginine vasopressin also known as vasopressin or antidiuretic hormone
AVR	aortic valve replacement
A&W	alive and well
AXR	abdominal X-ray
AZT	azidothymidine
Ba	barium
BaE	barium enema
BAER	brainstem auditory evoked responses
BAL	blood alcohol level
baso	basophil
BBA	born before arrival
BBB	blood brain barrier / bundle branch block
BBBB	bilateral bundle branch block
BBT	basal body temperature
BBx	breast biopsy
BC	birth control / bone conduction
BCC	basal cell carcinoma
BCG	bacilli (bacillus) Calmette–Guérin
b.d.	bis die (twice a day)
BDA	British Diabetic Association
BE	bacterial endocarditis / barium enema
BET	bacterial endotoxin test
BI	bone injury
BID	brought in dead
b.i.d.	bis in die (twice daily)
B/KA	below knee (amputation)
BM	bowel movement
BMI	body mass index
BMR	basal metabolic rate
BM (T)	bone marrow (trephine)

BMT	bone marrow transplant
BNF	British National Formulary
BNO	bowels not open
BO	bowels open
BOR	bowels open regularly
BP	blood pressure / British Pharmacopoeia / bypass
BPD	bronchopulmonary dysplasia
BPH	benign prostatic hyperplasia/benign prostatic hypertrophy
BPM	beats per minute
BPPV	benign paroxysmal positional vertigo
BRO	bronchoscopy
BS	blood sugar / bowel sounds / breath sounds
BSA	body surface area
BSE	bovine spongiform encephalopathy / breast self-examination
BSO	bilateral salpingo-oophorectomy
BSS	blood sugar series
BT	bedtime / bone tumour (Am. tumor) / brain tumour / breast tumour / bleeding time
BTS	blood transfusion service
BUC, Buc, bucc	buccal (pertaining to the cheek or mouth cavity)
BUN	blood urea nitrogen
BW	body weight
BX, Bx, bx.	biopsy
C	Celsius
c	with
C 1–7	cervical vertebra
CA, Ca, ca.	cancer / carcinoma / cardiac arrest / coronary artery
Ca	calcium
CABG	coronary artery bypass grafting
CACX, CaCx	cancer of the cervix
CAD	coronary artery disease
CAG	closed-angle glaucoma
CAH	chronic active hepatitis / congenital adrenal hyperplasia
CAL	computer-assisted learning
CAO	chronic airway obstruction / conscious, alert, orientated
CAPD	continuous ambulatory peritoneal dialysis
cap., capsul.	capsule
CAT	computed axial tomography
Cath	catheter/catheterization
CAVH	continuous arteriovenous haemofiltration (Am. hemofiltration)
CAVHD	continuous arteriovenous haemodialysis (Am. hemodialysis)
CBC	complete blood count
CBE	clinical breast examination
CBF	cerebral blood flow
CCCC	closed-chest cardiac compression
CCF	chronic cardiac failure / congestive cardiac failure

CCIE	counter current immuno electrophoresis
CCU	coronary care unit
CD	Crohn disease / cluster designation
CDH	congenital dislocation of the hip joint
CEA	carcino embryonic antigen
CF	cancer free / cardiac failure / cystic fibrosis
CFT	complement fixation test
CFTR	cystic fibrosis transmembrane regulator
CGL	chronic granulocytic leukaemia (Am. leukemia)
CGN	chronic glomerulonephritis
cGy	centigray (one hundredth of a gray)
CH	cholesterol
chemo	chemotherapy
CHD	coronary heart disease
CHF	congestive heart failure
CHI	creatinine height index
chol	cholesterol
CHOP	**c**yclophosphamide, **h**ydroxydaunorubicin, **O**ncovin and **p**rednisolone
CHR, chr	chronic
CI	cardiac index / cerebral infarction
CIBD	chronic inflammatory bowel disease/disorder
CIN	cervical intraepithelial neoplasia
CIS	carcinoma in situ
CJD	Creutzfeldt–Jakob disease
CK	creatine kinase
CKD	chronic kidney disease
CL	clubbing
CL/CP	cleft lip and cleft palate
CLD	chronic liver disease / chronic lung disease
CLL	chronic lymphocytic leukaemia (Am. leukemia)
CMF	cyclophosphamide, methotrexate, 5-fluorouracil
CMG	cystometrogram
CML	chronic myeloid leukaemia (Am. leukemia)
CMV	cytomegalovirus
CN	cranial nerve
CNS	central nervous system
CO	carbon monoxide / cardiac output / complains of
COAD	chronic obstructive airway disease
COD	cause of death
COLD	chronic obstructive lung disease
COPD	chronic obstructive pulmonary disease
COP	colloid osmotic pressure
C&P	cystoscopy and pyelogram
CP	cor pulmonale / cerebral palsy / chest pain
CPA	cardiopulmonary arrest / costophrenic angle
CPAP	continuous positive airways pressure
CPK	creatinine phosphokinase
CPN	community psychiatric nurse
CPPV	continuous positive-pressure ventilation
CPR	cardiopulmonary resuscitation
CR	complete response, complete remission
CrCl	creatine clearance

CRD	chronic renal disease
CRF	chronic renal failure
CRH	corticotropin-releasing hormone
C + S	culture and sensitivity (test)
CS, C-section, c/sect	caesarean section (Am. cesarean) c/sect
CSF	cerebrospinal fluid
CSH	chronic subdural haematoma (Am. hematoma)
CSM	cerebrospinal meningitis
CSOM	chronic suppurative otitis media
CSR	Cheyne–Stokes respiration / correct sedimentation rate
CSU	catheter specimen of urine
CT	cerebral tumour (Am. tumor) / clotting time / computed tomography / continue treatment / coronary thrombosis
CTS	carpal tunnel syndrome
CUG	cystourethrogram
CV	cardiovascular/cerebrovascular
CVA	cerebrovascular accident (stroke) / costovertebral angle
CVD	cardiovascular disease
CVP	central venous pressure
CVS	cardiovascular system/chorionic villus sampling
CVVH	continuous venovenous haemofiltration (Am. hemofiltration)
CVVHD	continuous venovenous haemodialysis (Am. hemodialysis)
Cx	cervical/cervix
CXR	chest X-ray
Cy	cyanosis
cyclic AMP	cyclic adenosine monophosphate
Cysto	cystoscopy
D	diagnosis
dB	decibel
DBP	diastolic blood pressure
D&C	dilatation and curettage
DC, d/c	decrease / direct current / discharge / discontinue
DCCT	diabetes control and complications trial
DCIS	ductal carcinoma in situ
DD	differential diagnosis / discharge diagnosis
DDA	Dangerous Drugs Act
DDAVP	desmopressin (synthetic vasopressin, deamino-8-D-arginine vasopressin)
ddC, DDC	Dideoxycytidine also called zalcitabine
ddI, DDI	didanosine/dideoxyinosine
DDx	differential diagnosis
D&E	dilatation and evacuation
Decub	decubitus (lying down)
Derm, derm	dermatology
DES	diethylstilbestrol
DEXA	dual-energy X-ray absorptiometry

DH	delayed hypersensitivity / drug history
DIC	disseminated intravascular coagulation
DIDMOAD	diabetes insipidus, diabetes mellitus, optic atrophy and deafness
Diff, diff	differential blood count (of cell types)
DIG dig	digitalis/digoxin
DIMS	disorders of initiating and maintaining sleep
DIOS	distal intestinal obstruction syndrome
DIP	distal interphalangeal
disp.	dispense
DIST, Dist	distal
DJK	degenerative joint disease
DKA	diabetics ketoacidosis
DLE	discoid lupus erythematosus / disseminated lupus erythematosus
DM	diabetes mellitus / diastolic murmur
DMD	Duchenne muscular dystrophy
dmft	decayed missing and filled teeth (deciduous)
DMFT	decayed missing and filled teeth (permanent)
D/N	day/night (frequency of urine)
DNA	deoxyribonucleic acid / did not attend
DNR	do not resuscitate
DOA	dead on arrival
DOB	date of birth
DOD	date of death
DOE	dyspnoea on exertion (Am. dyspnea)
DOES	disorders of excessive somnolence
DRE	digital rectal examination
DS	Down syndrome
D/S	dextrose and saline
DSA	digital subtraction angiography
DT	delirium tremens
DTP	diphtheria, tetanus and pertussis (vaccine)
DTR	deep tendon reflex
DU	duodenal ulcer
DUB	dysfunctional uterine bleeding
D&V	diarrhoea and vomiting
DVT	deep venous thrombosis
Dx	diagnosis
DXT	deep X-ray therapy
DXRT	deep X-ray radiotherapy
EBM	expressed breast milk
EBV	Epstein–Barr virus
ECF	extracellular fluid/extended care facility
ECFV	extracellular fluid volume
ECG	electrocardiogram
ECHO	echocardiogram/echocardiography
ECSL	extracorporeal shockwave lithotripsy
ECT	electroconvulsive therapy
ED	erectile dysfunction
EDC	expected date of confinement
EDD	expected date of delivery
EDV	end-diastolic volume
EEG	electroencephalography / electroencephalogram

EENT	eyes, ears, nose and throat
EFM	electronic fetal monitoring
EGD	esophagogastroduodenoscopy (Am.)
ELBW	extremely low birth weight
ELISA	enzyme-linked immunosorbent assay
Em	emmetropia (good vision)
EMB	endometrial biopsy
EMD	electromechanical dissociation
EMG	electromyogram / electromyography
EMI	elderly mentally infirm / **e**toposide-**m**ethotrexate-**i**fosfamide
EMU	early morning urine
EN	erythema nodosum
ENG	electronystagmogram/ electronystagmography
ENT	ear, nose and throat
EOG	electrooculogram
EOM	extraocular movement / extraocular muscles
eos	eosinophil(s)
EP	ectopic pregnancy
Epo	erythropoietin
EPSP	excitatory postsynaptic potential
ERCP	endoscopic retrograde cholangiopancreatography
ERF	established renal failure
ERG	electroretinogram
ERPC	evacuation of retained products of conception
ERT	estrogen replacement therapy (Am.)
ERV	expiratory reserve volume
ESM	ejection systolic murmur
ESP	end-systolic pressure
ESR	erythrocyte sedimentation rate
ESRD	end-stage renal disease
ESRF	end-stage renal failure
ESV	end-systolic volume
ESWL	extracorporeal shock wave lithotripsy
ET	embryo transfer / endotracheal / endotracheal tube
ET CPAP	endotracheal continuous positive airways pressure
ETD	eustachian tube dysfunction
ETF	eustachian tube function
ETT	endotracheal tube / exercise tolerance test
EUA	examination under anaesthesia (Am. anesthesia)
EUS	endoscopic ultrasound
EX	examination
EXP	expansion
Ez	eczema
F	Fahrenheit
FA	folic acid
FAS	fetal alcohol syndrome
FB	fasting blood sugar / finger breadth / foreign body

FBC	full blood count
FBE	full blood examination
FBS	fasting blood sugar
FDIU	fetal death in utero
Fe	iron
FESS	functional endoscopic sinus surgery
FET	forced expiratory technique
FEV	forced expiratory volume
FEV1	forced expiratory volume in 1 second
FFA	free fatty acids
FFP	fresh frozen plasma
FH	family history
FHH	fetal heart heard
FHNH	fetal heart not heard
FHR	fetal heart rate
FLP	fasting lipid profile
FMH	family medical history
FMRI	functional magnetic resonance imaging
FNA	fine needle aspiration
FNAB	fine needle aspiration biopsy
FOB	faecal occult blood (Am. fecal)
FOBT	faecal occult blood testing (Am. fecal)
FP	false positive
FRC	functional reserve capacity / functional residual capacity
FROM	full range of movement
FSH	follicle stimulating hormone
FSHRH	follicle stimulating hormone releasing hormone
FT	full term
FT_4	free thyroxine
FTI	free thyroxine index
FTND	full term, normal delivery
F/u	follow up
FUO	fever of unknown origin
FVC	forced vital capacity
FX, Fx, fx.	fracture
g	gauge
G	gravid (pregnant), e.g., gravida I, a first pregnancy
GA	general anaesthesia (Am. anesthesia) / general appearance
GABA	gamma-aminobutyric acid
GAD	generalized anxiety disorder
GB	gall bladder / Guillain–Barré (syndrome)
GC	gonococci
GCSF	granulocyte colony stimulating factor
GE	gastroenterology
GERD	gastroesophageal reflux disease (Am.)
GF	glomerular filtration / gluten-free
GFR	glomerular filtration rate
gGTP	gamma glutamyl transpeptidase
gGT	gamma glutamyl transferase
GH	growth hormone
GHIH	growth hormone inhibiting hormone

GHRH	growth hormone releasing hormone
GHRIH	growth hormone release-inhibiting hormone
GI	gastrointestinal
GIFT	gamete intrafallopian transfer
ging	gingiva (gum)/gingivitis
GIS	gastrointestinal system
GIT	gastrointestinal tract
GKI	glucose/potassium/insulin
GM	grand mal seizure
GN	glomerulonephritis
GNC	Gram-negative coccus
GNDC	Gram-negative diplococci
GnRH	gonadotropin releasing hormone
GP	general practitioner
GPC	Gram-positive coccus
grav	gravid (pregnant)
GS	general surgery / genital system
G&S/XM	group and save/cross-match
GTN	glyceryl trinitrate
gtt	guttae (drops)
GTT	glucose tolerance test
GU	gastric ulcer / genitourinary / gonococcal urethritis
GUS	genitourinary system
GVHD	graft versus host disease
GYN, Gyn	gynaecology (Am. gynecology)
H	hydrogen/hypodermic
HAART	highly active antiretroviral therapy (HIV treatment)
HAV	hepatitis A virus
HB	heart block
Hb, Hgb	haemoglobin (Am. hemoglobin)
HBAg	hepatitis B antigen
HBGM	home blood glucose monitoring
HBO	hyperbaric oxygenation
HBP	high blood pressure
HBsAg	hepatitis B surface antigen
HBV	hepatitis B virus
HC	head circumference
HCG, hCG	human chorionic gonadotrophin
H/ct, h.ct	haematocrit (Am. hematocrit)
HCV	hepatitis C virus
HCVD	hypertensive cardiovascular disease
HD	haemodialysis (Am. hemodialysis) / Hodgkin disease / Huntington disease
HDL	high density lipoprotein
HDN	haemolytic disease of newborn (Am. hemolytic)
HDV	hepatitis delta virus
HEENT	head, eyes, ears, nose and throat
HF	heart failure
HGH, hGH	human growth hormone
HGP	human genome project
HHNK	hyperglycaemic (Am. hyperglycemic) hyperosmolar non-ketonic

HHV	human herpes virus
Hib	*Haemophilus influenzae* type b
Hist, histo	histology (lab)
HIV	human immunodeficiency virus
HIVD	herniated intervertebral disc
H&L	heart and lungs
HL	Hodgkin lymphoma
HLA	human leucocyte antigen (Am. leukocyte)
HMG, hMG	human menopausal gonadotropin
HOCM	hypertrophic obstructive cardiomyopathy
HO	house officer
H&P	history and physical
HPC	history of present condition
HPEN	home parenteral and enteral nutrition
hpf	high power field
HPI	history of present illness
HPV	human papilloma virus
HR	heart rate
HRM	human resource management
HRT	hormone replacement therapy
HSA	human serum albumin
HSG	hysterosalpingography
HSV	*Herpes simplex* virus
5-HT	5-hydroxytryptamine
HT	hypertension
HTLV	human T-cell leukaemia / lymphoma virus (Am. leukemia)
HTN	hypertension
HTVD	hypertensive vascular disease
HUS	haemolytic uraemic syndrome (Am. hemolytic uremic syndrome)
HVD	hypertensive vascular disease
Hx	history
IABP	intraaortic balloon pump
IAP	immunosuppressive acid protein
IBC	iron-binding capacity
IBD	inflammatory bowel disease
IBS	irritable bowel syndrome
IC	intercostal/intracerebral/intracranial
ICA	islet cell antibody
ICF	intracellular fluid
ICH	intracerebral haemorrhage (Am. hemorrhage)
ICM	intercostal margin
ICP	intracranial pressure
ICS	intercostal space
ICSH	interstitial cell stimulating hormone
ICU	intensive care unit
ID, id	identity/intradermal/infectious disease
I&D	incision and drainage
IDDM	Insulin-dependent diabetes mellitus (Type 1)
IDL	intermediate-density lipoprotein
IFG	impaired fasting glycaemia (Am. glycemia)
IFN	interferon
Ig	immunoglobulin (eg, IgA, IgG)

IGT	impaired glucose tolerance
IHD	ischaemic heart disease (Am. ischemic)
IHR	intrinsic heart rate
IM, i/m	infectious mononucleosis/intramuscular
IMHP	intramuscular high potency
IMI	inferior myocardial infarction
IMP	impression
IMRT	intensity-modulated radiotherapy
IMV	intermittent mandatory ventilation
IN	internist (Am.)
Inf.	inferior
inf.MI	inferior myocardial infarction
INR	international normalized ratio
int	between/internal
I&O	intake and output
IOFB	intraocular foreign body
IOL	intraocular lens
IOP	intraocular pressure
in utero	within uterus
i.p.	intraperitoneal
IPD	idiopathic Parkinson disease
IPF	idiopathic pulmonary fibrosis
IPPA	inspection, palpation, percussion, auscultation
IPPB	intermittent positive-pressure breathing
IPPV	intermittent positive-pressure ventilation
IQ	intelligence quotient
IRDS	idiopathic respiratory distress syndrome
IRV	inspiratory reserve volume
ISQ	idem status quo (ie, unchanged)
IT	intrathecal
ITCP	idiopathic thrombocytopenia purpura
ITP	idiopathic thrombocytopenic purpura
ITT	insulin tolerance test
ITU	intensive therapy unit
IU	international units
IUC	idiopathic ulcerative colitis
IUCD	intrauterine contraceptive device
IUD	intrauterine death / intrauterine device
IUFB	intrauterine foreign body
IUGR	intrauterine growth retardation
IUP	intrauterine pregnancy
IV, i/v	intravenous
IVC	inferior vena cava / intravenous cholecystogram
IVD	intervertebral disc
IVF	in vitro fertilization/in vivo fertilization
IVH	intraventricular haemorrhage (Am. hemorrhage)
IVHP	intravenous high potency
IVI	intravenous infusion
IVP	intravenous pyelogram/intravenous pyelography
IVSD	interventricular septal defect
IVT	intravenous transfusion
IVU	intravenous urography

J	jaundice
JVD	jugular venous distension
JVP	jugular vein pressure / jugular venous pressure
K	potassium/kalium (K+)
KA	ketoacidosis
KCCT	kaolin-cephalin clotting time
KCO	transfer coefficient (K) for carbon monoxide
Kg	kilogram (1000 grams)
KJ	knee jerk
KLS	kidney, liver, spleen
KO	keep open
KS	Kaposi sarcoma
KUB	kidney, ureter, bladder (X-ray)
KVO	keep vein open
L	lymphadenopathy
(L)	left/lower
L 1–5	lumbar vertebrae
L&A	light and accommodation
LA	left arm / left atrium / local anaesthetic (Am. anesthetic)
La	labial (lips)
LAD	left axis deviation
LaG	labia and gingiva (lips and gums)
LAS	lymphadenopathy syndrome
LASIK	laser-assisted in situ keratomileusis
LAT, lat.	lateral
LAVH	laparoscopic-assisted vaginal hysterectomy
LBBB	left bundle branch block
LBM	lean body mass
LBW	low birth weight
LCCS	low cervical caesarean section (Am. cesarean)
LD	lethal dose / loading dose
LDH	lactic dehydrogenase
LDL	low density lipoprotein
L-dopa	levodopa (a drug used to treat Parkinson disease)
LE	lupus erythematosus
LFT	liver function test
LGA	large for gestational age
LH	luteinizing hormone
LHRH	luteinizing hormone releasing hormone
LIF	left iliac fossa
LIH	left inguinal hernia
LKKS	liver, kidney, kidney, spleen
LL	left leg / left lower / lower lobe
LLETZ	large loop excision of the transformation zone
LLL	left lower lid (eye) / left lower lobe (lung)
LLQ	left lower quadrant
LMM	lentigo maligna melanoma
LMN	lower motor neuron
LMP	last menstrual period

LN	lymph node
LNMP	last normal menstrual period
LOC	level of consciousness / loss of consciousness
LOM	limitation of movement
LOPP	Leukeran, Oncovin, procarbazine, prednisolone
LP	lumbar puncture
LPA	left pulmonary artery
LPN	licensed practical nurse (Am.)
LRI	lower respiratory infection
LS	left side / liver and spleen / lumbosacral / lymphosarcoma
LSB	long stay bed (geriatric)
LSCS	lower section caesarean section (Am. cesarean)
LSD	lysergic acid diethylamide
LSK	liver, spleen, kidneys
LSM	late systolic murmur
LTB	laryngotracheal bronchitis
LTC	long-term care
LTOT	long-term oxygen therapy
L&U	lower and upper
LUL	left upper lobe
LUQ	left upper quadrant
LV	left ventricle
LVDP	left ventricular diastolic pressure
LVE	left ventricular enlargement
LVEDP	left ventricular end-diastolic pressure
LVEDV	left ventricular end-diastolic volume
LVET	left ventricular ejection time
LVF	left ventricular failure
LVH	left ventricular hypertrophy
LVP	left ventricular pressure
L&W	living and well
Lymphos	lymphocytes
M	male/married/murmur
MA	mental age
MAB, mAb, -mab	monoclonal antibody
MABP	mean arterial blood pressure
MAC	mid-arm circumference / *Mycobacterium avium* complex
MAMC	mid-arm muscle circumference
mane	in the morning
MAOI	mono-amine oxidase inhibitor
MAP	mean arterial pressure/muscle action potential
MAV	migraine associated vertigo
MBD	minimal brain dysfunction
MCH	mean corpuscular (red cell) haemoglobin (Am. hemoglobin)
MCHC	mean corpuscular haemoglobin concentration (Am. hemoglobin)
MCL	mid-clavicular line

MCP	metacarpophalangeal	MSL	midsternal line
MCV	mean corpuscular (cell) volume	MSOF	multisystem organ failure
MD	maintenance dose / mitral disease / muscular dystrophy	MSSU	midstream specimen of urine
		MSU	midstream urine
MDD	major depressive disorder	MTA	mid-thigh amputation
MDI	metered dose inhaler	MTP	metatarsophalangeal
MDM	mid-diastolic murmur	MV	mitral valve
MDRTB	multidrug resistant tuberculosis	MVP	mitral valve prolapse
ME	myalgic encephalopathy	MVR	minute volume of respiration/mitral valve replacement
Med.	medial		
MEN	multiple endocrine neoplasia	My, my	myopia
meQ	milliequivalent		
mEq/L	milliequivalent per litre	N	nitrogen/normal
Metas, mets	metastasis	Na	sodium/natrium (Na$^+$)
MF	mycoses fungoides / myocardial fibrosis	NAD	nothing abnormal discovered / no acute distress / normal axis deviation
MFT	muscle function test		
MG	myasthenia gravis	NAG	narrow-angle glaucoma
MGN	membranous glomerulonephritis	NANB	non A, non B viruses
MH	medical history / menstrual history	NAP	neutrophil alkaline phosphatase
MHC	major histocompatibility complex	NAS, nas	nasal / no added salt
MHz	megahertz (megacycles per second)	NB	newborn
MI	mitral incompetence / mitral insufficiency / myocardial infarction	NBM	nil (nothing) by mouth
		NBS	normal bowel sounds / normal breath sounds
MIBG	meta-iodobenzyl guanidine	NCVs	nerve conduction velocities
MIC	minimum inhibitory concentration	ND	normal delivery / normal development
MID	multi-infarct dementia	NEC	necrotizing enterocolitis
MIMS	Monthly index of medical specialities / medical information management system	NED	no evidence of disease
		neg	negative
ML	middle lobe / midline	NFTD	normal full-term delivery
mL	millilitre	NG	nasogastric
MLT	medical laboratory technician / technologist	NGU	non-gonococcal urethritis
		NHL	non-Hodgkin lymphoma
MM	malignant melanoma	NHS	National Health Service (UK)
mm^3	cubic millimetre	NIDDM	non-insulin-dependent diabetes mellitus
mmHg	millimetres of mercury		
MMM	mitozantrone, methotrexate, mitomycin C	NIH	National Institute of health (USA)
mmol	millimole	NK	natural killer (cells)
MMR	measles, mumps and rubella (vaccine)	NKT	natural killer T-cell
MNJ	myoneural junction	NMR	nuclear magnetic resonance
MODY	maturity onset diabetes of the young	NMRI	nuclear magnetic resonance imaging
MOFS	multiple organ failure syndrome	NMSC	nonmelanoma skin cancer
mono	monocyte(s)	NO	nitric oxide
MOPP	**m**ustine, **O**ncovin (vincristine), **p**rocarbazine, **p**rednisolone	#NOF	fractured neck of femur
		NP	nasopharynx
MPJ	metacarpophalangeal joint	NPN	non-protein nitrogen
MPQ	McGill Pain Questionnaire	NPO, npo	non per os (nothing by mouth)
MR	mitral regurgitation	NREM	non-rapid eye movement (in sleep)
MRDM	malnutrition-related diabetes mellitus	NRS	numerical rating scale
MRI	magnetic resonance imaging	NS	nephrotic syndrome / nervous system / no specimen
mRNA	messenger ribonucleic acid		
MRSA	methicillin-resistant *Staphylococcus aureus*	NSAID	nonsteroidal antiinflammatory drug
MS	mitral stenosis / multiple sclerosis / muscle shortening / muscle strength / musculoskeletal/musculoskeletal system	NSFTD	normal spontaneous full-term delivery
		NSR	normal sinus rhythm
		NST	non-shivering thermogenesis
		NSU	nonspecific urethritis
MSAFP	maternal serum alphafetoprotein	NT	nasotracheal / nasotracheal tube
MSE	mental state examination		
MSH	melanocyte-stimulating hormone	N&T	nose and throat

NTP	normal temperature and pressure
N & V	nausea and vomiting
NVD	nausea, vomiting and diarrhoea (Am. diarrhea)
O	oxygen/oedema (Am. edema)
O&A	observation and assessment
OA	on admission/osteoarthritis
OAD	obstructive airway disease
OAG	open-angle glaucoma
OB	occult blood
Ob-Gyn	obstetrics and gynaecology (Am. gynecology)
Obst-Gyn	obstetrics and gynaecology (Am. gynecology)
OC	oral cholecystogram / oral contraceptive
OCD	obsessive compulsive disorder
OCP	oral contraceptive pill
OD	oculus dexter (right eye), oculo dextro (in the right eye) / overdose
o.d.	every day (omni die)
Odont	odontology
ODQ	on direct questioning
O/E, OE	on examination / otitis externa
OGD	oesophagogastroduodenoscopy
OGTT	oral glucose tolerance test
OH	occupational history / oral hygiene
OHS	open heart surgery
OM	olim mane (once daily in the morning) / otitis media
OOB	out of bed
OPA	outpatient appointment
OPD	outpatient department
Ophth	ophthalmology
OPT	Orthopantomogram (panoramic X-ray of the lower face)
OR	operating room
ORT	operating room technician
Ortho	orthopaedics (Am. orthopedics)
Orthop	orthopnoea (Am. orthopnea)
OS	oculus sinister (left eye), oculo sinistro (in left eye)
Os	mouth
OT	occupational therapy / old tuberculin / oxytocin
OTC	over the counter (remedies)
oto	otology (study of the ear)
OU	oculus unitas (both eyes together) / oculus uterque (for each eye)/oculus utro (in each eye)
P	phosphorus / posterior / pressure
PA	pernicious anaemia (Am. anemia) / postero-anterior / pulmonary artery
P&A	percussion and auscultation
PABA	para-aminobenzoic acid
PACG	primary angle closure glaucoma

PAD	peripheral artery disease
PADP	pulmonary artery diastolic pressure
PAH	pulmonary artery hypertension / pregnancy-induced hypertension
palp	palpable/palpation
PALS	paediatric (Am. pediatric) advanced life support
PAP	primary atypical pneumonia
Pap.	Papanicolaou smear test
Para	number of viable births, eg, Para 1 (unipara)
PAS	p-aminosalicylic acid
PAT	paroxysmal atrial tachycardia
PAWP	pulmonary artery wedge pressure
PBC	primary biliary cirrhosis
PBI	protein bound iodine
pc	post cibum (after meals/food)
PCA	patient-controlled analgesia
PCAS	patient-controlled analgesia system
PCN	penicillin
PCNL	percutaneous nephrolithotomy
PCOS	polycystic ovary syndrome
PCO2	partial pressure carbon dioxide
PCP	*Pneumocystis carinii* pneumonia
PCR	polymerase chain reaction
PCT	prothrombin clotting time
PCV	packed cell volume
PCWP	pulmonary capillary wedge pressure
PD	Parkinson disease / peritoneal dialysis
PDA	patent ductus arteriosus
PE	physical examination / pleural effusion / pulmonary embolism / pressure equalization
PEC	pneumoencephalogram
PED	paediatrics (Am. pediatrics)
PEEP	positive end expiratory pressure
PEF	peak expiratory flow
PEFR	peak expiratory flow rate
PEG	percutaneous endoscopic gastrostomy / pneumoencephalogram
PEJ	percutaneous endoscopic jejunostomy
PEM	protein-energy malnutrition
PERLAC	pupils equal, react to light, accommodation consensual
per os	by mouth
PERRLA	pupils equal, round, react to light, accommodation consensual
PET	positron emission tomography / preeclamptic toxaemia (Am. toxemia)
PF	peak flow
PFT	peak flow rate / pulmonary function test
PG	prostaglandin
PGL	persistent generalized lymphadenopathy
PH	past history / patient history / prostatic hypertrophy / pulmonary hypertension
pH	hydrogen-ion concentration
PID	pelvic inflammatory disease / prolapsed intervertebral disc

PIH	prolactin-inhibiting hormone / pregnancy-induced hypertension
PIP	proximal interphalangeal / peak inspiratory pressure
PIN	prostatic intraepithelial neoplasia
PIVD	protruded intervertebral disc
PKU	phenylketonuria
PM	postmortem
PMB	post-menopausal bleeding
PMH	past medical history
PMI	past medical history / point of maximum impulse
PML	progressive multifocal leucoencephalopathy (Am. leukoencephalopathy)
PMN	polymorphonuclear leucocytes (Am. leukocyte)
PMS	premenstrual syndrome
PMT	premenstrual tension
PMV	prolapsed mitral valve
PN	percussion note / peripheral nerve / peripheral neuropathy
PND	paroxysmal nocturnal dyspnoea (Am. dyspnea) / post nasal drip
PNS	peripheral nervous system
PO or p.o.	by mouth (per os) / post-operative
PO2	partial pressure oxygen
POAG	primary open-angle glaucoma
POLY	polymorphonuclear leucocytes (Am. leukocytes)
POP	plaster of Paris
pos	position
Post.	posterior
PPAM	pneumatic post-amputation mobility
PPD	packs per day / purified protein derivative (of tuberculin)
PPE	personal protective equipment
PPH	postpartum haemorrhage (Am. hemorrhage)
PPS	plasma protein solution
PPT	partial prothrombin time
PPV	positive-pressure ventilation
PR, p.r.	per rectum / plantar reflex / partial response
pre op	preoperative
PRH	prolactin releasing hormone
PRK	photorefractive keratectomy
PRL	prolactin
PRN, p.r.n.	pro re nata (as required)
PROG	progesterone
PROM	premature rupture of membranes
Prot.	protocol (a detailed plan)
PRV	polycythaemia rubra vera (Am. polycythemia)
procto	proctoscopy
pros	prostate
Prox.	proximal
PS	pulmonary stenosis / pyloric stenosis
PSA	prostate specific antigen

PSCT	pain and symptom control team
PSD	personal and social development
PSG	presystolic gallop
PSVT	paroxysmal supraventricular tachycardia
PT, pt	patient/physical therapy / prothrombin time / physical therapist (Am.)
PTA	prior to admission
PTC	percutaneous transhepatic cholangiogram / cholangiography
PTCA	percutaneous transluminal coronary angioplasty
PTD	permanent and total disability
PTH	parathormone / parathyroid hormone
PTR	prothrombin ratio
PTT	partial thromboplastin time
PTX	pneumothorax
PU	peptic ulcer / per urethra / pregnancy urine
PUO	pyrexia of unknown origin
PUVA	psoralen + ultraviolet light A
PV	per vagina
P&V	pyloroplasty and vagotomy
PVC	premature ventricular contraction
PVD	peripheral vascular disease
PVP	pulmonary venous pressure
PVS	persistent vegetative state
PVT	paroxysmal ventricular tachycardia
PX	physical examination
Px	past history / prognosis
q.d.s.	quater die sumendum (four times a day)
q.i.d.	quater in die (four times a day)
qn	each night (quaque nox)
(R)	right/respiration
RA	rheumatoid arthritis / right atrium
Ra	radium
RAD	radiation absorbed dose / right axis deviation
rad	radical
RAS	reticular activating system
RAST	radio-allergosorbent test
RBBB	right bundle branch block
RBC	red blood cell / red blood (cell) count
RBS	random blood sugar
RCC	red cell concentrate / red cell count
R-CHOPS	rituximab, cyclophosphamide, hydroxydaunorubicin, Oncovin and prednisolone
RCT	root canal treatment
RDA	recommended dietary allowance
RDDA	recommended daily dietary allowance
rDNA	recombinant deoxyribose nucleic acid
RDS	respiratory distress syndrome
RE	rectal examination
REM	rapid eye movement (in sleep)
RES	reticulo endothelial system
RF, RhF	renal failure / rheumatic fever / rheumatoid factor

RFLA	rheumatoid factor-like activity	SBE	subacute bacterial endocarditis
RFT	respiratory function tests	SBO	small bowel obstruction
Rh	Rhesus factor (in blood)	SBP	systolic blood pressure
RHD	rheumatic heart disease	SC, s.c.	subclavian/subcutaneous
RHL	right hepatic lobe	SCA	sickle-cell anaemia
RIA	radioimmunoassay	SCC	squamous cell carcinoma
RIF	right iliac fossa	SCD	sequential pneumatic compression device / sudden cardiac death
RIND	reversible ischaemic (Am. ischemic) neurologic deficit	SCID	severe combined immunodeficiency syndrome
RK	radial keratotomy / right kidney	SDH	subdural haematoma (Am. hematoma)
RL	right leg / right lung	SDS	same-day surgery
RLC	residual lung capacity	SED	skin erythema dose
RLD	related living donor	SEM	systolic ejection murmur
RLE	right lower extremity	SG	skin graft / specific gravity
RLL	right lower lobe	SGA	small for gestational age
RLQ	right lower quadrant	SGOT	serum glutamic oxaloacetic transaminase, now serum aspartate transferase
RM	radical mastectomy		
RML	right middle lobe (of the lung)	SGPT	serum glutamic pyruvic transaminase
RN	registered nurse	SF	synovial fluid
RNA	ribonucleic acid	SH	social history
R/O	rule out	SIADH	syndrome of inappropriate antidiuretic hormone
ROM	range of movement (exercises)		
ROS	review of symptoms	SIDS	sudden infant death syndrome
RP	radial pulse/retrograde pyelogram	SIG	sigmoidoscope/sigmoidoscopy
RPD	removable partial denture	SIMV	synchronized intermittent mandatory ventilation
RPE	retinal pigment epithelial (cells, layer)		
RPG	retrograde pyelogram	s.l.	sublingual
RPR	rapid plasma reagin	SLE	systemic lupus erythematosus
RQ	respiratory quotient	SLS	social and life skills
RR	recovery room / respiratory rate	SMD	senile macular degeneration
RR&E	round regular and equal	SNS	somatic nervous system
RRR	regular rate and rhythm	SOA	swelling of ankles
RS	respiratory system / Reye syndrome	SOB	short of breath / stools for occult blood
RSI	repetitive strain injury	SOBOE	short of breath on exertion
RSV	respiratory syncytial virus	SOS	swelling of sacrum
RT	radiologic technologist (Am.) / radiotherapy / radiation therapy / right	SP	systolic pressure
		SPECT	single-photon emission computed tomography
RTA	renal tubular acidosis / road traffic accident	SPF	sun protection factor
RUL	right upper lobe	SPP	suprapubic prostatectomy
RUQ	right upper quadrant	SR	sedimentation rate / sinus rhythm
RV	residual volume / right ventricle	SS, S/S	saline solution / signs and symptoms
RVF	right ventricular failure	SSM	superficial spreading melanoma
RVH	right ventricular hypertrophy	ST	sinus tachycardia / skin test
Rx	prescription, recipe	STD	sexually transmitted disease / skin test dose
		Strep	streptococci
s	without (sine)	STS	serological tests for syphilis
S1	first heart sound	STU	skin test unit
S2	second heart sound	Subcu	subcutaneous
SA	sarcoma / sinoatrial (node) / sinus arrhythmia / Stokes-Adams (attacks)	subling	sublingual / under the tongue
		Sup.	superior
SACD	subacute combined degeneration	SV	stroke volume
SAD	seasonal affective disorder	SVC	superior vena cava
SADS	sudden arrhythmic death syndrome	SVD	spontaneous vaginal delivery
SAH	subarachnoid haemorrhage (Am. hemorrhage)	SVI	stroke volume index
SB	seen by		

SVR	systemic venous resistance
SVT	supraventricular tachycardia
SWS	slow wave sleep
Sx	symptoms
syph.	syphilis
Sz	seizure
T	temperature / tumour (Am. tumor) / time
t	terminal
T 1–12	thoracic vertebrae
T_3, T_4	triiodothyronine, tetraiodothyronine (thyroid hormones)
T&A	tonsils and adenoids or tonsillectomy / adenoidectomy
T.A.	toxin-antitoxin
tab	tablet
TAH	total abdominal hysterectomy
TAS	transabdominal sonography
TB, Tb	tuberculosis (tubercle bacillus)
TBA	to be arranged
TBG	thyroid binding globulin
TBI	total body irradiation / traumatic brain injury
TBW	total body water / total body weight
T&C	type and cross-match
Tc	technetium
TCP	thrombocytopenia
TD	thymus dependent cells
TDM	therapeutic drug monitoring
t.d.s.	ter die sumendum (three times a day)
TED	thromboembolic deterrent (stockings)
TENS	transcutaneous electrical nerve stimulation
TFT	thyroid function test
TH	thyroid hormone (thyroxine)
THR	total hip replacement
TI	thymus independent cells
TIA	transient ischaemic attack (Am. ischemic)
TIBC	total iron-binding capacity
t.i.d.	ter in die (three times daily)
TIP	terminal interphalangeal
TIPS	transjugular intrahepatic portosystemic shunting
TJ	triceps jerk
TKR	total knee replacement
TKVO	to keep vein open
TLC	tender loving care / total lung capacity
TLD	thoracic lymph duct
TLE	temporal lobe epilepsy
TM	tympanic membrane
TMJ	temporomandibular joint
TMR	transmyocardial revascularization
TNF	tumour necrosis factor (Am. tumor)
TNM	tumour, node, metastases (Am. tumor)
TOP	termination of pregnancy
tPA	recombinant tissue-type plasminogen activator

TPHI	*Treponema pallidum* haemagglutination inhibition (Am. hemagglutination)
TPI	*Treponema pallidum* immobilization
TPN	total parenteral nutrition
TPR	temperature, pulse, respiration
TRH	thyrotrophin-releasing hormone
TRUS	transrectal ultrasound
TSA	tumour specific antigen (Am. tumor)
TSF	triceps skinfold thickness
TSH	thyroid stimulating hormone
TSS	toxic shock syndrome
TT	tetanus toxoid / thrombin clotting time
TTA	transtracheal aspiration
TTO	to take out (to home)
TUIP	transurethral incision of the prostate
TUR	transurethral resection (of prostate)
TURB	transurethral resection of bladder
TURP	transurethral resection of the prostate gland
TURT	transurethral resection of tumour (Am. tumor)
TV	tidal volume
TVH	total vaginal hysterectomy
TVS	transvaginal sonography
Tx	therapy/transfusion/treatment
T&X	type and cross-match
U	unit
UA	uric acid / urinalysis
UAC	umbilical artery catheter
UAO	upper airway obstruction
UC	ulcerative colitis / uterine contractions
UDO	undetermined origin
U&E	urea and electrolytes
UG	urogenital
UGH	uveitis, glaucoma and hyphaema syndrome (Am. hyphema)
UGI	upper gastrointestinal
UIBC	unsaturated iron-binding capacity
Ung.	ointment (unguentum)
U/O	urinary output
URI	upper respiratory (tract) infection
URT	upper respiratory tract
URTI	upper respiratory tract infection
US	ultrasonography / ultrasound / urinary system
USS	ultrasound scan
UTI	urinary tract infection
UVA	ultraviolet light A
UVB	ultraviolet light B
UVC	ultraviolet light C / umbilical venous catheter
VA	visual acuity
VAC	**v**incristine, **a**driamycin, **c**yclophosphamide
VAS	visual analogue scale
VC	vital capacity / vulvovaginal candidiasis
VCU, VCUG	voiding cystourethrogram
VD	venereal disease

VDRL	venereal disease research laboratory (test)	X-match	cross-match
VE	vaginal examination	XOP	exophoria
VF	ventricular fibrillation / visual field	XOT	exotropia
VHD	valvular heart disease	XR	X-ray
VLBW	very low birth weight	XRT	X-ray therapy / radiation therapy / radiotherapy
VLDL	very low density lipoprotein		
VMA	vanillyl-mandelic acid	yrs	age in years
VP	venous pressure		
VPC	ventricular premature contraction	ZE	Zollinger-Ellison (syndrome)
VRS	verbal rating scale	ZN	Ziel-Nielsen Stain
VS	vital signs		
VSD	ventricular septal defect		

Symbols

VT	ventricular tachycardia	♂	male
VUR	vesicoureteric reflux	♀	female
VWF	von Willebrand factor	*	birth
VV	varicose veins / vulva and vagina	α	alpha
		β	beta
WBC	white blood (cell) count / white blood cell	Γ	gamma
WCC	white cell count	Δ	delta/diagnosis
WNL	within normal limits	$\Delta\Delta$	differential diagnosis
WPW	Wolff–Parkinson–White (syndrome)	#	fracture
WR	Wasserman reaction (test for syphilis)	†	dead

GLOSSARY

The glossary contains a list of prefixes, suffixes and combining forms used in common medical terms. The meaning of each word component is given with an example of its use in a medical term. Use the list to decipher the meaning of unfamiliar words. Note that a dash is added to indicate whether the component usually precedes or follows the other elements of a compound word; for example, **ante-** precedes the word root *nat* as in **ante**natal, whilst **-ectomy** follows the root *arter* as in end*arter***ectomy**. Some word components are made from a root combined with a suffix; for example **-algia** contains the root **alg-** meaning pain and the suffix **-ia** meaning condition of. The vowels of combining forms are used or dropped by the application of the 'rules' described in the introduction of this book. Some roots are listed with more than one combining vowel, for example, **ren/i/o**; both vowels may be used in combination with the root as in **ren**ipelvic and **ren**ography.

Component	Meaning	Example
a-	without, not (an is added before words beginning with a vowel)	**a**phasia
-a	noun ending / a name	burs**a**
ab-	away from	**ab**duct
abdomin/o	abdomen	**abdomin**opelvic
-able	capable of / having ability to	palp**able**
ac-	pertaining to/to/toward	mani**ac**
acanth/o	spiny	**acanth**osis
acarin/o	mites of the order Acarina	**acarin**osis
acar/i/o	mites of the order Acarina	**acar**icide
acetabul/o	acetabulum	**acetabul**oplasty
acet/o	vinegar	*Aceto*bacter
aceton-	ketones/acetone	**aceton**aemia (Am. **aceton**emia)
achill/o	Achilles tendon	**achill**otomy
acid/o	acid	**acid**ophil
acin/i	sac-like dilatation	**acin**us
acne/o	acne vulgaris / point / peak	**acne**genic
acou-	hear/hearing	**acou**metric
-acousia	condition of hearing	dys**acousia**
acoust/o	hear/hearing/sound	**acoust**ic
acro-	extremities, point	**acro**megaly
acromi/o	acromion (point of the shoulder)	**acromi**oclavicular
act-	do, drive, act	**act**ion
actin/o	rays, eg. of sun / ultraviolet radiation	**actin**otherapy
acu-	hear/hearing/severe/sudden	**acu**te
-acusia	condition / sense of hearing	dys**acusia**
ad-	to/toward/in the direction of the midline/near	**ad**duct
adamant/o	dental enamel	**adamant**ine
aden/o	gland	**aden**oid
adenoid-	adenoids (nasopharyngeal tonsils)	**adenoid**ectomy
adip/o	adipose tissue / fat	**adip**osity
adnex/o	bound to / conjoined	**adnex**a
adrenal/o	adrenal gland	**adrenal**ectomy
adren/o	adrenal gland	**adren**ogenital
adrenocortic/o	adrenal cortex	**adrenocortic**al
-aem-	blood (Am. -em-)	an**aem**ia (Am. -an**em**ia)
-aemia	condition of blood (Am. -emia)	leuk**aemia**
aer/o	air/gas	**aer**ophagia
aesthe/s/i/o	sensation/sensitivity (Am. esthe/s/i/o)	an**aesthesio**logy (Am. an**esthesio**logy)

Component	Meaning	Example
aeti/o	cause (Am. eti/o)	**aetio**logy (Am. **etio**logy)
af-	to/towards/near	**af**ferent
ag-	to/towards/near	**ag**glutinate
agglutin/o	sticking / clumping together	**agglutin**ation
-ago	abnormal condition / disease	lumb**ago**
-agogic	pertaining to inducing / stimulating	dacry**agogic**
-agogue	an agent that promotes / induces	lact**agogue**
agora-	market place / open space	**agora**phobia
-agra	seizure / sudden pain	pod**agra**
-aise	comfort/ease	mal**aise**
-al^1	pertaining to	bronchi**al**
-al^2	used in pharmacology to mean a drug or drug action	antifung**al**
albin/o	white	**albin**ism
alb/i/o	white	**alb**us
album-	white	**album**in
albumin/o	albumin/albumen	**albumin**uria
aldosteron-	aldosterone	**aldosteron**ism
-algesia	condition of pain	an**algesia**
alges/i/o	sense of pain	**algesio**meter
-algia	condition of pain	neur**algia**
alg/e/i/o	pain	**alg**esthesia
aliment/o	to nourish	**aliment**ary
all/o	other / different from normal	**allo**genic
alopec	baldness / like the mange of (a fox)	**alopec**ia
alve/o	trough / channel / cavity	**alve**us
alveol/o	alveoli (of lungs)	**alveol**itis
ambi-	both / on both sides	**ambi**lateral
ambly/o	dull/dim	**ambly**opia
ameb/o (Am.)	ameba, a type of protozoan	**ameb**iasis
amel/o	dental enamel	**amelo**blast
-amine	nitrogen containing compound	catechol**amine**
amni/o	amnion / fetal membrane	**amnio**centesis
amnion/o	amnion / fetal membrane	**amnion**ic
amoeb/o	amoeba a type of protozoan (Am. ameb/o)	**amoeb**iasis (Am. **ameb**iasis)
amph/i	both / doubly / both sides	**amphi**gonadism
amyl/o	starch	**amyl**oid
an-	without / not	**an**encephalic
-an	pertaining to / characteristic of	ovari**an**
ana-	reversion / going backward / apart / up / again	**ana**plastic
ancyl/o	crooked/stiffening/fusing/bent	**ancylo**stomiasis
andr/o	male/masculine/man	**andr**ology
-ane	a saturated, open-chain hydrocarbon	meth**ane**
aneurysm/o	aneurysm	**aneurysmo**plasty
angi/o	vessel / blood vessel	**angio**plasty
an-iso-	unequal/dissimilar	**aniso**coria
ankyl/o	crooked/stiffening/fusing/bent	**ankyl**osis
an/o	anus	**ano**rectal
-ant	having the characteristic of / an agent that...	stimul**ant**
ante-	before in time or place / in front of / forward	**ante**natal
anter/o	front / in front of / anterior to	**antero**lateral
anthrac/o	coal dust / black	**anthrac**osis
anthrop/o	man/human	**anthropo**metry
anti-	against	**anti**fungal

Component	Meaning	Example
antr/o	antrum / maxillary sinus	**antro**tomy
anxi/o	anxiety	**anxio**lytic
aort/o	aorta	**aorto**rrhaphy
ap-	to / towards / near / separated from	**ap**position
-aph-	touch	hyper**aph**ia
-apheresis	removal	leuk**apheresis**
aphth/o	ulcer	**aphth**ous
apic/o	apex	**apic**al
ap/o	away from / detached / derived from / separate	**apo**physis
aponeur/o	aponeurosis (flat tendon)	**aponeuro**rrhaphy
append/ic/o	appendix	**appendic**ectomy
aqu/a/e/o	water	**aque**ous
-ar	pertaining to	lob**ar**
arachn/o	spider	**arachn**ophobia
arc/o	arch/bowed	**arc**us
-arch/e-	beginning	men**arche**
arrhen/o	male/masculine	**arrheno**blastoma
arter/i/o	artery	**arterio**sclerosis
arteriol/o	arteriole	**arteriolo**necrosis
arthr/o	joint	**arthro**desis
articul/o	joint	**articul**ate
-ary	pertaining to / connected with	pulmon**ary**
as-	to/towards/near	**as**sociation
-ase	an enzyme	amyl**ase**
-asia	state or condition	euthan**asia**
-asis	state or condition	elephanti**asis**
-asthenia	condition of weakness	my**asthenia**
asthen/o	weakness	**astheno**coria
astr/o	star-shaped/star	**astro**cyte
at-	to/towards/near	**at**traction
-ate	denoting a state or function / possessing / a chemical from a specific source / like	stimul**ate**
atel/o	imperfect/incomplete	**atelo**cardia
ather/o	atheroma, a fatty plaque lining a blood vessel	**athero**sclerosis
-ation	action/condition	ejacul**ation**
-atresia	condition of occlusion / closure / absence of opening	anal **atresia**
atret/o	closure of a normal opening / imperforation	**atreto**metria
atri/o	atrium	**atrio**ventricular
audi/o	hearing / sense of hearing	**audio**metry
audit/o	hearing / sense of hearing	**audit**ory
-aural	pertaining to the ear	mon**aural**
auricul/o	pinna of the ear or auricle	**auriculo**plasty
aur/i/o	ear/hearing	**auri**scope
auto-	self	**auto**lysis
aux/i/o	increase	**auxi**lytic
-auxis	increase	onych**auxis**
-ax	noun ending / a name	thor**ax**
axill/o	armpit	**axill**ary
ax/i/o	axis	**axi**petal
axon/o	axis / axon of neuron	**axon**al
azot/o	urea/nitrogen	**azot**aemia (Am. **azot**emia)
bat-	go/walk/stand	hypno**bat**ia
bacill/o	bacillus / a rod-shaped bacterium	**bacill**uria

Component	Meaning	Example
bacter/i/o	bacterium/bacteria	**bacterio**phage
balan/o	glans penis	**balan**itis
ballist/o	throw/movement	**ballisto**cardiograph
bar/i/o	pressure / weight	**baro**trauma
bartholin/o	Bartholin glands / greater vestibular glands of the vagina	**bartholin**itis
basi-	base/basic/alkaline	**basi**chromatin
baso-	base/basic/alkaline	**baso**phil
bathy-	deep	**bathy**pnoea (Am. **bathy**pnea)
bi-	two/twice/double/life	**bi**pedal
bili-	bile	**bili**ary
bilirubin/o	bilirubin	**bilirubin**uria
bin-	two each / double	**bin**ocular
bio-	life/living	**bio**logy
-blast	germ cell / immature cell / embryonic cell / developing stage	osteo**blast**
blast/o	germ cell / immature cell / embryonic cell / developing stage	retino**blast**oma
blenn/o	mucus	**blenn**oid
blephar/o	eyelid	**blephar**optosis
bol-	ball	**bol**us
brachi/o	arm	**brachi**al
brachy-	short	**brachy**gnathia
brady-	slow	**brady**cardia
brev/i	short	**brevi**flexor
bromidr/o	stench / smell of sweat	**bromidr**osis
bronch/i/o	bronchus / bronchial tube / windpipe	**broncho**scopy
bronchiol/o	bronchiole	**bronchiol**itis
bront/o	thunder	**bronto**phobia
bucca-	cheek	**bucca**l
bucc/o	cheek	**bucco**pharyngeal
bulb/o	bulb / medulla oblongata	**bulb**ar
burs/o	bursa (fluid-filled sac)	**burs**itis
byssin/o	cotton dust	**byssin**osis
cac/o	bad/ill/abnormal	**caco**cholia
caec/o	caecum (Am. cecum)	**caeco**cele (Am. **ceco**cele)
calcane/o	calcaneus / heel bone	**calcaneo**plantar
calc/i/o	calcium/lime/heel	**calci**penia
calcin/o	calcium	**calcin**osis
calcul/o	calculus / stone / little stone	**calcul**us
calic-	calyx (Am. calix) / a cup-shaped organ or cavity	**calic**ectasis
calor/i	heat	**calori**metry
calyc-	calyx (Am. calix) / a cup-shaped organ or cavity	**calyc**ulus
cancer/o	cancer (general term)	**cancero**phobia
canth/o	canthus (corner of the eye)	**cantho**plasty
capill/o	blood capillary / hair-like	**capill**ary
capit/o	head	**capit**ate
-capnia	condition of carbon dioxide	hyper**capnia**
caps-	container	**caps**itis
capsul/o	capsule	**capsul**ar
carb/o	carbon/bicarbonate	**carbo**hydrate
carcin/o	cancerous / malignant tumour of epithelial tissue	**carcin**oma
carcinomat-	carcinoma	**carcinomat**ous
-cardia	condition of the heart	tachy**cardia**

Component	Meaning	Example
cardi/o	heart	**cardio**logist
cari/o	rot/decay (of teeth)	**cario**genesis
carp/o	carpal / wrist bones	**carpo**ptosis
cary/o	nucleus	eu**caryo**tic
cat/a	down/negative/wrong/back	**cata**bolic
caud/o	tail / towards the tail / lower part of body	**caud**al
caus-	burn/corrosive	**caus**tic
caut-	burn	**caut**ery
cav-	hollow	**cav**ity
cec/o (Am.)	cecum	**ceco**cele
-cele	swelling/protrusion/hernia	vesico**cele**
celi/o	hollow/abdomen	**celio**scope
cell-	cell	**cell**ular
cellul-	cell	**cellul**ar
cel/o (Am.)	hollow/abdomen/celom	**celo**schisis
cement/o	cementum of a tooth	**cemento**clasia
cen/o	new/empty/common	**ceno**sis
-centesis	surgical puncture to remove fluid	amnio**centesis**
centi-	hundred / one hundredth	**centi**grade
centr/i/o	centre / central location	**centri**lobular
cephal/o	head	hydro**cephal**ic
cerat/o	horny/epidermis/cornea (synonym: kerat/o)	**cerato**cricoid
cerebell/o	cerebellum	**cerebell**ar
cerebr/i/o	cerebrum/brain	**cerebr**oma
cer/o	wax	**cer**oma
cerumin/o	cerumen / ear wax	**cerumin**ous
cervic/o	cervix	**cervic**al
-chalasis	slackening/loosening	blepharo**chalasis**
chancr-	chancre, a destructive sore	**chancr**oid
cheil/o	lip	**cheilo**plasty
cheir/o	hand	**cheiro**megaly
chem/i/c/o	chemical	**chemo**receptor
-chezia	condition of defaecation, especially of foreign substances	uro**chezia**
chil/o	lip (cheil/o now used)	**chilo**plasty
chir/o	hand	**chiro**pody
chlorhydr/o	hydrochloric acid	**chlorhydr**ia
chlor/o	green/chlorine	**chlor**oma
cholangi/o	bile vessel / bile duct	**cholangio**gram
cholecyst/o	gallbladder	**cholecysto**lithiasis
choledoch/o	common bile duct	**choledocho**lithiasis
chol/e/o	bile	**chol**uria
cholester/o	cholesterol	**cholester**osis
chondr/o	cartilage	**chondro**sarcoma
chord/o	string/cord	**chordo**tomy
chore/o	chorea / dance / jerky movement	**chore**a
chori/o	chorion / outer fetal membrane	**chorio**allantois
choroid/o	choroid layer of eye	**choroid**itis
chromat/o	colour	**chromat**opsia
-chromia	condition of haemoglobin / colour (Am. hemoglobin)	hypo**chromia**
chrom/o	colour	**chromo**cystoscopy
chron/o	time	**chron**ic
chrys/o	gold	**chryso**derma

Component	Meaning	Example
chyl/e/o	chyle, a fluid formed by lacteals (lymphatics) in the intestine, a product of fat digestion	**chylo**thorax
chym/o	chyme, a creamy material produced by digestion of food	**chymo**poiesis
cib/o	meal	**cib**us
-cidal	pertaining to killing	bacterio**cidal**
-cide	agent that kills / killing	acari**cide**
cili/o	cilia / ciliary body of eye / eyelash	**cili**ectomy
cinemat/o	movement/motion (picture)	**cinemato**graphy
cine/o	movement/motion	**cine**angiography
cinesi/o	movement/motion	**cinesi**ology
circum-	around	**circum**cision
cirrh/o	yellow/tawny	**cirrh**osis
cirs/o	varicose vein / varix	**cirs**ectomy
cis-	on the near side / this side	**cis** position
-cis-	cut/kill	ex**cis**ion
cistern/o	cistern / enclosed space (sub-arachnoid space)	**cisterno**graphy
-clasia	condition of breaking	osteo**clasia**
-clasis	breaking	osteo**clasis**
-clast	a cell that breaks	osteo**clast**
claustr/o	barrier/enclosed	**claustro**phobia
clavic/o	clavicle	**clavico**tomy
clavicul/o	clavicle	**clavicul**ar
-cle	small	vesi**cle**
cleid/o	clavicle	**cleido**tomy
clin/o	bend/incline	**clino**dactyly
clitor/i/o	clitoris	**clitor**ism
clon/o	clone of cells	mono**clon**al
-clonus	violent action	myo**clonus**
-clysis	infusion/injection/irrigation	veno**clysis**
co-	with/together	**co**factor
coagul/o	clotting	anti**coagul**ant
coccid/i	types of parasitic protozoa of the order Coccidia	**coccid**iosis
cocc/i/o	a berry-shaped bacterium/a coccus	**cocc**ogenous
-coccus	a berry-shaped bacterium	strepto**coccus**
coccyg/o	coccyx	**coccyg**eal
cochle/o	cochlea	**cochleo**vestibular
-coel(e)	hollow/abdomen	blasto**coel(e)**
coel/o	hollow/abdomen/ceolom (Am. celom)	**coel**om (Am. **cel**om)
col-	with/together	**col**lateral
coll/a	glue	**colla**gen
collagen/o	collagen	**collagen**ase
col/o	colon	**colo**stomy
colon/o	colon	**colon**ic
colp/o	vagina	**colpo**hysterectomy
com-	with/together	**com**mensal
coma/t/o	a deep sleep, a coma or state of unconsciousness	**coma**tose
con-	with/together	**con**centric
condyl/o	condyl	**condyl**ar
coni/o	dust	**coni**osis
conjunctiv/o	conjunctiva	**conjunctiv**itis
contra-	against/opposed/opposite	**contra**ception
-conus	cone-like protrusion	kerato**conus**
copr/o	faeces (Am. feces)	**copro**lith

Component	Meaning	Example
cor-	with/together	**cor**rosive
cord/o	a cord	**cordo**tomy
cor/e/o	pupil	**core**morphosis
-coria	condition of the pupils	aniso**coria**
corne/o	cornea/horny (consisting of keratin)	**corneo**blepharon
coron/o-	crown-like projection / encircling / coronary vessels of the heart	**coron**ary
corpor/o	body	**corpor**al
-cortex-	outer part / bark	adrenal **cortex**
cortic/o	adrenal cortex / cortex / outer region	**cortico**trophic
cost/o	rib	inter**cost**al
cox/o	hip / hip joint	**coxo**femoral
crani/o	cranium/skull	**cranio**tomy
cren/o	crenated/notched	**creno**cytosis
-crescent	crescent / sickle-shaped / shaped like a new moon	epithelial **crescent**
-crine	secrete	exo**crine**
crin/o	secrete	endo**crin**ology
-crit	separate / device for measuring cells	haemato**crit** (Am. hemato**crit**)
crur/o	leg	**crur**al
cry/o	relating to cold	**cryo**stat
crypt/o	hidden	**crypt**orchism
cubit/o	elbow	**cubit**us
culd/o	Douglas pouch / rectouterine pouch / cul-de sac	**culdo**scope
-cule	small	animal**cule**
cult-	cultivate	**cult**ure
cune/i	wedge (shape)	**cune**iform
cutane/o	skin	**cutane**ous
cut/i	skin	**cuti**cle
cyan/o	blue	**cyan**osis
cycl/o	ciliary body / circle	**cyclo**tomy
cyes/i/o	pregnancy	**cyesi**ology
-cyesis	pregnancy	pseudo**cyesis**
cylindr/o	cylinder	**cylindr**oid
cyll/o	deformity	thoraco**cyll**osis
cyn/o	dog	**cyn**ophobia
cyrt/o	curved / abnormal curvature	**cyrto**meter
cyst/i/o	bladder / a cyst	**cyst**ostomy
-cyte	cell	melano**cyte**
cyt/o	cell	**cyto**logy
-cytosis	condition of cells, usually an abnormal increase	erythro**cytosis**
dacry/o	tear / lacrimal apparatus	**dacry**olith
dacryocyst/o	lacrimal sac	**dacryocysto**tomy
dactyl/o	digits / fingers or toes	**dactylo**megaly
de-	down / away from / loss of / reversing	**de**calcification
deca-	ten	**deca**gram
deci-	one-tenth	**deci**litre
demi-	half	**demi**facet
dem/o	people	**demo**graphic
dendr/i/o	tree/tree-like (dendrite of neuron)	**dendri**tic
dentin/o	dentine of tooth (Am. dentin)	**dentino**genesis
dent/i/o	tooth	**dent**ist
derm/a/o	skin	**derm**abrasion
dermat/o	skin	**dermat**ology
descemet/o	Descemet membrane (of cornea)	**descemeto**cele

Component	Meaning	Example
-desis	fixation / to bind together by surgery / sticking together	arthro**desis**
desm/o	band/ligament	**desmo**pathy
deuter/o	second	**deuter**anopia
dextro-	right	**dextro**cardia
di-	two/twice/double	**di**coria
dia-	through/apart/across/between	**dia**physis
-dialysis	separate	haemo**dialysis** (Am. hemo**dialysis**)
diaphor/o	sweating (excessive)	**diaphor**esis
diaphragmat/o	diaphragm	**diaphragmat**algia
diastol-	diastole	**diastol**ic
didym-	twins	epi**didym**is
digit/o	finger / toe	**digito**plantar
dipl/o-	double	**dipl**opia
dips/o	thirst	poly**dips**ia
dis-	apart / reversal / separation / duplication / free from	**dis**location
disc/o	intervertebral disc	**disco**graphy
disk/o (Am.)	intervertebral disk	**disk**ectomy
dist/o	far from point of origin	**dist**al
diverticul/o	diverticulum	**diverticul**itis
doch/o	duct / to receive	chole**doch**itis
dolich/o	long	**dolicho**cranial
dolor/i/o	pain (dol, unit of pain)	**doloro**genic
-dorsal	pertaining to the back (of the body)	ventro**dorsal**
dors/i/o	the back (of the body) / dorsal	**dorso**ventral
-drome	a course / conduction / flowing	syn**drome**
drom/o	a course / conduction / flowing	**dromo**tropic
-duct-	a tube to lead material toward or away from a structure	ovi**duct**
duoden/o	duodenum	**duodeno**stomy
dur/o	dura mater / hard	epi**dur**al
dynam/o	force/power (of movement)	**dynam**ic
-dynia	condition of pain	pleuro**dynia**
dys-	difficult/disordered/painful/bad	**dys**phasia
e-	away from / out from / outside / without	**e**masculation
-e	noun ending / a name	trigon**e**
-eal	pertaining to	oesophag**eal**
ec-	away from / out from / outside / without	**ec**cyesis
ech/o	echo / reflected sound	**echo**lalia
ect-	out / outside / outer part	**ect**ethmoid
ecto-	out / outside / outer part	**ecto**derm
ectopia-	condition of displacement	**ectopia** lentis
ectop/o	displaced away from normal position	**ectop**ic
-ectasia	condition of dilation or stretching	pneumon**ectasia**
-ectasis	dilatation, stretching	bronchi**ectasis**
-ectomy	removal, excision	appendic**ectomy**
ectro-	congenital absence / miscarriage	**ectro**dactylia
edema- (Am.)	condition of swelling due to fluid	**edema**tous
ef-	out / away from	**ef**ferent
eikon/o	icon	**eikono**meter
elast/o	elastic / elastic tissue / elastin	**elasto**sis
electr/o	electrical	**electro**cardiograph
ele/o (Am.)	oil/fat	**ele**oma
ellipto-	shaped like an ellipse	**ellipto**cytosis

Component	Meaning	Example
em-	in	**em**pathy
-em- (Am.)	blood	an**em**ia
-ema	condition	myxed**ema**
embol/o	embolus/plug/blockage	**embol**ism
embry/o	embryo	**embry/o**genesis
-emesis	vomiting	haemat**emesis** (Am. hemat**emesis**)
emet/o	vomiting	**emet**ic
-emia (Am.)	condition of blood	an**emia**
emmetr/o	in due measure / normally proportioned	**emmetr**opia
-emphraxis	blocking / stopping up	salping**emphraxis**
en-	within / in	**en**sheathed
encephal/o	brain	**encephal**itis
endo-	within/inside/inner	**endo**scope
endocardi/o	endocardium	**endocardi**tis
endocrin/o	endocrine (gland)	**endocrin**ologist
endometri/o	endometrium of uterus (the lining of the uterus)	**endometri**osis
endotheli/o	endothelium	**endotheli**al
enter/o	intestine	**enter**itis
-ent	person/agent	dilu**ent**
ento-	within, inside	**ento**cranial
eosin/o	rosy-red / dawn coloured / eosin, a red acid dye	**eosin/o**phil
ep-	above / upon / on	**ep**arterial
epi-	above / upon / on / in addition	**epi**dermis
epiderm/o	epidermis	**epiderm**al
epididym/o	epididymis	**epididym/o**vasectomy
epiglott/o	epiglottis	**epiglott**itis
epilept/i/o	epilepsy	**epilept**iform
epipl/o	omentum	**epipl/o**plasty
episi/o	vulva/pudendum	**episi/o**tomy
epitheli/o	epithelium	**epitheli**al
equin/o	horse	**equin**e
-er	one who / a person / an agent	radiograph**er**
erg/o/n/o	work	**erg/o**nometer
-erysis	drag / draw / suck out	phaco**erysis**
erythem/o	reddening of the skin / flushed / erythema	**erythem/o**genic
erythr/o	red	**erythr/o**cyte
-esis	abnormal state / condition	ur**esis**
es/o	within/inwards	**es/o**deviation
esophag/o (Am.)	esophagus/gullet	**esophag/o**stomy
esthesi/o (Am.)	sensation	an**esthesi/o**logy
estr/o (Am.)	estrogen/female/estrus	**estr/o**genic
ethm/o	ethmoid bone	**ethm/o**idonasal
ethmoid/o	ethmoid bone	**ethmoid/o**palatal
eti/o (Am.)	causation (of disease)	**eti/o**logy
eu-	good/normal/easily	**eu**tocia
eury-	wide/broad	**eury**cephalic
ex-	out / out of / away from	**ex**ophthalmos
exo-	out / away from / outside	**exo**gastric
-externa	external	otitis **externa**
extr/a/o	outside of / beyond / outward	**extr/a**hepatic
faci/o	face	**faci/o**maxillary
faec/a/o	faeces (Am. feces)	**faec/a**lith (Am. **feco**lith)
falc/i	falx / sickle-shaped structure	**falc/i**form
fascicul/o	fascicle	**fascicul**ar

Component	Meaning	Example
fasci/o	fascia / fibrous tissue, eg, covering muscles	**fascio**tomy
febr/o	fever	**febr**ile
fec/o (Am.)	feces/waste	**fec**al
femor/o	femur/thigh	**femor**al
-ferent	carrying / to carry / to bear	ef**ferent**
fer/o	to carry / to bear	urini**ferous**
ferr/o	iron	**ferro**protein
fet/i/o (Am.)	fetus	**feto**metry
fibrill/o	muscular twitching	**fibrill**ation
fibrin/o	fibrinogen	**fibrino**lytic
fimbri/o	fringe	**fimbri**ate
fibr/o	fibre	**fibr**osis
fibul/o	fibula	**fibulo**calcaneal
-fida	split	spina bi**fida**
fil/o	thread	**filo**pressure
fissur-	split/cleft	**fissur**al
fistul/o	tube/pipe	**fistul**a
flagell/o	flagellum/whip	**flagell**osis
flav/o	yellow	**flavo**protein
-flect	bend	re**flect**
-flex-	bend	**flex**ion
fluor/o	fluorescent/luminous/flow	**fluoro**scopy
-flux	flow	re**flux**
foet/o	foetus (Am. fet/o)	**foet**al (Am. **fet**al)
follicul/o	small sac/follicle	**follicul**itis
fore-	before / in front of	**fore**brain
-form	having form / structure of	epilepti**form**
foss/o	depression	**foss**a
fove/o	pit / often used to mean the central fovea of the retina	**fove**a
fraen/o	fraenum or fraenulum / a restraining structure, eg, fraenulum of the lip	**fraen**al (Am. **fren**al)
fren/o (Am.)	frenum or frenulum / a restraining structure, eg, frenulum of the lip	**freno**plasty
front/o	front/forehead	**fronto**temporal
-fuge	agent that suppresses / gets rid of	lacti**fuge**
fund/o	bottom/base (of an organ)	**fund**us
fung/i	fungus	**fung**icide
furc/o	branching	bi**furc**ation
-fy	making or cause to become	ossi**fy**
galact/o	milk	**galacto**poiesis
gamet/o	gametes / sperm or eggs	**gameto**genesis
gangli/o	ganglion / swelling / plexus	**gangli**form
ganglion-	ganglion / swelling / plexus	**ganglion**ectomy
gastr/o	stomach	**gastro**pathy
-gen	agent that produces / precursor	pepsino**gen**
-genesis	capable of causing / pertaining to formation	spermato**genesis**
-genic	pertaining to formation/originating in	oestro**genic**
genicul/o	knee	**genicul**ar
geni/o	chin	**genio**glossal
genit/o	genitals / reproductive organs/produced by birth	**genit**al
gen/o	cause/produce/originate	**geno**phobia
-genous	arising from / produced by / producing	andro**genous**
ger/i/o	old age/the aged	**ger**iatric

Component	Meaning	Example
geront/o	old age/the aged	**geront**ology
gest/o	pregnancy	**gest**ation
gingiv/o	gum	**gingiv**itis
glauc/o	grey (Am. gray)	**glauc**oma
glen/o	socket of a joint / pit / glenoid cavity	**glen**oid
gli/a/o	glue-like / neuroglia, the supporting cells of the CNS	**gli**oma
glisson-	Glisson capsule (around the liver)	**glisson**itis
-globin	protein	myo**globin**
-globulin	protein	immuno**globulin**
-globus	globe / like a small ball	kerato**globus**
glomerul/o	glomerulus of kidney	**glomerul**itis
gloss/o	tongue	**gloss**ectomy
glott/o	glottis (the vocal apparatus and its opening)	**glott**al
gluc/o	glucose/sugar/sweet	**gluc**oneogenesis
glyc/o	glucose/sugar/sweet	**glyc**oprotein
glycogen/o	glycogen, a polysaccharide	**glycogen**osis
glycos-	sugar (an obsolete variant meaning glucose)	**glycos**uria
gnath/o	jaw	**gnath**oplasty
-gnomy	science or means of judging	patho**gnomy**
-gnos-	to know / known or knowledge of / judgment	**gnos**ia
-gnosia	condition of knowing / receiving / recognizing	hyper**gnosia**
-gnosis	to know / known or knowledge of / judgment	pro**gnosis**
gonad/o	gonads (the ovaries or testes)	**gonad**otrophin
gonecyst/o	seminal vesicle	**gonecyst**olith
gon/e/o	seed/semen/sperm/knee	**gono**coccus
goni/o	angle/corner	**goni**oscopy
gony/o	knee	**gony**oncus
-grade	to go	retro**grade**
-gram	X-ray / tracing / recording / one-thousandth of a kilogram (g)	mammo**gram**
granul/o	granule/granular	**granul**oma
-graph	usually recording instrument / a recording / an X-ray picture / a mathematical curve representing data	electrocardio**graph**
-graphy	technique of recording / making X-ray	electrocardio**graphy**
-gravida	pregnancy / a pregnant woman	primi**gravida**
gravid/o	pregnancy	**gravid**ocardiac
gryp/h	abnormal curvature / hooked	**gryp**osis
gynaec/o	gynaecology / female reproductive system / woman (Am. gynec/o)	**gynaeco**logy (Am. **gyneco**logy)
-gyne	woman/female	andro**gyne**
gynec/o (Am.)	gynecology / female reproductive system / woman	**gyneco**logical
gyn/o	gynaecology (Am. gynecology) / female reproductive system / woman	**gyn**opathy
-gyric	pertaining to circular motion	oculo**gyric**
haemangi/o	blood vessel (Am. hemangi/o)	**haemangi**oma (Am. **hemangi**oma)
haem/a/o	blood (Am. hem/a/o)	**haemo**globin (Am. **hemo**globin)
haemat/o	blood (Am. hemat/o)	**haemat**ology (Am. **hemat**ology
haemoglobin/o	haemoglobin (Am. hemoglobin)	**haemoglobin**uria (Am. **hemoglobin**uria)
halit/o	breath	**halit**osis
hallucin/o	hallucination	**hallucin**ogenic
hallux	great toe	**hallux** rigidus
hal/o	salts	**hal**ogen

Component	Meaning	Example
hapl/o	single/simple	**hapl**opia
hapt/o	touch	**hapt**ometer
hecto-	one hundred	**hecto**gram
helc/o	ulcer	**helc**osis
helic/o	helix / spiral form	**helic**oid
heli/o	sun	**heli**osis
helmint/h/o	worms	ant**helminth**ic
hem/a/o (Am.)	blood	**hemo**cytoblast
hemat/o (Am.)	blood	**hemat**ology
hemi-	half / on one side	**hemi**plegia
hepatic/o	hepatic bile duct	**hepatico**stomy
hepat/o	liver	**hepato**cyte
hept/a	seven	**hepta**chromic
herni/o	hernia	**herni**orrhaphy
heter/o	other/another/different	**hetero**sexual
hex-	six/hold/being	**hex**ose
hidraden/o	sweat gland	**hidraden**itis
hidr/o	sweat/perspiration	**hidr**osis
histi/o	histiocyte, a type of macrophage	**histio**cytosis
hist/o	tissue	**histo**logy
hol/o	entire/whole	**holo**crine
homeo-	alike/unchanging/constant/resembling	**homeo**stasis
homo-	the same / resembling	**homo**zygous
humer/o	humerus	**humero**radial
hyal/o	glass-like	**hyal**oid
hydatid/i/o	hydatid cyst	**hydatid**osis
hydr/a/o	water	**hydr**onephrosis
hygr/o	moisture	**hygro**blepharic
hymen/o	hymen	**hymeno**tomy
hy/o	hyoid bone	**hyo**mandibular
hyp-	below / below normal / under	**hyp**hidrosis
hyper-	above / above normal / excessive / over	**hyper**chromia
hypn/o	sleep	**hypno**tic
hypo-	below normal / under	**hypo**thyroidism
hypophys-	hypophysis / pituitary gland	**hypophys**ectomy
hyster/o	uterus/womb	**hyster**ectomy
-ia	condition of / abnormal condition / disease	poly**uria**
-iac	pertaining to	coel**iac** (Am. cel**iac**)
-ial	pertaining to	bronch**ial**
-ian	belonging to / characteristic of / supporter of / suffix that forms a noun	physic**ian**
-iasis	abnormal condition / process or condition resulting from / disease	lith**iasis**
-iatrics	a medical specialty	paed**iatrics** (Am. ped**iatrics**)
iatr/o	medical treatment / doctor	**iatro**genic
-iatry	treatment by a doctor / specialty (of doctor)	psych**iatry**
-ible	capable of / able	flex**ible**
-ic[1]	pertaining to	gast**ric**
-ic[2]	used in pharmacology to mean a drug or drug action	diure**tic**
-ical	pertaining to / dealing with	cytolog**ical**
ichthy/o	fish-like/dry/scaly	**ichthy**osis
-ician	person associated with / specialist	techn**ician**
-icle	small	ves**icle**

Component	Meaning	Example
-ics	art or science of	gene**tics**
-ictal	pertaining to seizure/attack	prei**ctal**
icter/o	jaundice	**ictero**genic
-ide	a binary chemical compound	glycos**ide**
idi/o	self / one's own / peculiar to an organism / unknown	**idio**pathic
-ify	make or produce / cause to become	acid**ify**
-igo	attack / abnormal condition	vert**igo**
il-	in/none	**il**legitimate
-ile	capable of / able to / relating to / belonging to	contract**ile**
ile/o	ileum	**ileo**colitis
ili/o	ilium/flank	**ilio**femoral
im-	in/within/none/not	**im**potence
immun/o	immune/immunity	**immuno**logy
in-	in/none/not	**in**cision
-in	used as suffix for various chemicals	glycer**in**
incud/o	incus (the anvil-shaped ear ossicle) / anvil	**incudo**malleal
-ine	pertaining to / a suffix used for chemicals derived or thought to be derived from ammonia	am**ine**
infer/o	below / beneath / inferior to	**infero**lateral
infra-	below / inferior to	**infra**mammary
inguin/o	groin	**inguin**al
insulin/o	insulin / islets of Langerhans	**insulino**genesis
inter-	between	**inter**costal
-interna	internal	otitis **interna**
intestin/o	intestine	**intestin**al
intra-	within/inside	**intra**nasal
intro-	into/within/inwards	**intro**flexion
intus-	in/into	**intus**susception
iod/o	iodine	**iod**ism
-ion	action / condition resulting from an action	abla**tion**
ion/o	ion / to wander	**ion**ic
-ior	pertaining to	poster**ior**
ips/e/i/o	the same / self	**ipsi**lateral
ir-	in/none/not	**ir**reducible
irid/i/o	iris	**irido**plegia
ir/o	iris	**ir**itis
ischi/o	ischium	**ischio**coccygeal
isch/o	holding back / reducing / suppressing	**isch**aemia (Am. **isch**emia)
-ism	process / state or condition / practice of / theory of	prostat**ism**
-ismus	spasm / process / state or condition	strab**ismus**
iso-	same/equal	**iso**graft
-ist	specialist	optometr**ist**
-ite	a substance produced through a process; an end product of a reaction	metabol**ite**
-itic	relating to or having something specified	syphil**itic**
-itis	inflammation	tonsill**itis**
-ity	state/condition	sever**ity**
-ium	metallic element	calc**ium**
-ive[1]	pertaining to / tendency	adhes**ive**
-ive[2]	used in pharmacology to mean a drug or drug action	antituss**ive**
-ize	use / subject to treatment or action / to make or treat / combine with	neutral**ize**

Component	Meaning	Example
-ject	throw	pro**ject**ile
jejun/o	jejunum	**jejuno**stomy
juxta-	adjoining/near	**juxta**position
kal/i	potassium (K⁺), from Latin kalium	**kal**iuresis
kary/o	nucleus	**karyo**gram
keratin/o	keratin (a protein present in skin, hair and nails)	**keratin**ous
kerat/o	epidermis/cornea/horny	**kerato**plasty
kern-	nucleus (of nerve cells)	**kern**icterus
ket/o/n	ketones / ketone bodies / carbonyl group	**keton**uria
kin/e/o	motion/movement	**kin**esis
kinesi/o	motion/movement	**kinesio**logy
-kinesis	a motion/movement	irido**kinesis**
kinet/o	motion/movement	**kineto**cardiography
kilo-	one thousand	**kilo**calorie
klept/o	thief/stealing	**klepto**mania
-kymia	condition of involuntary twitching of muscle / a wave of contraction in a muscle	myo**kymia**
kyph/o	crooked / hump / forward curvature of the thoracic spine	**kyph**osis
labi/o	lip	**labio**plasty
labyrinth/o	labyrinth of ear	**labyrinth**itis
lachrym/o	tear / tear ducts / lacrimal apparatus	**lachrym**al
lacrim/o	tear / tear ducts / lacrimal apparatus	**lacrimo**nasal
lact/i/o	milk	**lacti**ferous
laevo-	left (Am. levo-)	**laevo**cardia (Am. **levo**cardia)
-lalia	condition of talking	dys**lalia**
lal/o	speech	**lalo**plegia
lamell/a	thin leaf or plate	**lamell**ar
lamin/o	lamina / thin plate / part of vertebral arch	**lamin**ectomy
lapar/o	abdomen/flank	**laparo**tomy
-lapaxy	empty / wash out / evacuate	litho**lapaxy**
-lapse	fall/slide/sag	pro**lapse**
laryng/o	larynx	**laryng**ectomy
later/o	side	**latero**torsion
lei/o	smooth	**leio**dermia
leiomy/o	smooth muscle	**leiomy**oma
-lemma	sheath/covering	sarco**lemma**
lent/i	lens	**lenti**conus
-lepsy	seizure/fit	epi**lepsy**
lept/o	thin/fine/slender	**lepto**meningitis
leth-	fatal/causing death	**leth**al
leuc/o	white	**leuco**cyte (Am. **leuko** cyte)
leukaem/o	leukaemia (Am. leukemia)	**leukaem**ic (Am. **leukem**ic)
leukem/o (Am.)	leukemia/leukaemia	**leukemo**gen
leuk/o	white	**leuko**blast
levo- (Am.)	left	**levo**cardia
-lexia	condition of speech/words	dys**lexia**
lien/o	spleen	**lieno**cele
-ligation	tying off of a vessel with a suture	vaso**ligation**
lingu/a/o	tongue	**linguo**gingival
lip/o	fat / fatty tissue	**lip**oma
-listhesis	slipping	spondylo**listhesis**
-lith	stone	uretero**lith**

Component	Meaning	Example
-lithiasis	abnormal condition of stones	uretero**lithiasis**
lith/o	stone	**litho**trite
lob/o	lobe	**lob**ar
lochi/o	vaginal discharge (lochia)	**lochio**rrhagia
loc/o	place	**loc**us
logad-	white of the eye	**logad**ectomy
-logist	specialist who studies	cardio**logist**
log/a/o	words/speech/study/thought	**loga**phasia
-logy	study of	laryngo**logy**
loph/o	ridge/tuft	**loph**odont
lord/o	bend forward / forward curvature of the lumbar spine	**lord**osis
lox/o	oblique/slanting	**lox**ophthalmos
-lucent	to shine	radio**lucent**
lumb/o	loin / lower back	**lumbo**costal
lump-	lump/swelling	**lump**ectomy
lute/o	yellow / corpus luteum of ovary	**luteo**trophic
lymph/a/t/o	lymph	**lymph**oma
lymphaden/o	lymph node (lymph gland)	**lymphaden**itis
lymphangi/o	lymph vessel	**lymphangio**graphy
lymphocyt/o	lymphocyte	**lymphocyt**osis
lymphomat-	lymphoma	**lymphomat**osis
lyo-	water soluble / solvent / dissolve	**lyo**philic
lys/o	break down / disintegration / dissolving	**lys**in
-lysis	break down / disintegration / dissolving	auto**lysis**
-lytic	pertaining to break down / disintegration	haemo**lytic** (Am. hemo**lytic**)
macro-	large	**macro**phage
macul/o	spot / blotch	**maculo**papular
mal-	bad / diseased or impaired	**mal**nutrition
-malacia	condition of softening	myo**malacia**
malac/o	softening	**malac**ic
malign-	bad/harmful	**malign**ant
malleol/o	malleolus (the process on the side of the ankle)	**malleol**ar
malle/o	malleus (the hammer-shaped ear ossicle) / hammer	**malle**otomy
mamill/i/o	nipple	**mamill**iplasty
mamm/a/o	breast / mammary gland	**mamm**ography
mammill/i/o	nipple	**mammill**itis
mandibul/o	mandible (lower jaw bone)	**mandibulo**plasty
mani-	mental disorder / madness	**mani**ac
-mania	condition of mental disorder / psychosis (extreme excitement)	nympho**mania**
man/o	pressure	**man**ometry
manus-	hand	**manus** extensa
mast/o	breast / mammary gland	**mast**algia
mastoid/o	nipple-shaped / mastoid process / mastoid air cells	**mastoid**ectomy
maxill/o	maxilla (upper jaw bone)	**maxillo**facial
meat/o	meatus / opening / external orifice, eg, of the urethra	**meat**otomy
medi/o	middle/midline	**medi**al
-media	condition of being in the middle	otitis **media**
medull/o	inner part / medulla	adrenal **medulla**
mega-	abnormally large	**mega**colon
megal/o	abnormally large	**megalo**glossia
-megaly	enlargement	acro**megaly**

Component	Meaning	Example
melan/o	melanin / dark pigment	**melan**oma
melanomat-	melanoma	**melanomat**osis
melit/o	sugar/honey	**melit**uria
mel/o	limb/cheek	**mel**agra
melon/o	cheek	**melon**oplasty
mening/i/o	meninges, the protective membranes of the CNS	**mening**itis
menisc/o	meniscus/crescent-shaped	**menisc**ocyte
men/o	menses / menstruation / monthly flow	**men**orrhagia
ment/o	chin/mind	**ment**oplasty
mes/o	middle/intermediate	**mes**oderm
meta-	change in form, position or order / after / next / between	**meta**plasia
metacarp/o	metacarpus/metacarpal or metacarpal bone	**metacarp**al
metatars/o	metatarsus/metatarsal or metatarsal bone	**metatars**algia
-meter	measuring instrument / a measure	audio**meter**
metr/a/i/o	uterus/womb	endo**metri**osis
-metrist	person who measures	audio**metrist**
-metry	process of measuring	audio**metry**
micro-	small/one-millionth	**micro**glia
mid-	middle	**mid**brain
-mileusis	carving, shaping	kerato**mileusis**
milli-	one-thousandth	**milli**litre
-mimesis	simulation/imitation	patho**mimesis**
-mimetic	simulation of a specific effect	sympatho**mimetic**
-mimia	condition of expressing through gestures	macro**mimia**
mi/o	make smaller / less	**mi**osis
-mission	to send	e**mission**
mito-	thread-like/mitosis	**mito**tic
mono-	one/single	**mono**somy
monocyt/o	monocyte	**monocyt**openia
-morph	shape/form	ecto**morph**
morph/o	shape/form	**morph**ogenesis
mort/o	death	**mort**al
-motor-	moving / action / set in motion	oculo**motor**
muc/o	mucus	**muc**ous
multi-	many	**multi**gravida
muscul/o	muscle	**muscul**ocutaneous
mut/a	change (genetic change)	**mut**agen
my-	(from myein) to close/squint	**my**opia
mycet/o	fungus	**mycet**oid
myc/o	fungus	broncho**myc**osis
mydr-	widen or enlarge	**mydr**iatic
myelin/o	myelin / myelin sheath	**myelin**ated
myel/o	bone marrow / spinal cord / myelocyte	**myel**oma
myelomat/o	myeloma	**myelomat**osis
my/o	muscle	**my**oglobin
myocardi/o	myocardium (heart muscle)	**myocardi**opathy
myomat/o	myoma (muscle tumour)	**myomat**osis
myop-	short-sighted	**myop**ia
myos/o	muscle	**myos**itis
myring/o	eardrum / tympanic membrane	**myring**otome
myx/o	mucus/mucoid tissue (embryonic connective tissue)	**myx**adenitis
myxomat-	myxoma	**myxomat**osis

Component	Meaning	Example
nano-	one-billionth / a quantity multiplied by (10^{-9})	**nano**metre (Am. **nano**meter)
narc/o	stupor/numbness	**narco**tic
nas/o	nose	**naso**pharyngitis
nasopharyng/o	nasopharynx	**nasopharyngo**scope
-natal	pertaining to birth	ante**natal**
nat/o	birth	neo**nato**logy
natr/i	sodium (Na⁺), from Latin natrium	**natri**uresis
necr/o	death / death of tissue	**necr**osis
neo-	new/recent	**neo**plasia
nephr/o	kidney	**nephr**itis
neur/o	nerve (rarely tendon)	**neuro**logy
neuron/o	neuron	**neuron**al
neutr/o	neutral	**neutro**phil
nid-	nest / focus of	**nid**al
noc/i	harm	**noci**ceptor
noct/i	night/darkness	**noct**uria
nod/o	knot/swelling	**nod**ule
nom/o	distribute/law/custom	**nomo**topic
non-	without/no	**non** compos mentis
normo-	normal	**normo**cytosis
nos/o	disease	**noso**logy
not/o	back	**noto**chord
nucle/o	nucleus	**nucleo**protein
nulli-	none	**nulli**para
nyctal/o	night/darkness	**nyctal**opia
nyct/o	night/darkness	**nyct**algia
nymph/o	labia minora / nymphae	**nympho**mania
-nyxis	perforation/pricking/puncture	kerato**nyxis**
obstetr-	midwifery/obstetrics	**obstetr**ician
occipit/o	occiput, the posterior region of the skull	**occipito**cervical
occlus/o	shut/close up	**occlus**ion
oct/a/i/o-	eight	**octi**gravida
ocul/o	eye	bin**ocul**ar
odont/o	tooth/teeth	orth**odont**ics
odyn/o	pain	**odyno**phagia
-oedema	swelling due to fluid (Am. edema)	myx**oedema** (Am. myx**edema**)
oesophag/o	oesophagus/gullet (Am. esophago)	**oesophago**stomy (Am. **esophago**stomy)
oestr/o	oestrogen (a female sex-hormone) / oestrus (Am. estr/o)	**oestr**ogenic (Am. **estr**ogenic)
-oid	resembling	lip**oid**
-ola	small	arteri**ola**
-ole	small	arteri**ole**
olecran/o	elbow/olecranon (the bony projection of the ulna)	**olecran**arthropathy
ole/o	oil	**oleo**granuloma
olfact/o	sense of smell / smell	**olfact**ory
olig/o	deficiency/few/little	**olig**uria
-olisthesis	slipping	spondyl**olisthesis**
-oma	tumour (Am. tumor) / swelling	sarc**oma**
oment/o	omentum (peritoneal fold of stomach)	**omento**plasty
om/o	shoulder	**omo**clavicular
omphal/o	navel / umbilicus / umbilical cord	**omphalo**genesis
onc/o	tumour (Am. tumor) / mass	**onco**logy
-one	hormone	progester**one**

Component	Meaning	Example
onych/o	nail	**onycho**dystrophy
oo-	egg	**oo**cyte
oophor/o	ovary	**oophor**ectomy
-opaque	obscure	radi**opaque**
-op-	seeing / looking at	presby**op**ia
ophthalm/o	eye	**ophthalmo**scope
-ophthalmos	eye	ex**ophthalmos**
-opia	condition of vision / defective vision	ambly**opia**
opistho-	backward/behind	**opistho**gnathism
-opsia	condition of vision / defective vision	hemiachromat**opsia**
-opsy	to view / process of viewing	bi**opsy**
optic/o	vision / eye / optic nerve	**optic**al
opt/o	vision/eye	**opto**metry
orbit/o	orbit (the bony cavity of the eye)	**orbito**nasal
-or	a person or agent / a device	don**or**
orchid/o	testicle/testis	**orchido**pathy
orch/i/o	testicle/testis	**orchio**plasty
-orexia	condition of appetite	an**orexia**
organ/o	organ	**organo**genesis
or/o	mouth	**or**al
orth/o-	correct/normal/straight	**orth**optics
-ory	pertaining to	sens**ory**
os-	bone / a mouth / an orifice	**os** uteri
osche/o	scrotum	**oscheo**plasty
-ose	carbohydrate / sugar / starch / full of / pertaining to / having the form of	gluc**ose**
-osis	abnormal condition / disease of / abnormal increase	leucocyt**osis** (Am. leukocyt**osis**)
osm/a/o	odour / smell / osmosis	**osmo**dysphoria
osphresi/o	odour/smell/olfaction (the sense of smell)	**osphresio**logy
osse/o	bone	**osse**ous
oss/i	bone	**ossi**cle
ossicul/o	ear ossicles / ear bones	**ossicul**ectomy
ost/e/o	bone	**osteo**arthritis
ot/o	ear	**oto**logy
-ous	pertaining to	urinifer**ous**
ovari/o	ovary	**ovario**tomy
ov/i/o	egg/ovum	**ovi**duct
-oxia	condition of oxygen	hyp**oxia**
ox/i/o	oxygen	**oxi**metry
oxy-	oxygen/sharp/quick	**oxy**tocic
oxysm/o	sudden	par**oxysm**al
pachy-	thick	**pachy**dermia
paed/o	child (Am. ped/o)	**paed**iatric (Am. **ped**iatric)
palae/o	old/primitive (Am. pale/o)	**palaeo**cortex (Am. **paleo**cortex)
palat/o	palate	**palato**plasty
pale/o (Am.)	old/primitive	**paleo**cortex
palm/o	palm	**palm**ar
palpebr/a	eyelid	**palpebr**itis
pan-	all	**pan**carditis
pancreatic/o	pancreatic duct	**pancreatico**enterostomy
pancreat/o	pancreas	**pancreato**lysis
pannicul/o	fatty layer, eg, of abdomen	**panni****cul**itis
pant/o	all/entire	**panta**trophy
papill/i/o	nipple-like / optic disc / optic papilla	**papillo**retinitis

Component	Meaning	Example
para-	beside / near / beyond / accessory to / wrong / abnormal / resembling / apart from	**para**nephric
-para	to bear / bring forth offspring / a woman who has borne viable young	primi**para**
parasympath/o	parasympathetic nervous system	**parasympatho**mimetic
parathyr/o	parathyroid gland	**parathyro**trophic
parathyroid/o	parathyroid gland	**parathyroid**ectomy
-paresis	slight paralysis	hemi**paresis**
-pareunia	sexual intercourse	dys**pareunia**
parotid/o	parotid gland	**parotid**itis
-parous	pertaining to production of live young	nulli**parous**
pars-	part / a division of a larger organ or structure	**pars** optica retinae
-partum	birth/labour	post-**partum**
parturi-	childbirth/labour/parturition	**parturi**ent
patell/o	patella / knee cap	**patello**femoral
-pathia	condition of disease	psycho**pathia**
pathic	pertaining to disease	idio**pathic**
path/o	disease	**patho**logist
-pathy	disease/emotion	gastro**pathy**
-pause	stopping	meno**pause**
pect-	chest/breast/thorax	**pect**us
pector/o	chest/breast/thorax	**pector**al
pedicul/o	lice	**pedicul**osis
ped/i/o (Am.)	foot/child	**ped**iatrics
pelli-	skin/hide	**pelli**cle
pelv/i/o	pelvis	**pelvi**meter
pend/o	to hang	**pend**ulous
-penia	condition of deficiency or lack of	erythro**penia**
pen/o	penis	**pen**itis
peps-	digestion	dys**peps**ia
-pepsia	condition of digestion	brady**pepsia**
pepsin/o	pepsin (an enzyme)	**pepsin**ogen
pept/o	digestion/pepsin/peptone	**pept**ic
per-	through/completely/excessive	**per**cutaneous
perone/o	fibula	**perone**al
peri-	around	**peri**corneal
pericardi/o	pericardium	**pericard**itis
perine/o	perineum	**perineo**rrhaphy
periton/e/o	peritoneum	**periton**itis
petr/o	stone/rock	osteo**petr**osis
-pexis	surgical fixation / fix in place / storage	glyco**pexis**
-pexy	surgical fixation / fix in place / storage	arthro**pexy**
phac/o	lens	**phaco**scopy
phae/o	dusky/dark (Am. phe/o)	**phae**ochromocyte (Am. **pheo**chromocyte)
-phagia	condition of eating / swallowing	poly**phagia**
phag/o	eating / consuming / a phagocyte	**phago**cytic
-phagy	eating or swallowing	copro**phagy**
phak/o	lens	**phak**itis
phalang/o	phalanx/finger/toe	**phalang**eal
phall/o	penis	**phall**ic
phaner/o	visible/manifesting	**phanero**genic
phant-	an illusion / imaginary / hallucination	**phant**osmia
pharm/ac/o	drug/medicine	**pharmaco**logy

Component	Meaning	Example
pharyng/o	pharynx	**pharyng**itis
-phasia	condition of speaking/speech	dys**phasia**
phas/i/o	speech	a**phasio**logy
phe/o (Am.)	dusky/dark	**pheo**chromocyte
-phil	love/affinity for / a cell type with affinity for something	neutro**phil**
-philia	condition of love/affinity for something / an increase in (eg, number of cells)	neutro**philia**
-phily	condition of love / affinity for something	necro**phily**
phim/o	to muzzle or constrict	**phim**osis
phleb/o	vein	**phleb**ectomy
-phobia	condition of irrational fear / aversion	hydro**phobia**
-phonia	condition of having voice	a**phonia**
phon/o	speech/sound/voice	**phono**cardiograph
-phony	sound / type of speech	tracheo**phony**
-phore	a carrier	chromato**phore**
-phoresis	movement in a specified way / bearing / carrying / driving ions	electro**phoresis**
-phoria	condition of mental state / feeling / bearing / deviation of the eyes (heterophoria)	eu**phoria**
phor/o	mental state / bearing / carrier (eg, of disease)	**phoro**logy
phosph/o	phosphate / phosphorus / phosphoric acid	**phospho**lipid
phot/o	light	**photo**sensitive
phrenic/o	diaphragm / mind / phrenic nerve	**phrenic**ectomy
phren/i/o	diaphragm / mind / phrenic nerve	**phreno**gastric
-phthisis	wasting away	neuro**phthisis**
-phylaxis	protection	pro**phylaxis**
-phyma	tumour/boil/swelling (Am. tumor)	rhino**phyma**
phys/i/o	nature / physical things / physiology	**physio**therapy
-physis	growth	hypo**physis**
-phyt/e/o	plant / fungus / a pathological plant-like growth	dermato**phyte**
pico-	small / a quantity multiplied by 10^{-12}	**pico**gram
pil/o	hair	**pilo**sebaceous
pineal/o	pineal body / pineal gland	**pineal**ocyte
pituitar-	pituitary gland	hypo**pituitar**ism
placent/o	placenta	**placento**graphy
-plakia	condition of broad / flat (patch)	leuko**plakia**
-plania	condition of wandering, eg, a cell moving position	leucocyto**plania** (Am. leukocyto**plania**)
plan/o	flat	**plano**cellular
plant/i	sole of foot	**plant**ar
-plasia	condition of growth due to formation of cells	hyper**plasia**
-plasm	formative substance / growth	cyto**plasm**
plasma-	plasma cell / plasma the fluid matrix of blood	**plasma**therapy
plasm/o	anything moulded, shaped or formed / formative substance/growth/plasma	**plasmo**cyte
-plastic	pertaining to formation of cells or moulding of tissues	neo**plastic**
-plasty	surgical repair / reconstruction	kerato**plasty**
platy-	flat	**platy**onychia
-plegia	condition of paralysis / stroke	para**plegia**
pleo-	more	**pleo**cytosis
plethysm/o	volume	**plethysmo**graph
pleur/o	pleural membranes / rib / side	**pleuro**dynia
-plexia	condition arising from a stroke or other occurrence	apo**plexia**

Component	Meaning	Example
plex/o	network of nerves, blood or lymph vessels	**plex**us
-plexy	strike/paralyze	apo**plexy**
-ploid(y)	chromosome sets in a cell	di**ploid**
pluri-	several/more	**pluri**glandular
-pnea (Am.)	breathing	a**pnea**
pne/o	breath/breathing	**pne**ogram
pneum/a/o	gas/air/lung/breathing	**pneum**othorax
pneumat/o	gas/air/lung/breathing	**pneumat**ometry
pneumon/o	lung	**pneumon**ectomy
-pnoea	breathing (Am. pnea)	dys**pnoea** (Am. dys**pnea**)
pod/o	foot	**pod**iatry
pogon/o	beard	**pogon**iasis
-poiesis	formation	erythro**poiesis**
-poietin	substance that forms	erythro**poietin**
poikil/o	varied/irregular	**poikilo**cyte
polio-	grey matter (of the CNS, Am. gray)	**polio**myelitis
pollex	thumb	**pollex** flexus
poly-	many / too much	**poly**uria
polyp/o	polyp / small growth	**polyp**ectomy
pont/o	pons (part of metencephalon of the brain)	**ponto**cerebellar
por/o	passage / pore	osteo**porosis**
port/o	portal vein	**port**ography
post-	after/behind	**post**-ganglionic
poster/o	back of body / behind / posterior to	**postero**superior
posth/o	prepuce/foreskin	balano**posth**itis
-prandial	pertaining to a meal	post**prandial**
-praxia	condition of purposeful movement or conduct	a**praxia**
-praxy	mechanical treatment of deformities	ortho**praxy**
pre-	before / in front of	**pre**tracheal
preputi/o	prepuce/foreskin	**preputi**otomy
presby/o	old man / old age	**presby**opia
primi-	first	**primi**gravida
-privia	condition of loss or deprivation	calci**privia**
pro-	before / favouring / in front of	**pro**drome
proct/o	rectum/anus	**proct**algia
progest/o	progesterone	**progest**ogen
prosop/o	face	**prosop**oplegia
prostat/o	prostate gland	**prostat**ism
prosth-	adding (a replacement part)	**prosth**odontics
prote/o	protein	prote**ase**
proto-	first	**proto**diastole
protoz/o	protozoa	**protoz**oiasis
proxim/o	near	**proxim**al
prurit/o	itching	**prurit**ic
pseudo-	false	**pseudo**plegia
psych/o	mind	**psych**osis
psychr/o	cold	**psychro**algia
-ptosis	falling/displacement/prolapse	blepharo**ptosis**
-ptotic	pertaining to falling / displacement / prolapse / affected with a ptosis	nephro**ptotic**
ptyal/o	saliva	**ptyalo**graphy
-ptysis	spitting / coughing up	pyo**ptysis**
pub/i/o	pubis / pubic region	**pub**ovesical
pudend-	pudendum/vulva	**pudend**al

Component	Meaning	Example
puerper/o	puerperium / time of childbirth	**puerper**al
pulm/o	lung	**pulmo**aortic
pulmon/o	lung	**pulmon**ary
pupill/o	pupil	**pupillo**metry
purul/o	pus-filled	**purul**oid
pustul/o	infected pimple / pustule	**pustul**osis
pyel/o	the renal pelvis (the space in which urine collects in the kidney)	**pyelo**lithotomy
pykn/o	compact/thick/frequent	**pykn**osis
pyle/o	portal (vein)	**pyle**phlebitis
pylor/o	pylorus	**pylor**ic
py/o	pus	**pyo**genic
pyret/o	heat/fire/burning/fever	**pyret**ic
pyrex/o	heat/fire/burning/fever	**pyrex**ial
pyr/o	heat/fire/burning/fever	**pyro**gen
quadr/i/u-	four	**quadr**iplegia
quinque-	five	**quinque**cuspid
quint-	five	**quint**an
rachi/o	backbone / spine / vertebral column	**rachio**pathy
radic/o	spinal nerve root	**radic**otomy
radicul/o	spinal nerve root	**radicul**itis
radi/o	radioactivity/radiation/X-ray/radius	**radio**therapy
re-	back/contrary/again	**re**position
rect/o	rectum	**recto**sigmoid
ren/i/o	kidney	**reno**graphy
reticul/o	net-like/ reticulum	**reticulo**cytosis
reticuloendotheli/o	reticuloendothelial system	**reticuloendotheli**um
retin/o	retina	**retino**blastoma
retro-	backwards/behind	**retro**verted
rhabd/o	rod/rod-shaped	**rhabd**oid
rhabdomy/o	striated muscle	**rhabdomy**oma
rhe/o	electric current / flow of fluid	**rhe**ology
rheumat/o	rheumatism	**rheumat**ism
rhin/o	nose	**rhino**plasty
rhiz/o	root / spinal nerve root	**rhizo**tomy
rhod/o	red	**rhod**opsin
rhytid/o	wrinkle	**rhytido**plasty
roentgen/o	X-ray / Roentgen ray	**roentgeno**graphy
rostr/i	superior / a rostrum / a beak	**rostr**al
-rrhage	bursting forth / excessive flow	haemo**rrhage** (Am. hemo**rrhage**)
-rrhagia	condition of bursting forth / excessive flow	oto**rrhagia**
-rrhaphy	stitching/suturing	teno**rrhaphy**
-rrhea (Am.)	excessive discharge/flow	rhino**rrhea**
-rrhexis	breaking/rupturing	ovario**rrhexis**
-rrhoea	excessive discharge / flow (Am. -rrhea)	rhino**rrhoea**
(r)rhythm/o	rhythm	ar**rhythm**ia
rubr-	red	**rub**or
rug/o	wrinkle/fold/ridge	**rug**a
racchar/o	sugar/sweet	**racchar**olytic
saccul/o	saccule of the inner ear	**saccul**ar
sacr/o	sacrum	**sacro**coccygeal
salping/o	eustachian (auditory) tube / fallopian tube	**salpingo**stomy
sanguin/o	blood/bloody	**sanguino**lent

Component	Meaning	Example
sapr/o	decay / decayed matter	**sapr**odontia
sarc/o	flesh / connective tissue	**sarc**oid
-sarcoma	malignant (fleshy) tumour of connective tissue (Am. tumor)	Kaposi **sarcoma**
sarcomat/o	sarcoma, a malignant tumour (Am. tumor) of connective tissue	**sarcomat**osis
scapul/o	scapula	**scapulo**clavicular
scat/o	faeces / faecal matter (Am. feces)	**scato**logy
-schisis	cleaving/splitting/parting	palato**schisis**
schist/o	cleaving/splitting/parting	**schisto**cephalus
schistosom/o	a parasitic worm of the genus *Schistosoma*	**schistosom**iasis
schiz/o	split/cleft/divided	**schizo**trichia
scint/i	scintillation / spark / flash of light	**scinti**scan
scirrh/o	hard	**scirrh**us
scler/o	hard / sclera (the white of the eye)	**sclero**tome
-sclerosis	abnormal condition of hardening	arterio**sclerosis**
scoli/o	crooked / twisted / lateral curvature of the spine	**scoli**osis
-scope	instrument to view / examine	endo**scope**
-scopic	pertaining to examining / viewing	micro**scopic**
-scopist	specialist who examines or uses a viewing instrument	endo**scopist**
-scopy	visual examination / examination	endo**scopy**
scot/o	darkness/scotoma	**scot**opia
scotoma-	scotoma / blind spot	**scotoma**graph
scrot/o	scrotum	**scroto**cele
seb/o	sebum / sebaceous gland	**sebo**lith
-sect(ion)	cut	re**section**
secundi-	second	**secundi**gravida
semi-	half/partly	**semi**comatose
semin/i	semen/testis/testicle	**semin**oma
sen/i	old	**sen**ile
sens/o	sense	**senso**motor
sensor/i	sense/sensation	**sensor**ium
-sepsis	infection	a**sepsis**
septi-	seven	**septi**para
septic/o	sepsis/infection/putrefaction	**septic**aemia (Am. **septic**emia)
sept/o	septum, eg, nasal septum	**septo**tomy
sequestr-	sequestrum, a portion of dead bone	**sequestr**ectomy
ser/o	serum	**sero**positive
sex/i	six	**sex**idigital
sialaden/o	salivary glands	**sialaden**itis
sial/o	saliva / salivary gland or duct	**sialo**graphy
sider/o	iron	**sidero**penia
sigmoid/o	sigmoid colon	**sigmoido**scopy
silic/o	glass/silica	**silic**osis
sinistr/o	left / left side	**sinistro**cardia
sin/o	sinus	**sino**atrial
sinus-	sinus	**sinus** venosus
sinus/o	sinus	**sinus**itis
-sis	abnormal condition / action / state of	symbio**sis**
-sitia	condition of appetite for food	eu**sitia**
sit/o	food	**sito**phobia
-sol	solution	cyto**sol**
somatic/o	body	**somatico**splanchnic

Component	Meaning	Example
somat/o	body	**Somato**trophic
-some	body	lyso**some**
somn/i/o	sleep	**somn**ial
son/o	sound / ultrasound	ultra**sono**graphy
-spadia(s)	condition of drawing out / cleft or rent of the male urethra	hypo**spadia**
-spasm	involuntary contraction of muscle	blepharo**spasm**
spasm/o	spasm / involuntary muscle contraction	**spasm**odic
spermat/o	sperm	**spermato**genesis
sperm/i/o	sperm	**spermi**cidal
sphen/o	sphenoid bone / wedge-shaped	**spheno**mandibular
spher/o	sphere-shaped / round	**sphero**phakia
sphincter/o	sphincter / ring-like muscle	**sphinctero**plasty
sphygm/o	pulse	**sphygmo**manometer
-sphyx-	pulsation	a**sphyx**ia
spin/o	spine/backbone	**spino**cerebellar
spirill/i	spiral-shaped bacteria of the genus *Spirillum*	*Spirillum minus*
spir/o	to breathe	**spiro**metry
spirochaet/o	spirochaete (a spiral-shaped bacterium)	**spirochaet**e
spirochet/o (Am.)	spirochete (a spiral-shaped bacterium)	**spirochet**e
splanchnic/o	splanchnic nerve	**splanchnic**ectomy
splanchn/i/o	viscera / splanchnic nerve	**splanchn**ic
splen/o	spleen	**splen**ectomy
spondyl/o	vertebra	**spondyl**itis
spongi/o	sponge	**spongi**form
spor/o	spore	**sporo**mycosis
squam/o	scale/scale-like	**squam**ous
-stalsis	contraction	peri**stalsis**
stapedi/o	stapes (the stirrup-shaped ear ossicle) / stirrup	**stapedio**tenotomy
staphyl/o	*Staphylococcus* / a grape-like cluster / the uvula	**staphylo**cocci
staphylococc/o	*Staphylococcus*	**staphylococc**al
-stasis	stopping / controlling / cessation of movement	haemo**stasis** (Am. hemo**stasis**)
-stat	an agent / device that prevents change, regulates or stops	cryo**stat**
-static	pertaining to stopping / controlling / standing or without motion	haemo**static** (Am. hemo**static**)
-staxis	dripping, eg, of blood	epi**staxis**
stear/i/o	fat	**steari**form
steat/o	fat	**steat**oma
sten/o	narrow/constricted	**steno**coriasis
-stenosis	abnormal condition of narrowing	urethro**stenosis**
sterc/o	faeces (Am. feces)	**sterc**olith
ster/e/o	solid/three-dimensional	**stereo**scopic
stern/o	sternum / breast bone	**sterno**costal
steth/o	chest/breast	**stetho**scope
-sthenia	condition of strength / full power	mya**sthenia**
sthen/o	strength / full power	a**sthen**ic
-stitial	a space or position / pertaining to standing	inter**stitial**
stomat/o	mouth	**stomat**itis
stom/o	a mouth / a mouth-like opening	**stom**al
-stomy	to form a new opening or outlet / a communication / an opening	colo**stomy**
strabism/o	a squint / strabismus	**strabism**ic
strab/o	a squint / strabismus	**strab**ismus

Component	Meaning	Example
strat/i	layer	**strat**iform
strept/o	*Streptococcus* / a twisted chain	**strepto**cocci
streptococc/o	*Streptococcus*	**streptococc**al
striat/o	a mark / stripe	**striat**ed
styl/o	stake / styloid process (of the temporal bone)	**stylo**mastoid
sub-	beneath/under	**sub**cutaneous
sud/or/i	sweat/perspiration	**sudor**esis
super/o	superior/above/excess	**supero**lateral
supra-	superior/above/excess	**supra**hepatic
sy-	with/together	**sy**stole
sym-	with/together	**sym**melia
sympath/o	sympathetic nervous system / sympathetic nerves	**sympatho**lytic
symphysi/o	symphysis (a fibro-cartilaginous joint), eg, the symphysis pubis	**symphysio**tomy
syn-	together / in association / with	**syn**chronous
synapt-	synapse	**synapt**ic
syncop-	faint / cut off	**syncop**ic
syndesm/o	ligament / connective tissue	**syndesm**ectomy
syndrom/o	running together	**syndrom**ic
-synechia	condition of adhering together	blepharo**synechia**
synovi/o	synovia / synovial fluid/membranes	**synovi**al
syphil/o	syphilis	**syphil**oma
syring/o	tube/cavity	**syringo**myelia
system/o	system	**system**ic
systol-	systole	**systol**ic
tachy-	fast	**tachy**cardia
tact-	touch	**tact**ile
tal/o	ankle / ankle bone	**tal**ar
tars/o	tarsus, tarsal or tarsal bone / ankle bone / eyelid / connective tissue plate in the eyelid	**tars**algia
-taxia	condition of ordered movement	a**taxia**
tax/o	ordered movement, arrangement or classification	**tax**ology
tectori/o	covering/roof-like	**tectori**al
tel-	tela or web	**tel**angiectasis
-tela	a web-like membrane	epi**tela**
tele-	far away / operating at a distance	**tele**cardiography
telo-	end/complete	**telo**phase
tempor/o	temple (the lateral region on either side of the head above the zygomatic arch)	**temporo**mandibular
tendin/o	tendon	**tendino**plasty
tend/o	tendon	**tendo**tome
ten/o	tendon	**teno**rrhaphy
tenont/o	tendon	**tenonto**phyma
-tension	pressure	hyper**tension**
ter-	three	**ter**valent
terat/o	monster-like / a deformed embryo or fetus	**terato**genic
terti-	third	**terti**gravida
testicul/o	testicle/testis	**testicul**ar
test/o	testicle/testis	**testo**sterone
tetra-	four	**tetra**ploid
thalam/o	thalamus (part of cerebral cortex)	**thalamo**tomy
thalass/o	the sea	**thalass**aemia (Am. **thalass**emia)
than/at/o	death	**thanato**phobia
thec/o	sheath / a covering, eg, the dura mater	**thec**al

Component	Meaning	Example
thel/e/o	nipple	**thele**plasty
-therapy	treatment	physio**therapy**
-thermia	condition of heat	hypo**thermia**
therm/o	heat	**therm**ography
-thermy	state of heat / process of heating	cystodia**thermy**
thio-	sulphur	**thio**cyanate
thoracico-	thorax	**thoracico**abdominal
thorac/o	thorax	**thoraco**tomy
-thorax	thorax/chest	pneumo**thorax**
thromb/o	thrombus/clot	**thromb**osis
thrombocyt/o	platelet/thrombocyte	**thrombocyto**penia
thymic/o	thymus gland	**thymico**lymphatic
thym/o	thymus gland	**thym**ic
thyr/o	thyroid gland	**thyr**otrophic
thyroid/o	thyroid gland	hypo**thyroid**ism
tibi/o	tibia	**tibi**ofibular
-tic	pertaining to, equivalent in meaning to -ic	necro**tic**
tine/o	ringworm/like a gnawing worm	*Tinea pedis*
-tion	state or condition/process	resec**tion**
-tocia	condition of birth / labour (Am. labor)	eu**tocia**
toc/o	labour/birth (Am. labor)	**toc**ology
-tome	a cutting instrument	myringo**tome**
tom/o	a slice / section	**tomo**graphy
-tomy	incision into	laparo**tomy**
-tonia	condition of tension / tone	a**tonia**
ton/o	stretching/tension/tone	**tono**meter
tonsill/o	tonsil	**tonsill**ectomy
top/o	place / particular area	**topo**logy
tort/i	twisted	**torti**collis
-toxic	pertaining to poisoning	nephro**toxic**
toxic/o	poison	**toxico**logy
tox/i/o	poison	**tox**ic
trabecul/o	trabecula / anchoring strand of connective tissue / the trabecular meshwork of the eye	**trabecul**ectomy
trachel/o	neck / uterine cervix	**trachel**oplasty
trache/o	trachea	**trache**ostomy
trans-	across/through	**trans**urethral
-trauma	an injury or wound	baro**trauma**
-tresia	condition of having an opening / perforation	a**tresia**
tri-	three	**tri**cuspid
trichin/o	*Trichinella spiralis* (a parasitic nematode worm)	**trichin**iasis
trich/o	hair	**trich**osis
trigon/o	trigone / triangular space, eg, at the base of the bladder	**trigon**itis
-tripsy	act of crushing	litho**tripsy**
-tripter or -triptor	instrument designed to crush or fragment, eg, using shock waves	litho**triptor**
-trite	instrument designed to crush or fragment	litho**trite**
-trity	act of crushing (syn. lithotripsy)	litho**trity**
-trope	influencing / a cell influencing something / influenced by	gonado**trope**
-trophic	pertaining to nourishment / stimulation	adreno**trophic**
troph/o	nourishment/food/stimulation	**troph**oblast
-trophy	nourishment / development / increase in cell size	a**trophy**

Component	Meaning	Example
-tropia	condition of turning / deviation / heterotropia / strabismus	hyper**tropia**
-tropic	pertaining to affinity for / stimulating / changing in response to a stimulus / turning towards	thyro**tropic**
-tropin	a hormone that has a stimulating effect on a target organ	gonado**tropin**
-tubal	pertaining to a tube	ovario**tubal**
tub/o	fallopian tube / oviduct / tube / uterine tube	**tub**oplasty
turbin/o	top-shaped / turbinate bone (nasal concha)	**turbin**ectomy
tuss/i	cough	anti**tuss**ive
tympan/o	tympanic membrane / middle ear	**tympan**oplasty
-type	a classification/type of	pheno**type**
typhl/o	caecum (Am. cecum)	**typhl**ocele
-ula	small/little	ling**ula**
ulcer/o	ulcer / sore / local defect in a surface	**ulcer**ogenic
-ule	small	ven**ule**
uln/o	ulna	**uln**oradial
ul/o/e	scar/gingiva (gums)	**ul**oid
ultra-	beyond	**ultra**sonography
-ulum	small	coag**ulum**
-ulus	small	sacc**ulus**
-um	a thing / a structure / noun ending / a name	ov**um**
un-	not / opposite of / release from	**un**differentiated
ungu/o	nail	**ungu**al
uni-	one	**uni**lateral
uran/o	palate	**uran**orrhaphy
urat/o	urates / salt of uric acid (found in calculi)	**urat**uria
urea-	urea	**urea**poiesis
-uresis	excrete in urine / urinate	lith**uresis**
ureter/o	ureter	**ureter**ostenosis
urethr/o	urethra	**urethr**oscopy
-uria	condition of urine / urination	poly**uria**
uric/o	uric acid	**uric**ometer
urin/a/o	urine	**urin**ometer
ur/o	urine / urinary tract	**ur**ology
urticar/i	nettle rash / hives	**urticar**ia
-us	a thing / a structure / noun ending / a name	bronch**us**
uter/o	uterus	**uter**otubal
utricul/o	utricle of the inner ear	**utricul**us
uve/o	uvea (the pigmented parts of the eye)	**uve**itis
uvul/o	uvula	**uvul**optosis
vagin/o	vagina	**vagin**itis
vag/o	vagus nerve (the 10th cranial nerve)	**vag**otomy
valv/o	valve	**valv**otomy
valvul/o	valve	**valvul**otome
varic/o	varix (a dilated vein) / varicose vein	**varic**otomy
vascul/o	vessel	**vascul**ar
vas/o	vessel / vas deferens	**vas**ectomy
vel/o	soft/veil	**vel**opharyngeal
venacav/o	vena cava (a great vein)	**venacav**ography
ven/e/i/o	vein	**ven**esection
vener/o	sexual intercourse	**vener**eal
ventricul/o	ventricle of the heart or brain	**ventricul**ography

Component	Meaning	Example
ventr/i/o-	ventral / belly side of the body / in front of	**ventro**dorsal
verm/i	worm	**vermi**cide
-version	turning	retro**version**
vertebr/o	vertebra	**vertebr**al
vesic/o	bladder/blister	**vesico**prostatic
vesicul/o	seminal vesicle	**vesicul**itis
vestibul/o	vestibule / vestibular apparatus / a space leading to the entrance of a canal, eg, in the ear	**vestibulo**tomy
vibri/o	comma-shaped bacterium of the genus *Vibrio*	**vibrio**cidal
vibr/o	vibration	**vibro**cardiogram
vir/o/u	virus/virion	**viro**lactia
viscer/o	viscera / internal organs (esp. of the abdomen)	**viscero**peritoneal
vit/o	life	**vit**al
vitre/o	glass / the vitreous body of eye	**vitreo**retinal
viv/i	life	**vivi**section
vol/o	palm	**vol**ar
vulv/o	vulva	**vulv**itis
xanth/o	yellow	**xanth**oma
xen/o	strange/foreign	**xeno**graft
xer/o	dry	**xer**ophthalmia
xiph/i/o	xiphoid process	**xiphi**costal
-y	process / condition / noun ending / a name	apoplex**y**
-yl-	a substance	but**yl**ene
zo/o	animal	**zo**oid
zyg/o	joined	**zygo**dactyly
zygomatic/o	zygomatic arch	**zygomatico**temporal
zygot-	zygote / fertilized egg	**zygot**ic
-zyme	enzyme/fermentation	lyso**zyme**
zym/o	enzyme/fermentation	**zym**osis

INDEX

Note: Page numbers followed by *b, t,* or *f* refer to boxes, tables, or figures, respectively.